W9-BRT-607

CARDIOVASCULAR DRUGS IN THE PERIOPERATIVE PERIOD

Editors

Pierre Foëx, MA, DPhil, FRCA, FANZCA
Nuffield Professor of Anesthesia
Nuffield Department of Anesthetics
Radcliffe Infirmary, Oxford University,
Oxford, United Kingdom

Gaisford G Harrison, MD, DSc (Med), FFARCS (Eng)
Emeritus Professor of Anesthesia
(formerly Head of Department of Anesthesia,
University of Cape Town and Groote Schuur Hospital)
Cape Town, South Africa

Lionel H Opie, MD, DPhil, FRCP
Professor of Medicine and
Director
Cape Heart Centre
University of Cape Town
Cape Town, South Africa

with contributions by:
J L Atlee, S J Howell, N W Lawson, B J Leone, J D Meyer,
Jr., T J Monaco, Jr., M G Mythen, D M Philbin, H-J Priebe,
J Ramsay, D A Schwinn, L Wollman

Foreword by Julien F. Biebuyck

Authors' Publishing House,
New York

Lippincott-Raven Publishers
Philadelphia, New York
1999

Every effort has been made to check generic and trade names, and to verify drug doses as correct according to the standards accepted at the time of publication. The ultimate responsibility lies with prescribing physicians, based on their professional experience and knowledge of the patient, to determine dosages and the best course of treatment for the patient. The reader is advised to check the product information currently provided by the manufacturer of each drug to be administered to ascertain any change in drug dosage, method of administration, or contraindications. In no case can the institutions with which the authors are affiliated or the publisher be held responsible for the views expressed in the book, which reflects the combined opinions of several authors. Please call any errors to the attention of the authors.

ISBN: 0-620-23099-1

Copyright © 1999 by Authors' Publishing House, New York.

All rights reserved. No part of this publication may be reproduced, stored in a retrieval system or transmitted in any form or by any means, mechanical, photocopying, recording, or otherwise, without the prior written permission of the publishers, Authors' Publishing House, 2 Spook Rock Road, Tallman, New York, 10982-0015.

Printed in South Africa by
The Rustica Press, Ndabeni, Western Cape
D6392

John L Atlee, MS (Pharm), MD, FACA, FACC
Professor of Anesthesiology
Medical College of Wisconsin;
Department of Anesthesiology
Froedtert Memorial Lutheran Hospital
Milwaukee, USA

Pierre Foëx, MA, DPhil, FRCA, FANZCA
Nuffield Professor of Anaesthesia
Nuffield Department of Anaesthetics
Radcliffe Infirmary and University of Oxford
Oxford, UK

Gaisford G Harrison, MD, DSc (Med), FFARCS, FANZCA
Emeritus Professor of Anaesthesia and Fellow
University of Cape Town
South Africa

Simon J Howell, MA, MRCP, FRCA, MSc
Consultant Senior Lecturer
University Department of Anaesthetics
Bristol General Infirmary
Bristol, UK

Noel W Lawson, MD
Professor and Chairman
Department of Anesthesiology
and Perioperative Medicine
Health Sciences Center
Columbia, USA

Bruce J Leone, MD
Senior Associate Consultant with Mayo Clinic Jacksonville
Jacksonville
Florida, USA

Joseph D Meyer Jr., MD, PhD
Assistant Professor
Department of Anesthesiology
and Perioperative Medicine
Health Sciences Center
Columbia, USA

Thomas J Monaco, Jr., MD
Associate in Anesthesiology and Critical Care Medicine
Critical Health Systems of North Carolina
Raleigh, North Carolina, USA

Lionel H Opie, MD, DPhil, FRCP
Professor of Medicine and
Director, Cape Heart Center
Medical School
University of Cape Town
South Africa

Michael (Monty) G. Mythen, MB, BS, FRCA, MD
Consultant Anaesthetist,
Department of Anaesthesia,
University College London, UK

Daniel M Philbin, MD
Professor and Vice-Chairman
Department of Anesthesiology
University of Massachusetts Medical Center
Massachusetts, USA

Hans-Joachim Priebe, MD
Professor of Anesthesia
Klinikum der Albert-Ludwigs Universität Freiburg
Germany

James Ramsay, MD
Associate Professor of Anesthesia
Emory University Hospital
Atlanta, Georgia, USA

Debra A Schwinn, MD,
Assistant Professor of Anesthesiology and Pharmacology,
Division of Cardiac Anesthesiology
Department of Anesthesiology
Duke University Medical Centre
Durham, NC, USA

Lisa Wollman, MD
Staff Anesthesiologist and Intensivist
Massachusetts General Hospital;
Instructor in Anesthesia
Harvard Medical School
Massachusetts, USA

FOREWORD

Anesthesiologists and intensivists in North America, like their colleagues in Cardiology and Internal Medicine, have long admired and enjoyed Lionel Opie's excellent handbook, "Drugs for the Heart"[1], now in its fourth edition. Professor Opie's elegant presentation of cellular events and their linkage to drug action and related myocardial function, has helped all of us better to understand these complex inter-relationships.

Professor Opie is now joined by well-known practising anesthesiologists in three continents in editing a handbook which targets specifically perioperative cardiac pharmacology, and the way in which pre-existing cardiac disease and cardiac drugs influence function in the presence of anesthetic agents. I have always exhorted medical students preparing for a career in Anesthesiology, and also resident and fellow trainees planning clinical rotations, that "you cannot know too much Cardiology" to be a true consultant in the discipline. I could equally add that it is impossible to know "too much cardiac pharmacology"! Anesthesiologists are always justifiably more concerned about cardiac diagnosis and therapy than any other patient condition in the preoperative assessment clinic, in the operating rooms, and in the postoperative critical care units. This handbook should be useful in all three of these patient care environments. In addition, the organization of each chapter will appeal to trainees preparing for their certifying examinations.

The authors of these chapters represent a collection of clinicians in the fields of anesthesiology and cardiac anesthesia who have endeavored to integrate the physiologic responses of the normal and diseased heart, with the pharmacologic effects of cardiovascular agents in the anesthetized patient. As surgical techniques improve and the armamentarium for medical management of cardiovascular diseases strengthens, patients with increasingly complex and severe cardiovascular illnesses become candidates for surgical procedures, so that it is critical for the anesthesiologist who will be dealing with these patients in the future to understand the actions of new cardiac drugs and their interactions with anesthetics.

I believe that we are indeed fortunate that Lionel Opie has now directed his superb leadership as a researcher and teacher in cardiology to our discipline. We are equally fortunate that Pierre Foëx brings to the reader his respected and experienced British-European-North American views, and that Gaisford Harrison has also applied his extensive clinical, applied pharmacology research, and editorial background to the development of this volume.

JULIEN F BIEBUYCK, MB, ChB, DPhil, FRCA, FANZCA
Eric A Walker Professor and Chairman
Department of Anesthesia
Senior Associate Dean for Academic Affairs
Penn State University College of Medicine
The Milton S Hershey Medical Center
Hershey, PA 17033
USA

1. Opie, LH. *Drugs for the Heart*, 4th Edition. W.B. Saunders Company, Philadelphia, 1995.

PREFACE

Perioperative cardiac morbidity is the leading cause of death following anesthesia and surgery. Almost one quater of patients presenting for these procedures suffer from cardiac disease, of which hypertension is the most prevalent, and ischemic heart disease associated with the highest mortality. Approximately two-thirds of such patients will be on chronic medication. These bald statements highlight the need for the anesthesiologist to have, in particular, an understanding of and familiarity with cardiovascular drugs. This is essential, not only for the direct acute use of these agents during the perioperative period, but also for the anticipation and management of any interactions between the anesthetic agents and adjuvants and chronic cardiovascular drug medication which the patient may be taking. In this regard the current philosophy is that such treatment, when optimal, should not be interfered with, or interfered with as little as possible, by the procedures of anesthesia and surgery.

The aim and format of this book is to provide the anesthesiologist with a portable compendium and ready reference, for practical and clinically important information on the applied pharmacology of cardiovascular drugs. The first six chapters deal with drugs themselves – dynamics and kinetics, the receptors, ion channels and signal systems through which they act, and the effects of anesthetic agents themselves on the heart and circulation. The remaining six chapters deal with the application of these principles to specific conditions and clinical situations. Inherent in such an arrangement is a modicum of overlap between the pharmacological and clinically orientated groups of chapters. This we accept, knowingly, because each chapter is planned to stand alone for rapid consultation and immediate practical application, a process that would be defeated by excessive cross-referencing.

The contributing authors have been chosen for their expertise in their particular topics and, in our efforts to avoid any parochialism, come from four countries: the USA, UK, Germany and South Africa.

For the reader, a final admonition. This book is designed for the operating room, the ICU, and the ward. Not the bookshelf. It is our hope that you will use it that way.

Pierre Foëx
Gaisford G Harrison
Lionel H Opie

CONTENTS

Autonomic Receptors and Signal Systems as Sites of Action of Cardiovascular Drugs

Lionel H. Opie

During the perioperative period, there may be numerous changes in cardiovascular control. Any operation, of itself, is a stress that induces adrenergic activation, to which must be added the effects of anesthesia and the risks of fluid and electrolyte imbalance. All of these factors may induce perioperative changes in the cardiovascular status. It is on this background that cardiovascular drugs are called to act.

Always, before asking "Which drug and Why?", we need to consider the physiological background to cardiovascular drug action. The ultimate controlling cellular signal is usually the calcium ion that in turn regulates the contraction cycle. This chapter will outline the function of the autonomic nervous system and its receptors, as well as cardiovascular signal systems, as possible sites for drug action (Table 1-1).

AUTONOMIC NERVOUS SYSTEM

Cardiovascular control is exerted at several levels, including the autonomic nervous system and the periphery. Messages that play a major role in regulating the circulation, reach the heart from the central nervous system along the *autonomic pathways*, which function independently of the conscious nervous system. The two divisions of the autonomic nervous system have opposite functions (Figs 1-1 and 1-2). First, the *adrenergic* or *sympathetic nervous system* is able to release its excitatory messengers, epinephrine and norepinephrine (adrenaline and noradrenaline) in "sympathy with" states of excitation, such as waking up, the start of exercise or perioperative stress (Fig 1-1). Second, the *parasympathetic system* acts alongside the adrenergic nervous system to release its own transmitter, acetylcholine. Alternate names for this system, activated by sleep or anesthesia, are the *cholinergic or vagal nervous system* (Fig 1-2).

**Table 1-1. Levels of autonomic control and sites of cardio-
vascular drug action**

Site of autonomic action	Physiological control	Drug examples
Central activation	Increased by peri-operative "stress", facilitated by A II; decreased by sleep, mental depression, anesthesia	Decreased by tranquilizers, antidepressants, anesthetic agents, ACE inhibitors
Vasomotor centre	Responds to central activation and baroreflexes; two centres interact	Acute vasodilation causes reflex adrenergic-angiotensin activation
Autonomic ganglia	Respond to discharge rates of vasomotor centres by release of ACh	Ganglion blockers eg trimethaphan compete with ACh; atropine not effective, poor penetration
Neurotransmission	Increased by A II & E, decreased by ACh (M_2), adenosine, NO	Tricyclic antidepressants and monoamine oxidase inhibitors (MAOIs) act here
Cholinergic receptors	Parasympathetic	Atropine blocks
Beta-adrenergic receptors	adrenergic, NE and E	Beta-agonists or antagonists
Alpha-adrenergic receptors	adrenergic, NE	Alpha-agonists and antagonists
Excitation-contraction coupling in myocardium	Beta-adrenergic, degree of Ca channel opening, cytosolic Ca	Inhibited by beta-blockers, calcium antagonists, experimental block of Ca release channel of SR
Myocardial contraction cycle	Cytosolic Ca, sensitivity of troponin-C to Ca, cAMP	Digitalis, Ca sensitizers, agents increasing cAMP including PDE inhibitors
Vascular Smooth Muscle (VSM) contraction	Ca entry; IP_3 releases Ca in response to A II, endothelin and α_1-adrenergic activity	Phenylephrine, high dose E, NE, A II
VSM relaxation	Ca entry inhibition; decreased IP_3 release; contraction inhibited by cAMP and cGMP	Ca antagonists; cGMP↑ by nitrates or SNP; decrease of IP_3 by ACE inhibitors or α1 or ET blockers; increase of cAMP by beta$_2$ agonists or adenosine

A II = angiotensin II; NE = norepinephrine; E = epinephrine;
cAMP = cyclic AMP; cGMP = cyclic GMP; M = muscarinic;
ACE = angiotensin converting enzyme;
SR = sarcoplasmic reticulum;
NO = nitric oxide, SNP = sodium nitroprusside;
IP_3 = inositol trisphosphate; ET = endothelin; ↑ = increase

Adrenergic and Cholinergic Effects

Each system has a certain intensity of stimuli flowing down
(neural traffic) from its vasomotor center in the medulla to
the terminal neurons (or varicosities) which lie close to the
effector cells of the organ to be controlled. The preganglionic sympathetic fibers terminate in the ganglia are sepa-

rated by synapses from the postganglionic cell bodies of the next neurons. Acetylcholine is the messenger across the synaptic gap, so that the impulse continues along the postganglionic fibers to end in the terminal varicosity. There the autonomic "first messengers", chiefly norepinephrine, noradrenaline or acetylcholine, travel across the final synaptic gap to the receptors on the external membrane of the heart cell or the vascular smooth muscle cell.

In the case of the sympathetic nervous system, the sympathetic ganglia specifically supplying the postganglionic fibers to the heart are the left and right stellate ganglia (Fig 1-1). Further preganglionic sympathetic fibers exit from the spinal chord further down, running to the adrenal medulla. There these fibers liberate acetylcholine at the synapses with medullary cells, which act as the postgangiolionic cells of this system to release epinephrine (adrenaline) into the circulation.

In the case of the parasympathetic system, the ganglia are situated rather close to or within the organ to which the impulses are travelling, so that the postganglionic fiber is rather short. In the heart, the postganglionic parasympathetic fibers innervate chiefly the sinoatrial and atrioventricular nodes, with some innervation also of the atria and ventricles. The messenger released by this system is acetylcholine.

Release of Norepinephrine from Terminal Adrenergic Nerves

During the sympathetic adrenergic response, norepinephrine is released from the *terminal varicosities*, lying on min-

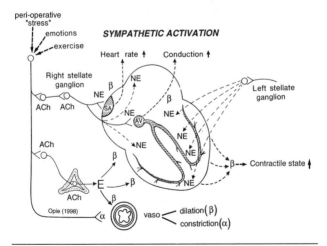

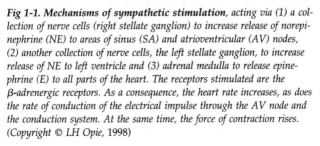

Fig 1-1. Mechanisms of sympathetic stimulation, *acting via (1) a collection of nerve cells (right stellate ganglion) to increase release of norepinephrine (NE) to areas of sinus (SA) and atrioventricular (AV) nodes, (2) another collection of nerve cells, the left stellate ganglion, to increase release of NE to left ventricle and (3) adrenal medulla to release epinephrine (E) to all parts of the heart. The receptors stimulated are the β-adrenergic receptors. As a consequence, the heart rate increases, as does the rate of conduction of the electrical impulse through the AV node and the conduction system. At the same time, the force of contraction rises. (Copyright © LH Opie, 1998)*

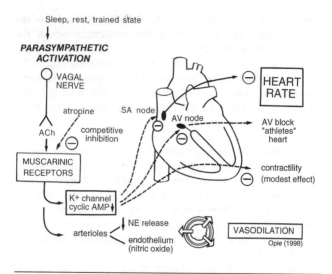

Fig 1-2. The parasympathetic or cholinergic system, acting via the muscarinic receptors, has inhibitory effects on the heart. The major site of action of parasympathetic control of the heart appears to be the sinoatrial node, where it reduces the heart rate in contrast to sympathetic stimulation. Other lesser parasympathetic effects include inhibition of the AV node and a mild inhibitory effect on contractile force. In trained athletes, parasympathetic activity increases to slow the heart rate. In overtraining, the AV node can be inhibited to block the conduction of the impulse from the SA node to the ventricles, an example of AV block. (Copyright © LH Opie, 1998)

ute end-branches of the neurons of the adrenergic nervous system. Norepinephrine is synthesized in these varicosities via dopa and dopamine and ultimately from the amino acid, tyrosine, which is taken up from the circulation. Such synthesis takes place only in the sympathetic nerve terminals, not in the ordinary myocardial cells. The norepinephrine thus synthesized is stored within the terminals in *storage granules* (or *vesicles*) to be released on stimulation by an adrenergic nervous impulse. Thus, when central stimulation increases during excitement or exercise, an increased number of adrenergic impulses liberate an increased amount of norepinephrine from the terminals. Most of the released norepinephrine is taken up again by the nerve terminal varicosities to re-enter the storage vesicles or to be metabolized. At least some of the released norepinephrine interacts with the specific vascular α-receptors and another fraction enters the circulation to account for the increased blood norepinephrine levels found during states of excitement or stress or exercise.

Neuromodulation. This is the process whereby the release of norepinephrine from the terminal neurons in response to a given degree of sympathetic stimulation, is either increased or decreased in response to a variety of controlling agents collectively called the neuromodulators (Fig 1-3). Negative neuromodulators, decreasing the release of norepinephrine, include the local messengers adenosine and nitric oxide formed during exercise. At night, when there is increased cholinergic activity, norepinephrine release is also lessened by the muscarinic presynaptic receptors. Pharmacologically, an important negative modulator is

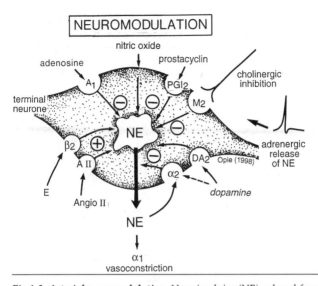

Fig 1-3. Arterial neuromodulation. Norepinephrine (NE), released from the storage granules of the terminal neurones into the synaptic cleft, has predominantly vasoconstrictive effects acting via postsynaptic α_1-receptors. In addition, presynaptic α_2-receptors are stimulated to allow feedback inhibition of its release to modulate any excess release of NE. Parasympathetic cholinergic stimulation releases acetylcholine (ACh), which stimulates the muscarinic (M_2) receptors to inhibit the release of NE and thereby indirectly to cause vasodilation. Circulating epinephrine (E) stimulates vasodilatory β_2-receptors. Angiotensin II, formed ultimately in response to renin released from the kidneys is also powerfully vasoconstrictive acting both by inhibition of NE release and directly on arteriolar receptors. AII = angiotensin II. Note that in the myocardium, released NE acts chiefly on α_1-receptors. (Copyright © LH Opie, 1998)

dopamine, acting chiefly by the DA_2 presynaptic receptor and to a lesser extent on the α_2 presynaptic receptor.

Of the positive neuromodulators, stimulating the release of norepinephrine, the most powerful is *angiotensin-II*, the circulating vasoconstrictor that helps to control the blood pressure (Lyons et al, 1997). When the blood pressure falls, as may inadvertently occur in the perioperative period, renin is released from the kidneys, ultimately to form circulating angiotensin-II (A II) and thereby to promote vasoconstriction and to restore the blood pressure. A II also directly causes vasoconstriction by acting on the post-synaptic angiotensin-II (AT_1) receptors on the vascular sarcolemma.

Adrenergic Facilitation by Angiotensin II

Besides promoting release of norepinephrine from the terminal neurons, A II facilitates the adrenergic stimulation at several levels (Fig 1-4). During chronic therapy with angiotensin converting enzyme (ACE) inhibitors, which lessen formation of A II, the outflow of sympathetic stimuli to the muscles also decreases (Grassi et al, 1997).

Pre- and post-synaptic α-adrenergic receptors. Norepinephrine inhibits its own release by negative feedback inhibition. Norepinephrine released into the synaptic cleft, acts on the inhibitory presynaptic (prejunctional) α_2-adrenergic receptors. In contrast, the post-synaptic α_1-adrenergic receptors are situated on the myocyte sarcolemma.

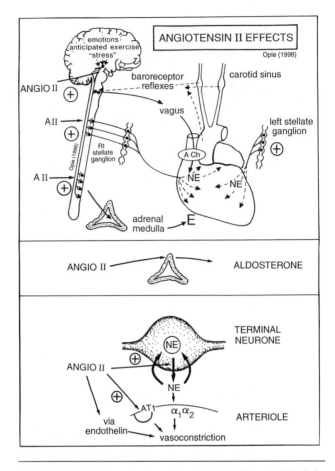

*Fig 1-4. Multiple sites of action of angiotensin II (angio II) includ-
ing central activation, facilitation of ganglionic transmission, release of aldosterone from the adrenal medulla, release of norepinephrine (NE) from
terminal sympathetic varicosities with inhibition of re-uptake and direct
stimulation of vascular angiotensin II (AT$_1$) receptors. Angiotensin II also
releases vasoconstrictory endothelin from the endothelium. The major net
effects are powerful vasoconstriction and sympathetic facilitation. (Copyright © LH Opie, 1998)*

RECEPTORS AND SIGNALS IN CONTRACTILE MYOCARDIUM

The tight molecular fit between the stimulant molecule
(agonist) and the receptor gives rise to the key and lock
model. Two major types of adrenergic receptors have been
defined by the specific nature of the cardiovascular reactions evoked by infused catecholamines. Those receptors
concerned with enhanced contractility and heart rate are
called β-adrenergic receptors and those concerned with
increasing the tone of arterioles are the α-adrenergic receptors. Cholinergic receptors respond to their messenger, acetylcholine and in general have the opposite effect to
adrenergic stimulation. For example, β-adrenergic stimulation increases heart rate, whereas cholinergic stimulation
decreases it. Cholinergic receptors are also called muscarinic
receptors, because they respond to the complex chemical
compound, muscarine, derived from certain mushrooms.

Sympathetic stimulation. Both β and α-adrenergic receptors are activated (Table 1-2). When the sympathetic nerves to the heart, but not to the peripheral circulation, are stimulated, β-adrenergic effects predominate (Fig 1-1). There follows a marked increase of heart rate, left ventricular pressure and the indices of left ventricular contractile activity. The blood pressure rises abruptly because much greater cardiac output has been ejected into the same vascular bed. During exercise, when such β-adrenergic stimulation of the heart is accompanied by a mixture of peripheral effects, α-adrenergic vasoconstriction tends to be offset by β-adrenergic and by autoregulatory local metabolic vasodilation.

Table 1-2. Comparative cardiovascular effects of α- and β-adrenergic receptor stimulation

	α-mediated	β-mediated
Electrophysiological effects	±	Conduction ◊ Pacemaker ◊ Heart rate ◊
Myocardial mechanics	±	Contractility ◊ Stroke volume ◊ Cardiac output ◊ Systolic BP ↑
Myocardial metabolism	±	O_2 uptake ◊ ATP use ◊
Coronary arterioles	Variable constriction (α_1 and α_2 mediated)	Direct dilation ↑ Indirect dilation ◊ (metabolic)
Peripheral arterioles	Constriction ◊ SVR ◊ BP ◊	Modest dilation SVR ↓ Diastolic BP may fall

± = little or no effect; ↑ = increase; ◊ = marked increase; SVR, systemic (peripheral) vascular resistance; BP, blood pressure

Intracellular signal systems explain the opposite effects of sympathetic and parasympathetic stimulation on heart rate, myocardial contraction and arteriolar tone. These signals link receptor occupation to the change in biological function (Fig 1-5), such as heart rate, myocardial contraction or vasoconstriction or vasodilation. When β-adrenergic receptors are occupied, the membrane bound enzyme adenylate cyclase is stimulated into activity by one of a superfamily of proteins, the stimulatory G protein G_S (Lefkowitz, 1995). The result is conversion of ATP into cyclic AMP, the second messenger, that in turn promotes calcium entry into the myocardial cell by increasing the opening of the calcium channel (Fig 1-5). Enhanced release of stored calcium from the sarcoplasmic reticulum follows next, so that cytosolic calcium rises more and the force of contraction increases.

Parasympathetic stimulation leads to an opposite series of events (Fig 1-5). Occupation of the muscarinic (M_2) receptor by the neurotransmitter acetylcholine interacts with the inhibitory G protein, G_i to decrease activity of adenylate cyclase (Neubig, 1994). There is less formation of cyclic AMP and a sequence of events opposite to those achieved by β-adrenergic stimulation. The end result is decreased

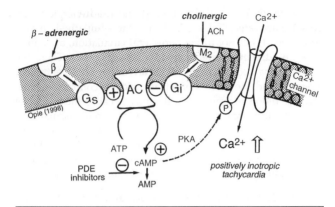

Fig 1-5. Adrenergic and cholinergic receptors. These are the β-adren-ergic receptor (β) and the cholinergic muscarinic (M₂) receptor, the latter for acetylcholine (ACh). The β-adrenergic receptor is coupled to adenyl cyclase (AC) via the activated stimulatory G-protein G$_s$. Consequent for-mation of cAMP activates protein kinase A (PKA) to phosphorylate (P) the calcium channel to increase calcium entry. Activity of adenyl cyclase can be decreased by the inhibitory subunits of the ACh-associated inhibi-tory G-protein, G$_i$. Cyclic AMP is broken down by phosphodiesterase (PDE) so that PDE-inhibitor drugs have a sympathomimetic effect. (Copyright © LH Opie, 1998)

contractile force. This cholinergic sequence may not be as important as anticipated in ventricular muscle because of (i) the relative sparseness of muscarinic receptors and (ii) the inhibitory sequence may be most evident when activity of adenylate cyclase is increased by prior β-adrenergic stimu-lation. Thus cholinergic activity can act as a break to excess to adrenergic stimulation of the myocardium. There is also a second messenger for the parasympathetic system, cyclic GMP, which is formed when acetylcholine interacts with guanylate cyclase. In general, cyclic GMP has opposite effects on the heart to cyclic AMP. Of note, cyclic GMP also serves as the second messenger of the nitric oxide messen-ger system (see later).

Receptor Desensitization, Uncoupling and Downregulation

With continued stimulation of a receptor by the agonist molecule, loss of response often follows (Raymond et al, 1990). This phenomenon is complex and the terminologies not clear. *Desensitization* is any factor decreasing the recep-tor response and includes three processes. The initial step is molecular uncoupling of the receptor from its effector sys-tem. Next is *internalization*, when receptors lose their sur-face alignment and enter the interior of the cell. Such internalized receptors may remain in that situation or may be re-incorporated into the cell membrane or, if they stay there or undergo breakdown. The latter explains true downregulation. Clinically, the phenomenon of loss of response to persistent stimulation of the beta-adrenergic receptor is well documented, for example after some hours of infusion of dobutamine. This phenomenon is best called drug *tolerance*, which avoids the question of the precise molecular mechanism involved.

SINUS NODE PACEMAKER ACTIVITY

Spontaneous pacemaking is a complex event, dependent on at least four currents (Irisawa et al, 1993), thereby providing fail-safe mechanisms to prevent sinus arrest, potentially a cause of sudden cardiac death. Of the four currents, (Fig 1-6), at least two respond to adrenergic stimulation. Thus *β-adrenergic stimulation* increases the heart rate at least in part because increased formation of cyclic AMP, the second messenger, enhances the rate of spontaneous pacemaking (Fig 1-7). In addition, there is increased firing of the current I_f which is the same current as that found in Purkinje fibers.

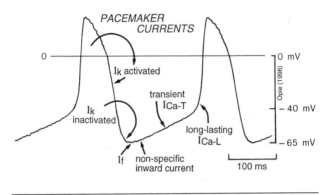

Fig 1-6. Pacemaker currents in SA node. There are four proposed different pacemaker currents. The repolarizing potassium current I_k is activated by full depolarization. Then, as the voltage decreases, it becomes inactivated and decays. At that time inward currents begin to flow, namely I_b (nonspecific background current, not shown) and probably I_f (inward current evoked by hyperpolarization). Later the voltage range for activation of the transient inward calcium current I_{Ca-T} is reached. Even later, the threshold for activation of the action potential itself is attained so that there is rapid depolarization, typical of the upstroke of the action potential of the SA node, involving the long-lasting calcium channel, I_{Ca-L}. For details see Hagiwara et al (1988). (Copyright © LH Opie, 1998)

Cholinergic stimulation slows the pacemaker rate by at least four mechanisms, two of which involve decreased formation of cyclic AMP (Levy and Martin, 1995). Acting at the preganglionic level, neuromodulation by M_2 receptor stimulation lessens the release of norepinephrine. Secondly, the postganglionic M_2 receptor decreases the formation of cyclic AMP by adenylate cyclase because there is lessened activity of G_S and increased activity of G_i. Thirdly, cholinergic stimulation of the M_2 receptor acts via another G protein (Fig 1-8) to help open a specific type of K^+ channel (K_{ACh}). The result is increased outward flow of K^+ ions, with a relatively greater positive charge outside the cell membrane and a relatively greater negative charge within the membrane of the sinus node cells. That is, there is *hyperpolarization* (Irisawa et al., 1993). This is event leads to decreased pacemaker activity because, starting from a greater negative charge within the cell, the inward potassium current and other pacemaking currents require more time to reach the threshold at which spontaneous depolarization and firing of the pacemaker takes place. Fourthly,

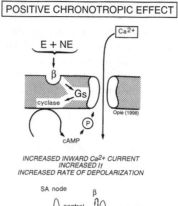

Fig 1-7. Mechanism of adrenergic positive chronotropic effect. Epinephrine (E) and norepinephrine (NE) stimulate β-adrenergic receptors (β) in the sinoatrial node to increase the calcium currents and the current I_f as shown in Fig 1-6. The result is more rapid depolarization and tachycardia. For P, see Fig 1-5. (Copyright © LH Opie, 1998)

the newly described nitric oxide messenger system may also be at work. The proposal is that cholinergic M_2 stimulation leads to formation of nitric oxide, that in turn promotes the formation of cyclic GMP (Han et al, 1995).

Of the above mechanisms, the first and second chiefly lessen the degree of increase of heart rate achieved by β-adrenergic stimulation. The other two mechanisms can

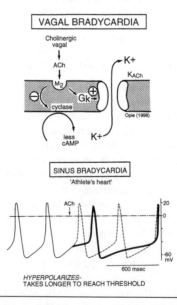

Fig 1-8. Mechanism of cholinergic bradycardia. Stimulation of the muscarinic receptor (subtype M_2) leads to two events. First, adenyl cyclase is inhibited (Fig. 1-7). Secondly, the acetylcholine (ACh) sensitive potassium channel is opened, in response to the G_K protein. Hyperpolarization slows the SA node. (Copyright © LH Opie, 1998)

work independently of the sympathetic tone. For example, at night, when vagal tone is high and adrenergic tone is low there is a marked slowing of heart rate, probably due to the two mechanisms that act independently of cyclic AMP.

Vascular Control

Of particular importance is the diameter of the small arteries (arterioles) that control the peripheral (systemic) vascular resistance, a major component of the afterload against which the heart works. The peripheral vascular resistance also helps to set the blood pressure. Control of this site is by vasoconstrictors and dilators that act in opposing ways (Fig 1-9). Such control cannot be simplified just into the opposing effects of the sympathetic and parasympathetic systems (Reviewed by Opie, 1998). Although α_1-adrenergic receptors cause vasoconstriction, almost paradoxically β_2-receptors cause vasodilation acting by increasing cyclic AMP in vascular smooth muscle. The latter change directly inhibits the contractile proteins in this tissue, to cause vasodilation rather than the expected vasoconstriction. Thus norepinephrine may be both vasoconstrictive by α_1-adrenergic stimulation and vasodilator via β_2-receptors. Hypothetically, norepinephrine released from the nerve terminals is more likely to interact with α_1-adrenergic receptors and circulating norepinephrine with β_2-receptors. Circulating epinephrine is only vasodilatory.

Parasympathetic stimulation causes vasodilation by a variety of mechanisms, including neuromodulation to

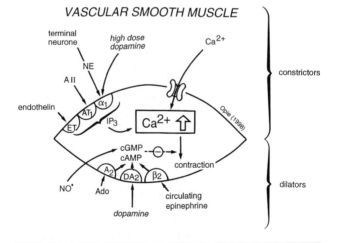

VASCULAR SMOOTH MUSCLE

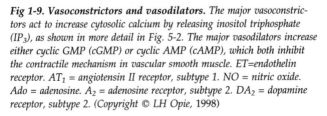

Fig 1-9. Vasoconstrictors and vasodilators. *The major vasoconstrictors act to increase cytosolic calcium by releasing inositol triphosphate (IP$_3$), as shown in more detail in Fig. 5-2. The major vasodilators increase either cyclic GMP (cGMP) or cyclic AMP (cAMP), which both inhibit the contractile mechanism in vascular smooth muscle. ET=endothelin receptor. AT$_1$ = angiotensin II receptor, subtype 1. NO = nitric oxide. Ado = adenosine. A$_2$ = adenosine receptor, subtype 2. DA$_2$ = dopamine receptor, subtype 2. (Copyright © LH Opie, 1998)*

decrease release of vasoconstrictory norepinephrine. Experimentally, large amounts of acetylcholine act to release vasodilatory nitric oxide from the inner lining of the blood vessels (endothelium), provided that the endothelium is not damaged. Signals emanating from the endothelium play a major role in regulation of vascular tone. For example, during exercise the shear stress of the increased blood flow induces the release of vasodilatory nitric oxide. Conversely, the damaged endothelium releases vasoconstrictory endothelin.

Overall Adrenergic Effects on Vascular Bed

Adrenergic stimulation has very complex overall effects on various vascular beds and on the cardiovascular system. In vascular smooth muscle, the α_1-mediated vasoconstrictive affects of norepinephrine are opposed by circulating epinephrine which is simultaneously released, for example during exercise and which stimulates vasodilatory β_2-receptors. In arterioles of the splanchic bed, epinephrine also stimulates α_1-adrenergic receptors to cause vasoconstriction, thereby helping to divert blood from non-muscular to muscular tissues. Although norepinephrine can stimulate the vasodilatory β_2-receptors, the reasons for its overall vasoconstrictive effect are thought to be that: (1) the α_1-receptors are anatomically closer than the β_2-receptors to the sites of norepinephrine release from the terminal neurons and (2) the α_1-adrenergic receptors may be greater in number or activity than the vasodilatory β-receptors. Furthermore, the overall effects of sympathetic stimulation on the arterioles differ from individual to individual. In those who are hypertensive or may be prone to develop hypertension, vasoconstrictive effects of norepinephrine appear to predominate. In contrast, during exercise in normal subjects, vasoconstriction is overridden by vasodilatory β_2-receptor stimulation. But even when these receptors are experimentally blocked, there is still an increase in muscle blood flow during exercise limited to those muscles that are actually used, whereas flow falls in those that are not being used. Thus the crucial factor is the production of vasodilatory local metabolites by the exercising muscles. A prominent factor seems to be the flow-induced release of nitric oxide from the vascular endothelium.

VASODILATORY LOCAL MESSENGERS

During periods of perioperative stress, adrenergic outflow is increased. Stimulation of the heart by β-receptors leads to an increase frequency and force of contraction, yet simultaneously α-adrenergic stimulation will tend to constrict the resistance arterioles (Fig 1-9). Therefore, such stress would be associated with an inevitable rise of blood pressure. In contrast, during physiological aerobic exercise, the blood pressure rises much less than expected. The reason why this happens is because (1) vasodilatory messengers are locally formed during muscle metabolism and act on the arterioles to vasodilate and (2) epinephrine released during exercise induces vasodilatory β_2-receptor stimulation, so that the peripheral vascular resistance falls during exercise. Similar changes are thought to account for the increase in coronary blood flow, also occurring during exercise.

Adenosine Signaling

Adenosine is one of these local messengers, being formed from the breakdown of the high-energy phosphate compound ATP during vigorous exercise or during hypoxia. It can act on three receptor subtypes (Fig 1-10). A_1-receptors and A_3-receptors act on the heart muscle, while A_2-receptors mediate peripheral vasodilation (Stiles, 1992). Adenosine is both a direct vasodilator by its actions on the adenosine A_2-receptor on vascular smooth muscle cells and by inhibiting the release of norepinephrine (Fig 1-3). Adenosine is formed from the breakdown of ATP both physiologically (as during an increased heart load) and pathologically (as in hypoxia or ischaemia). Adenosine diffuses from myocardial cells to act on coronary arterial smooth muscle to cause vasodilation. The mechanism of the latter effect is reasonably well understood and involves (1) the stimulation of vascular A_2-receptor and, hence, adenylate cyclase with formation of vasodilatory cyclic AMP (Fig 1-9), (2) negative

ADENOSINE RECEPTORS

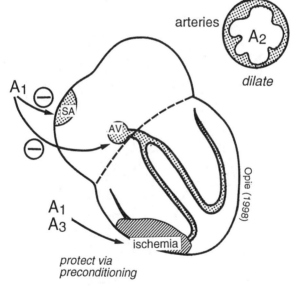

Fig 1-10. Adenosine receptors. The two basic subtypes are the adenosine-1 and adenosine-2 receptors. The former are found in the nodes and contractile myocardium. By inhibiting the formation of cyclic AMP (Fig 1-3), they decrease the heart rate, inhibit re-entrant nodal tachycardias and have a negative inotropic effect. A_2 receptors promote vasodilation by several mechanisms, including simulation of vascular cyclic AMP (Fig 1-9). A_3 myocardial receptors, recently described, play a role with A_1 receptors in ischemic preconditioning. SA = sinoatrial node; AV = atrial ventricular ndoe. Note different roles of the three subtypes. (Copyright © LH Opie, 1998)

neuromodulation with decreased release of NE from nerve terminals and (3) opening of the ATP-sensitive potassium channel (see later in this chapter).

Adenosine also acts on nodal tissue of the heart (Pappano and Mubagwa, 1992, Stiles, 1992), where A_1-receptors couple to the acetylcholine-sensitive potassium channel promoting the current I_{kACh} (also called I_{kADO}) to stimulate channel opening and thereby to exert inhibitory effects on the sinus and AV nodes. The latter inhibition is the basis for the use of adenosine in the treatment of supraventricular nodal reentry arrhythmias (Fig 7-11). The A_1-receptors also appear to mediate the chest pain of angina pectoris. The newly discovered A_3-receptors may play a protective role (together with A_1 receptors) in the experimental phenomenon of ischemic preconditioning (Tracey et al, 1997).

Nitric Oxide as Messenger with Cyclic GMP as Target

Nitric oxide is a newly defined messenger of considerable cardiovascular importance (Kelly et al, 1996, Moncada and Higgs, 1993), manufactured by the vascular endothelium (Fig 1-11). Nitric oxide vasodilates in at least two ways. It lessens the release of norepinephrine from terminal neurons (Fig 1-3). Nitric oxide also stimulates the formation of cyclic GMP by soluble guanylate cyclase (Fig 1-9). Cyclic GMP vasodilates through a mechanism thought to involve a

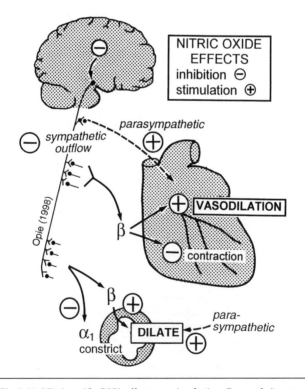

Fig 1-11. Nitric oxide (NO) effects on circulation. Proposed sites at which the local messenger nitric oxide can alter autonomic effects on the cardiovascular system, with venodilation and inhibition of contraction as end results. (Copyright © LH Opie, 1998)

cGMP-sensitive protein kinase (PKG) and a decrease of cytosolic calcium. Physiologically, nitric oxide can be synthesized both in the vascular endothelium and in the nerve terminals of the nitric oxide releasing nerves (*nitroxidergic nerves*), as well as in other sites in the nervous system. Such nerves, releasing nitric oxide, cause vasodilation in contrast to the vasoconstrictive sympathetic nerves. There are therefore several vasodilatory effects. Nitric oxide not only acts as a local messenger to convey signals from the endothelium to vascular smooth muscle, but it also exerts protective effects on the vascular endothelium by inhibition of platelet aggregation.

The stimulus to the release of nitric oxide from the endothelium during exercise is not fully known. Hypothetically, a low tissue oxygen tension, occurring as oxygen is used during exercise, could stimulate the synthesis of nitric oxide. Alternatively, the increased rate of blood flow during exercise causes a mechanical effect on the endothelium (shear stress) that liberates nitric oxide.

Until recently, it was thought that nitric oxide played no role in the regulation of myocardial cell function. Yet, in ventricular myocytes, production of nitric oxide enhances the negative inotropic effect of acetylcholine and decreases the positive inotropic effects of β-stimulation. Therefore, the nitric oxide system, it is proposed, may negatively modulate the cardiac effects of adrenergic stimulation, in keeping with the hypothesis that cyclic GMP opposes cyclic AMP in its myocardial actions. In this sense the nitric oxide path would have an effect ancillary to that of the cholinergic system, which also promotes the formation of cyclic GMP. Pathologically, considerable excess of nitric oxide can be synthesized in myocardial cells by the enzyme iNOS, where i = inducible and NOS = nitric oxide synthase. Such excess nitric oxide inhibits contraction in some serious disease states, such as septic shock.

Pharmacological Vasodilation

Pharmacological blockade of vascular agonist receptors

The three major vascular agonists are angiotensin II, endothelin and α_1-adrenergic catecholamines. In keeping with their basic vasoconstrictive properties of each, the result of pharmacological receptor blockade of each receptor is vasodilation. Thus indirect inhibition of angiotensin II by means of the angiotensin converting enzyme (ACE) inhibitors, or by the angiotensin II AT_1 receptor blockers such as losartan, is often used in the vasodilatory therapy of hypertension or heart failure. Endothelin receptor blockade may become of use in the therapy of heart failure; in hypertension endothelin blockade reduces the blood pressure (Krum et al, 1998). α_1-Adrenergic receptor blockade is used much more in the therapy of hypertension than of heart failure, because in the latter condition the long term results are no different from placebo, for reasons poorly understood.

Adenosine

Because adenosine is so rapidly broken down by adenosine deaminase, intravenous adenosine is very short lived in its action which is a therapeutic advantage when the circulation is compromised. Drugs acting on the adenosine system include dipyridamole, which inhibits the breakdown of adenosine to cause vigorous coronary vasodilation and caffeine or theophylline which antagonize adenosine at its receptors.

Nitrates

Nitrates as a group are compounds that are converted in the vascular wall to nitric oxide, a powerful vasodilator. Nitric oxide donors, such as sodium nitroprusside, do not need such conversion. The problem with the nitrate group of vasodilators is the development of severe tolerance so that intermittent therapy or dose step-up is often required.

Dopamine

Dopamine is vasodilator by virtue of presynaptic inhibition of the release of norepinephrine by DA_1-receptors and by virtue of the action on postsynaptic vasodilatory DA_2-receptors (Goldberg and Rajfer, 1985). The mechanism may be by stimulation of vascular adenylate cyclase and formation of cyclic AMP (Fig 1-9). In high doses, dopamine becomes vasoconstrictive by stimulation of postsynaptic α_1-adrenergic receptors.

Phosphodiesterase inhibitors

These agents, such as milrinone, inhibit the breakdown of vascular cyclic AMP, which is vasodilatory. Cyclic AMP also accumulates in the myocardium, with a positive inotropic effect. This combination of effects is called *inodilation*. In ischemia, the downside is that the cyclic AMP may be arrhythmogenic.

ENDOTHELIAL DYSFUNCTION

An important current concept is that the vascular endothelium can be damaged by a several major diseases, including atherosclerosis, diabetes mellitus and hypertension (Celermajer, 1997). The endothelium thus damaged releases less nitric oxide than the normal endothelium, which not only means less vasodilation, but also loss of the protective effects of nitric oxide such as inhibition of platelet aggregation (Fig 1-12). Instead the damaged endothelium releases an excess release of the vasoconstrictor *endothelin*. The result is that during exercise, the coronary arteries tend to constrict rather than dilate as they would normally, as shown by direct measurement of the coronary lumen. The stimulus to the release of vasodilatory nitric oxide during exercise is not fully known. Hypothetically, a low tissue oxygen tension, occurring as oxygen is used during exercise, could stimulate the synthesis of nitric oxide. Alternatively, the

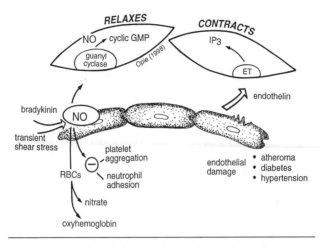

Fig 1-12. Role of endothelium in the regulation of vascular smooth muscle tone. The healthy endothelium (left) releases vasodilator nitric oxide (NO) in response to bradykinin and transient sheer stress. The damaged endothelium releases vasoconstrictory endothelin (ET). For role of IP₃ see Fig 5-2. (Copyright © LH Opie, 1998)

increased rate of blood flow during exercise could cause a mechanical effect on the endothelium (shear stress) to liberate nitric oxide. An important current hypothesis is that the ACE (angiotensin converting enzyme) inhibitors have a vascular protective effect, acting by increased formation of *bradykinin* (Fig 1-12) which elicits the release of protective nitric oxide from the vascular endothelium.

BAROREFLEXES AND CONTROL OF BLOOD PRESSURE

When the blood pressure (BP) rises excessively, pressure-sensitive cells in the aortic arch and the carotid artery respond by conveying impulses to a central coordinating site, the vasomotor center. The center then sends out vagal stimuli to decrease heart rate, which in turn will lower the cardiac output so that the BP then falls to the normal range (Fig 1-4):

> Increased blood pressure → baroreceptors → vasomotor center → vagal stimulation → decreased heart rate → decreased cardiac output → BP falls to appropriate levels.

This sequence explains the *reflex bradycardia* that can be expected during an acute elevation of arterial blood pressure as a result of stimulation of the baroreceptors in response to peripheral α_1-adrenergic vasoconstriction resulting from excess stimulation by an α_1-agonist such as norepinephrine or by the administration of methoxamine.

An interesting application of the principles of baroreflex control is the use of *carotid sinus massage* in the therapy of some types of supraventricular tachycardias. External manual stimulation of the mechanoreceptors in the carotid sinus provokes the afferent stimuli, which travel to the vagal nucleus to stimulate the efferent limb so that there is increased vagal inhibition of both sinus and atrioventricular nodes, which in turn helps to terminate the tachycardia.

CONTROL OF CELL CALCIUM

Once the cardiac impulse has travelled from the pacemaker cells of the sinus node to the ventricular cells, the next event of critical importance is the voltage-induced increased opening of the calcium channels of contractile cells of the ventricles. Thereafter follows a series of intracellular movements of calcium ions, leading to the myocardial contraction-relaxation cycle (Fig 1-13). The wave of excitation is linked to myocyte contraction by the process of *excitation-contraction coupling* (Opie, 1997). Contraction must be followed by relaxation, which results from uptake of calcium ions into the sarcoplasmic reticulum (SR). Only small amounts of calcium ions actually enter and leave the cell with each cardiac cycle. The major calcium ion movements are from the intracellular calcium stores to the cytosol and back again. The sarcolemma maintains a vast gradient of calcium ion concentration from the extracellular value of about 10^{-3}M (1 mM, 1 mmol/litre) to intracellular values, which can increase from diastolic values of about 10^{-7}M up to systolic values of 10^{-5}M during maximal contraction.

Calcium Ion Movements

The normal SR spontaneously releases small packets of calcium called the *calcium sparks* (Wier et al, 1997). The key event that converts the sparks into a substantial release of calcium from the SR, is the sudden arrival of calcium ions that have entered the myocyte by the opening of the L-type calcium channels in response to depolarization. This process is the *calcium-induced release of calcium* from the SR (Fabiato,

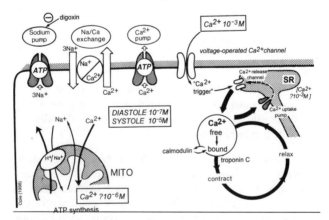

Fig 1-13. Calcium ion fluxes in the myocardium. *Note much higher extracellular (10^{-3} mol/l) than intracellular value and a hypothetical mitochondrial value of about 10^{-6} mol/l. The mitochondria could act as a buffer against excessive changes in the free cytosolic calcium concentration. For details of digoxin action, see Fig 10-4 (page 298). MITO, mitochondria.*
SR= sarcoplasmic reticulum. (Copyright © LH Opie, 1998)

1985, Santana et al, 1996) as follows. The major intracellular calcium store is in the sarcoplasmic reticulum (Fig 1-13). In response to the relatively large amounts of calcium ions are liberated, there is an increasing interaction of calcium ions with the contractile protein troponin-C. When the ambient calcium concentration is low, troponin-C has a molecular structure that inhibits the interaction between actin and myosin. As the cytosolic calcium increases, the molecular structure of troponin-C changes and this inhibition is removed. The interaction of actin and myosin is facilitated and contraction takes place. When the release of calcium ions from the sarcoplasmic reticulum ceases, then the rise of cytosolic calcium comes to an end and contraction ceases. To initiate relaxation, the cytosolic calcium is rapidly taken up by the calcium pump of the sarcoplasmic reticulum. This hypothesis has received strong support from the molecular characterization of the receptor on the sarcoplasmic reticulum that releases calcium (Berridge, 1993). A lesser amount of calcium is moved out of the cell. As the cytosolic calcium concentration falls, relaxation is initiated as troponin-C starts to inhibit actin and myosin once more.

To balance the small amount of calcium entering the heart cell with each depolarization, a similar quantity of calcium ions leave the cell by one of two processes. First, internal calcium can be exchanged for external sodium ions by Na^+/Ca^{2+} exchange (Fig 1-13). Second and of lesser importance, a sarcolemmal calcium pump that is ATP-consuming, can transfer calcium outwards into the extracellular space against a concentration gradient. The exchange between mitochondrial and cytosolic calcium is relatively slow when compared to that between the sarcoplasmic reticulum and the cytosol. Hence mitochondria do not participate in the beat-to-beat control of calcium ion movements. Nevertheless, during conditions of cellular cytosolic calcium overload, to be discussed later in this chapter, mitochondria may help to protect the cell by storing some of the excess calcium.

Contraction in Vascular Smooth Muscle

Many of the cellular events are similar to those already described in the cardiac contraction cycle: the entry of calcium, the calcium-induced calcium release from the sarcoplasmic reticulum, the rise in cytosolic free calcium ion concentration, the interaction of calcium with the myosin ATPase, the subsequent uptake of calcium into the sarcoplasmic reticulum and the discharge of excess calcium via calcium exit channels.

β-receptor stimulation causes the myocardium to contract and the peripheral vessels to dilate by different mechanisms (Figs 1-5 and 1-9). Depolarization is not essential for the initiation of the contractile cycle in vascular smooth muscle because it can be set off by the rise of calcium released from the sarcoplasmic reticulum by inositol trisphosphate (IP_3), the second messenger of several vasoconstrictory stimuli. In peripheral vascular muscle, troponin-C is absent from the actin filaments, so that calcium ions must regulate the myosin-actin interaction by a different calcium regulator which is calmodulin. Calcium ions combine with calmodulin to form calcium-calmodulin, which promotes phosphorylation of the light chains of the myosin heads to initiate vascular contraction.

ION CHANNELS AND DRUG ACTION

Channels are pore-forming macromolecular proteins that span the sarcolemmal lipid bilayer to allow a highly selective pathway for ion transfer into the heart cell when the channel changes from a closed to an open state (Katz, 1993). Ion channels have two major properties: gating and permeation (Fig 1-14). Guarding each channel are two or more hypothetical gates that control its opening. Ions can permeate through the channel only when both gates are open. In the case of the sodium and calcium channels, which are best understood, the activation gate is shut at the normal resting membrane potential and the inactivation gate is open, so that the channels are *voltage-gated.* Depolarization opens the activation gate.

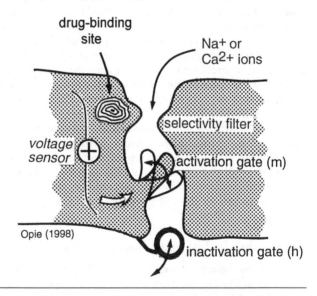

Fig 1-14. Channel pore model, showing activation and inactivation gates. The selectivity filter allows a specific ion to enter. The voltage sensor is a highly charged segment (helix) of the membrane-spanning domain responding to the voltage changes during depolarization and repolarization. The sensor "tells" the activation and inactivation gates to open and close. (Copyright © LH Opie, 1998)

Channels are not simply open or closed. Rather, the open state is the last of a sequence of many molecular states, varying from a fully closed to a fully open configuration. Therefore, it is more correct to speak of the *probability of channel opening*.

Sodium Channels

One of the first events in response to the onset of depolarization of phase 0 of the action potential is opening of the sodium channel when the voltage reaches -70 to -60 mV, which its *threshold of activation* (Fig 1-15).

The sodium current flows inward very rapidly during the first millisecond of depolarization. The inactivation gates turn off the current flow more slowly and have two time constants. The first time constant is less than 1 msec, switching off the sodium current very rapidly. The second component is much slower at about 4 sec and may account for the combined but constantly decreasing sodium inflow during the later stages of the action potential (current $I_{Na(s)}$). Some of this continued sodium inflow may be caused by the operation of the sodium-calcium exchanger with inward passage of sodium ions in response to a build-up of internal calcium.

The sodium channel is selectively inhibited by sodium channel blockers, for example by a highly toxic poison, tetrodotoxin (TTX) derived from the Japanese puffer fish, by their binding to an external membrane site on the channel. (Yet, when correctly prepared in a speciality restaurant in Japan, this fish is considered a great delicacy.) The number of molecules of TTX that bind to the surface is an indirect measure of the density of the sodium channels, which is about 16 per square micrometer. TTX also binds very specifically to neural sodium channels. Therefore, it cannot be used as an antiarrhythmic agent in humans because of the risk of central nervous system poisoning.

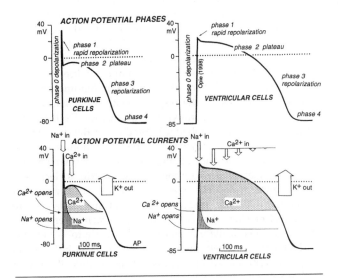

Fig 1-15. Action potential phases and currents. The four phases of the cardiac action potential (top panel) and the underlying currents (bottom panel) with Purkinje cells on the left and ventricular cells on the right. The rapid entry of sodium ions accounts for the initial phase of rapid depolarization of the action potential. Calcium ions enter chiefly by the slow calcium channel. After entry of positively charged sodium and calcium ions, the cell is fully depolarized. Then potassium channels open. The outward flow of positively charged potassium ions largely explains repolarization. Finally the cell re-enters the state of polarization. Purkinje cells, adapted for fast conduction of the cardiac impulse, have phase 0 that is relatively more prominent than in ventricular cells. The latter, adapted for contraction, have a more prominent plateau phase with more prolonged calcium ion entry. (Copyright © LH Opie, 1998)

If the potential difference from within to without the cell is removed by artificially increasing the extracellular potassium to depolarizing hyperkalemic values, then the sodium channel will not open. The result is inhibition of cardiac contraction with cardiac arrest (cardioplegia). Antiarrhythmic agents that inhibit the sodium channel are known as Class I antiarrhythmics and include lidocaine, quinidine and others.

Calcium Channels

Calcium ions must enter the cardiac myocyte via the calcium channel (Fig 1-15) to initiate the process of excitation-contraction coupling. There are two major subpopulations of sarcolemmal calcium channels relevant to the cardiovascular system, namely the T-channels and the L-channels. The *T-(transient) channels* open at a more negative voltage, having short bursts of opening and do not interact with conventional calcium antagonist drugs (Hagiwara et al, 1988). The T-channels presumably account for the earlier phase of the opening of the calcium channel, which may also give them a special role in the early electrical depolarization of the sinoatrial node and hence of initiation of the heart beat (Fig 1-6). Although T-channels are found in atrial cells, their existence in normal ventricular cells is controversial.

The sarcolemmal *L-(longlasting) channels* are the standard calcium channels found in the myocardium. These are also the channels that are involved in calcium-induced calcium release and are subject to inhibition by the usual calcium antagonist drugs (see Chapter 5). The molecular sites to which the calcium channel antagonist drugs bind are located in those transmembrane-spanning helices that are close to the pores. There are four major binding sites on L-type channels, being the respective sites of action of nifedipine (and other dihydropyridine agents, the DHPs), verapamil, diltiazem and mibefradil. Binding of the drug to the pore sites results in calcium channel inhibition. The common action of all calcium antagonists is vascular smooth muscle relaxation. In addition, the heart rate is decreased by the three non-DHP agents, verapamil, diltiazem and mibefradil. Of these 3 agents, verapamil and diltiazem are L-channel blockers that closely resemble each other in their clinical actions, while mibefradil binds chiefly to T- but also to L-channels. Mibefradil is claimed to have little or no negative inotropic effects because of the relative absence of T-channels on ventricular cells.

Potassium Channels

Although at least 10 potassium channel proteins have been identified, their function in the heart is relatively simple, namely to promote the efflux of potassium ions from heart cells (Carmeliet, 1992). By this action in depolarized cells, repolarization is enhanced and the cardiac action potential is thereby terminated (Fig 1-16). The major current concerned is called K_v or simply K. Efflux of potassium from polarized heart cells helps to maintain the resting membrane potential and the current concerned is K_{ir}, where $_{ir}$ = inward rectifier.

OUTWARD K⁺ CURRENTS

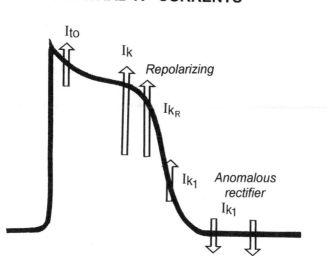

Fig 1-16. Outward potassium currents. These currents promote repolarization. For abbreviations, see text. (Copyright © LH Opie, 1998)

These potassium currents are still often called K and K_1 respectively. Another important potassium current is the transient outward current I_{to}, which flows especially at the end of the phase of rapid depolarization, to start of the process of repolarization.

The inward or anomolous rectifier potassium current, K_{ir} or K_1

This current is subject to inward rectification. Normally the relationship between the voltage and current is a straight line (Ohm's law). When a current can pass through the channel in both directions, but the flow in one direction is greater, then this selective process is called *rectification*. The channel rectifies in an inward direction when the voltage drops below the equilibrium potential for potassium (at about -90 mV). At a molecular level, the concept is that the inward current "unplugs" an internal divalent ion such as magnesium that would normally block the channel pore. Because of the marked deviation of the voltage-current relationship for this channel, the current is also called the *anomalous rectifier*. Outward rectification occurs when the major current flow is in the outward direction but voltage is more positive than zero. Thus, K_{ir} can contribute to the final stages of repolarization and it then reverses to become an inward current that helps maintain full diastolic depolarization. In the sinus node, this current is absent.

Voltage-operated K^+ channel, K_v or K

This channel, also called the *delayed rectifier*, conducts the current K_v that physiologically makes a major contribution to repolarization. Inactivation of this current also plays a crucial role in the initiation of spontaneous depolarization in the sinus node (Fig 1-6). The superfamily that includes this channel is sometimes called the *Shaker family* because the delayed rectifier was first cloned in a mutant of the fruitfly, Drosophila. When this channel is genetically absent from the fruitfly, exposure to ether provokes spasms of muscular shaking. Defects in the molecular structure of K_r and K_s, the rapid and slow components of this current, are important in an inherited human disorder called the long QT-syndrome that predisposes to certain potentially fatal arrhythmias. (Attali, 1996). Drugs that inhibit this channel prolong repolarization and hence the refractory period, namely the class III drugs such as amiodarone and sotatol (See Ch 7).

ATP-sensitive potassium channel and K channel openers

This channel is an example of a ligand (Latin *ligare*, to bind) operated potassium channel which can be opened by a chemical molecular signal that binds to a receptor site near the channel protein (Fig 1-17). There are two binding sites, one the SUR site (SUR = sulfonylureas, epitomized by the oral antidiabetic agent, glibenclamide) and the other for ATP (Ashford et al, 1994). The important regulatory role of internal ATP explains the name, the K_{ATP} *channel*. There appears to be no physiological role for this channel in cardiac myocytes. In general, this channel is closed in physiological conditions when ATP is high. During ischemia, as ATP breaks down with formation of ADP and adenosine, opening of

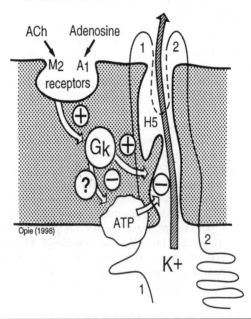

Fig 1-17. Ligand-gated potassium channels. These channels are part of the inward rectifier superfamily. This cartoon shows the proposed control mechanisms in response to acetylcholine (ACh) and adenosine, both of which slow the heart rate. M_2, muscarinic receptor subtype 2; A_1, adenosine receptor subtype 1; G_k, G-protein controlling activity of this potassium channel. (Copyright © LH Opie, 1998)

this K^+ channel is promoted. The outward passage of K^+ ions and their accumulation on the outside of the cell, causes loss of normal membrane polarization with a decreased contractile response and an induced state of inactivity or rest. It is supposed that adenosine, released in ischemia, helps to open this channel and thereby protects against subsequent ischemia, the phenomenon being called preconditioning.

The function of K_{ATP} in vascular smooth muscle is much more clear. There, in response to the formation of adenosine, this channel opens and participates in coronary vasodilation. Adenosine formed during myocardial hypoxia or during vigorous muscular work is thought to diffuse from the cardiac myocyte to the K_{ATP} channel on vascular smooth muscle cells, to relieve the inhibition by ATP and to allow channel opening. The egress of potassium ions causes hyperpolarization that, in turn, leads to vasodilation by inactivation of the calcium channels. (This vasodilatory mechanism is distinct from the interaction of adenosine with I_{kADO}, described in a previous section of this chapter, although both mechanisms lead to hyperpolarization).

Potassium channel openers is a term that usually refers to vasodilators that act by promoting K_{ATP} opening. Examples are pinacidil, cromakalim, minoxidil, and diazoxide. Nicorandil is a mixed nitrate-potassium opener. By mechanisms not fully understood, these drugs tend to protect ischemic myocardial cells. On the contrary, the inhibition K_{ATP} by the anti-diabetics sulfonylureas may promote coronary vasoconstriction. Sulfonylureas also lessen ischemic loss of potassium and inhibit early ischemic ventricular arrhythmias.

Chloride Channels

In the past, chloride currents were thought to play an insignificant electrophysiologic role in the heart, especially since one of the proposed chloride currents was more correctly identified as a potassium current, I_{to}. There are no less than five distinct cardiac chloride currents (Ackerman and Clapham, 1993). The most important is $I_{Cl(cAMP)}$ the chloride current activated by catecholamines. This shortening of the action potential duration is crucial during β-adrenergic stimulation when the whole heart "speeds up". By promoting influx of chloride ions with negative charges there is in effect an outward current that helps to shorten the action potential duration. Without this chloride current β-adrenergic stimulation would widen the action potential by enhanced opening of the calcium channel. There are no cardiovascular drugs that specifically act on this channel.

VENTRICULAR ACTION POTENTIAL

The characteristic appearance of the ventricular action potential (Fig 1-15) can now be interpreted in greater detail in terms of opening and closing of sodium, calcium and potassium channels that have just been discussed. Data obtained by computer modeling help to define the contribution of each of these channels. The rapid phase of depolarization of the action potential *(phase 0)* is the result of opening of the sodium channels. Sodium conductance first increases very rapidly, as does the flow of the inward current (I_{Na}) to peak within 1 msec and then to fall off equally rapidly. This flash of inward sodium movement, carrying positive charges, fully depolarizes the cell causing the rapid upstroke, or phase 0. It is on this phase that the class 1 antiarrhythmics, the sodium channel blockers, act.

In the meantime, the much slower L-calcium channels have already started to open. These are the sites of action of the standard calcium antagonists. As the sodium current fades away, it is replaced by flow of the L-type calcium current (I_{Ca} or I_{si}, slow inward current), which forms most of the plateau. From the peak of depolarization, the overshoot is lost *(phase 1)* and in the case of atrial and Purkinje tissue and subepicardial ventricular cells, the transient outward potassium current, I_{to}, flows at this stage. In the remaining ventricular myocardium, I_{to} is not so strong (Sicouri and Antzelevitch, 1991). Therefore phase 1 is much better defined in atrial and Purkinje fibers than in the ventricular myocardium (exception: epicardial cells). I_{to} is relatively inhibited in hypertrophied cells, which probably explains their prolonged action potential duration. There are, however, no clinically available drugs that inhibit this current.

As soon as *phase 1* has passed, a relatively flat plateau forms *(phase 2)*, which merges into the phase of rapid repolarization *(phase 3)*. Phase 3 of the action potential determines the duration of the action potential. It is complex in origin. First, as a result of the initial depolarization *(phase 0)*, potassium currents are activated after a delay (I_k and I_{k1}), thereby helping to terminate the action potential. The second proposal is that the calcium channel closes in response to a raised internal calcium, so that there is no more influx of calcium. Third, the inward current generated by sodium-calcium exchange ceases and becomes an outward current (see subsequent section). Fourth, an inward flow of negatively charged chloride ions might contribute to action potential shortening, especially during catecholamine stimulation. It is on the repolarizing potassium currents of phase three that the class 3 antiarrhythmic agents such as amiodarone act, to prolong the action potential duration.

Once the action potential is over, the resting membrane potential is restored and maintained *(phase 4)*. During this diastolic phase of electrical rest, the activity of the sodium-potassium pump and the various exchange systems restore any remaining ionic balance across the sarcolemma. In atrial and ventricular cells, once the resting membrane potential has been regained it remains stable throughout diastole, so that these cells cannot fire spontaneously.

Purkinje Action Potential

The action potential of the Purkinje fibers differs substantially from that of endocardial ventricular cells chiefly because of a prominent transient outward current, I_{to}, that is activated to form phase 1 and continues to flow to make the action potential duration shorter than in the ventricular myocardium. In injured Purkinje cells, spontaneous diastolic depolarization can occur (phase 4) by complex mechanisms. Such depolarization is known as *phase 4 depolarization* and is a slow process when compared with the rapid depolarization of phase 0. Purkinje depolarization occurs as result of the current I_f that is inhibited by the class 2 drugs, the beta-adrenergic blockers.

RESTITUTION OF MYOCARDIAL IONIC BALANCE

As a direct result of the rapid repetitive opening of the sodium channel followed by the slower opening of the calcium channel, a series of action potentials in the cardiac myocyte will lead to an early gain of sodium ions and a later gain of calcium ions. Both of these ionic imbalances can be corrected by operation of the *sodium-calcium exchanger* (Nicoll et al, 1990). Thus, it is proposed that the sodium-calcium exchanger acts *during* the action potential itself, adequately to restitute the ionic imbalances created by the sequential opening of the sodium and channels (Blaustein, 1988). During the repolarization phase of the action potential there is a net but albeit small loss of potassium ions. To pump these ions back into the cell against a large concentration gradient requires the activity of the sodium pump (Fig 1-13).

Sodium-potassium Pump

The resting heart cell sarcolemma is relatively impermeable to sodium ions but becomes highly permeable with the opening of the sodium gate initiated by depolarization. Even more sodium ions enter during the later phase of the action potential plateau by sodium-calcium exchange. All such sodium ions must eventually be returned to the extracellular space, or else the cell will be overloaded with sodium, with the further threat of absorption of water by osmosis, which could burst the overloaded cells. Most of this influx of sodium across the sarcolemma is corrected by the activity of the sodium-potassium pump. A lesser component is linked to the sodium-calcium exchange system when it transiently functions to extrude sodium from the cell during the early phase of the action potential.

The sodium-potassium pump uses energy to extrude sodium out of the cell and potassium into the cell against the electrochemical gradients (Eisner and Smith, 1992). Although commonly called the *sodium pump*, more accurate names are the sodium-potassium pump, or the Na^+/K^+-ATPase. The pump is activated by internal sodium or external potassium and uses energy in the form of ATP that is complexed to magnesium. Binding sites for ATP, Na^+, K^+ and digitalis have been identified.

$$3 \text{ (Na}^+\text{) in} \quad \rightarrow \quad 3 \text{ (Na}^+\text{) out}$$
$$2 \text{ (K}^+\text{)} \quad \rightarrow \quad 2 \text{ (K}^+\text{) in}$$
$$MgATP^{2-} \quad \rightarrow \quad MgADP^{1-} + P_i^{2-} + H^+$$

One ATP molecule is used per transport cycle. The ions are first secluded within the pump protein, then extruded to either side. One positive charge must leave the cell for each three sodium ions exported because only two potassium ions are imported. Thus, the pump is electrogenic because an unbalanced negative charge is left behind, tending to make the inside of the cell negatively charged.

Digoxin and other inotropic drugs

Digitalis-type compounds, including digoxin and ouabain, inhibit the sodium-potassium pump to increase internal sodium (Fig 10-4, p 298). Thereby they indirectly promote sodium-calcium exchange with an increase in internal calcium and a positive inotropic effect. In addition, digitalis stimulates the vagal nerve to lessen the heart rate. It also decreases the neurohumoral activation found in heart failure, which some experts believe may be more important than improving the contractile state of the myocardium.

Sympathomimetic drugs such as dobutamine act by stimulating the beta-adrenergic receptor and thereby increasing the myocardial concentration of cyclic AMP. *Phosphodiesterase inhibitors* increase cyclic AMP by lessening its breakdown. All agents that increase cyclic AMP also run the risk of increased arrhythmias, so that they are more suited for short than for long term use. *Calcium-sensitizing drugs*, not yet clinically approved, act to increase the sensitivity of the contractile mechanism to ambient levels of calcium (Lee and Allen, 1997).

SUMMARY

1. *The autonomic nervous system* links the regulation of the heart and circulation, so that they work in concert. The activity of the autonomic nervous system links the heart rate and contractile response of the heart to the requirements of the peripheral tissues via the peripheral circulation. The two major branches of the autonomic nervous system are the adrenergic and the cholinergic systems. The adrenergic system liberates two neurotransmitters, epinephrine and norepinephrine, whereas the cholinergic neurotransmitter is acetylcholine. Each of these neurotransmitters has a different pattern of effect on the heart and circulation. Epinephrine and norepinephrine both stimulate β-adrenergic receptors in the heart to increase heart rate and force of contraction. On the peripheral arterioles there are opposing effects. Epinephrine dilates the arterioles by acting on their β-adrenergic receptors, whereas norepinephrine locally released from the terminal neurones has a powerful arteriolar vasoconstrictory effect, the result of vascular α_1-adrenergic stimulation.

2. *β-adrenergic stimulation*. Calcium ions are also taken up

more rapidly by the SR. Beta-receptor stimulation is linked to formation of the second messenger, cyclic AMP, through a complex path that involves the stimulation of adenylate cyclase by the G-protein G_s. Cyclic AMP acts on protein kinase C so that more calcium ions enter cardiac cells, the rate and force of contraction increase, as does the rate of relaxation. Drugs that block this receptor, the β-adrenergic blockers, inhibit the formation of the second messenger, with negative chronotropic, dromotropic, inotropic and lusitropic (relaxing) effects.

3.   *Receptor uncoupling* occurs in response to prolonged receptor stimulation and is reversible. The next step is internalization of the receptor, still reversible and then receptor degradation with irreversible loss. These events explain why, during prolonged β-adrenergic stimulation by dobutamine, there is a progressive loss of the inotropic response.

4.   *Cholinergic stimulation* inhibits the formation of cyclic AMP both by decreasing the release of norepinephrine from the sympathetic nerve terminals (negative neuromodulation) and by stimulating the formation of the inhibitory G-protein, G_I. In addition, cyclic GMP acts as a second messenger that directly opposes cyclic AMP.

5.   *Arteriolar vascular tone* regulates the peripheral (systemic) vascular resistance and represents the balance between vasoconstrictory and vasodilatory stimuli. A common messenger system links the receptors of the physiological vasoconstrictors, angiotensin II, endothelin and α-adrenergic stimulation to an increased cytosolic calcium level in vascular smooth muscle cells. Of the vasodilators, much current interest focuses on the newly described messenger system that links nitric oxide, derived from the vascular endothelium, to guanylate cyclase and the formation of vasodilatory cyclic GMP. The latter signal decreases cytosolic calcium.

6.   *Adenosine* signalling is complex and multiple, leading to effects as diverse as bradycardia or AV-block, negative inotropy, vasodilation and preconditioning. Vasodilation results from a triple action: (1) negative neuromodulation with decreased release of norepinephrine; (2) direct stimulation of vascular A_2 receptors that are linked to the formation of vasodilatory cyclic AMP; (3) and opening of the ATP-sensitive potassium channels.

7.   *Dopamine* receptors have a dual function, namely direct vasodilation (DA_1) and indirect vasodilation by inhibition of the release of norepinephrine from terminal neurones (DA_2 receptors).

8.   *Calcium ion movements.* In the myocardium, calcium ions intimately govern the cross-bridge interactions of the contraction-relaxation cycle. The calcium ions concerned are released from the storage sites in the sarcoplasmic reticulum (SR) in response to voltage-induced

depolarization and opening of the sarcolemmal L-channels. In vascular smooth muscle, depolarization is not required to initiate contraction, which can be set off by calcium released from the sarcoplasmic reticulum in response to inositol trisphosphate, the second messenger of the three physiological vasoconstrictors (α_1-adrenergic activity, endothelin and angiotensin II). Both the cyclic nucleotides, cyclic AMP and cyclic GMP are vasodilatory, in contrast to their opposing effects on myocardial force of contraction. Thus formation of cyclic AMP explains part of the adenosine vasodilation.

9. *Sodium and calcium channels* open in response to voltage stimulation. The consecutive opening of inward conducting sodium and calcium and then outward potassium channels, accounts for the typical pattern of the cardiac action potential. Voltage works on a voltage sensor to open the activation gates. The sodium channel can exist in one of three hypothetical states: resting, activated and open and inactivated. Sodium channel inhibiting drugs such as the antiarrhythmic lidocaine (lignocaine) stabilize the inactivated state. The calcium channel likewise can exist in one of three states. The opening probability of this channel is increased in response to phosphorylation, the ultimate result of β-adrenergic stimulation. Calcium channel antagonist drugs increase the probability of this channel being closed, with decreased rate and force of contraction and peripheral vasodilation.

10. *Potassium channels* are of two types. One group responds to voltage in response to depolarization to allow outward flow of potassium ions to help terminate the action potential duration. Another group is a superfamily that responds to specific molecular ligands that bind to the channel to regulate opening. Examples of this superfamily include the potassium channels in the sinus node that respond to cholinergic or adenosine receptor stimulation by hyperpolarization, to decrease the rate of spontaneous depolarization; and the ATP-sensitive potassium channel that opens in vascular smooth muscle in response to depletion of ATP or formation of adenosine, as occurs in exercise.

11. *Exchangers and pumps.* These help to regulate cytosolic calcium levels. The sodium-calcium exchanger extrudes the small amount of calcium that has entered the myocardial cell with each action potential during each wave of depolarization. The sodium ions that are exchanged for calcium ions, enter as the calcium ions leave and must then be pumped out by the energy-requiring sodium pump (the sodium-potassium ATPase). This pump is the site of inhibition by digitalis, which exerts a positive inotropic effect by the indirect rise of cytosolic calcium.

REFERENCES

Ackerman MJ and Clapham DE. Cardiac chloride channels. *Trends Cardiovasc Med* 1993; 3:23–28.

Ashford MJL, Bond CT, Blair TA et al. Cloning and functional expression of a rat heart K_{ATP} channel. *Nature* 1994; 370:456–459.

Attali BA. New wave for heart rhythms. *Nature* 1996; 384:24–25.

Berridge MJ. Inositol triphosphate and calcium signalling. *Nature* 1993; 361:315–325.

Blaustein MP. Sodium/calcium exchange and the control of contractility in cardiac muscle and vascular smooth muscle. *J Cardiovasc Pharmacol* 1988; 12 (Suppl 5):S56–S58.

Carmeliet E. Potassium channels in cardiac cells. *Cardiovasc Drugs Ther* 1992; 6:305–312.

Celermajer DS. Endothelial dysfunction: Does it matter? Is it reversible? *JACC* 1997; 30:325–333.

Eisner DA and Smith TW. The Na-K pump and its effectors in cardiac muscle. In: Fozzard HA., ed. *The Heart and Cardiovascular System,* 2nd Edition. New York: Raven Press, 1992:863–902.

Fabiato A. Calcium-induced release of calcium from the sarcoplasmic reticulum. *J Gen Physiol* 1985; 85:189–320.

Goldberg LI and Rajfer SI. Dopamine receptors: Applications in clinical cardiology. *Circulation* 1985; 72:245.

Grassi G, Cattaneo BM, Seravalle G et al. Effects of chronic ACE inhibition on sympathetic nerve traffic and baroreflex control of circulation in heart failure. *Circulation* 1997; 96:1173–1179.

Hagiwara N, Irisawa H and Kameyama M. Contribution of two types of calcium currents to the pacemaker potentials of rabbit sinoatrial node cells. *J Physiol* 1988; 395:233–253.

Han X, Shimoni Y and Giles WR. A cellular mechanism for nitric oxide-mediated cholinergic control of mammalian heart rate. *J Gen Physiol* 1995; 106:45–65.

Irisawa H, Brown HF and Giles W. Cardiac pacemaking in the sinoatrial node. *Physiol Rev* 1993; 73:197–227.

Katz AM. Cardiac ion channels. N Engl J Med 1993; 328:1244–1251.

Kelly RA, Balligand J-L and Smith TW. Nitric oxide and cardiac function. *Circ Res* 1996; 79:363–380.

Krum H, Viskoper RJ, Lacourciere Y et al. The effect of an endothelin-antagonist, bosentan, on blood pressure in patients with essential hypertension. *New Engl J Med* 1998; 388:784–790.

Lee JA and Allen DG. Calcium sensitisers. *Cardiovasc Res* 1997; 36:10–20.

Lefkowitz RJ. Clinical implications of basic research. G proteins in medicine. *New Engl J Med* 1995; 332:186–187.

Levy MN and Martin PJ. Autonomic neural control of cardiac function. In: Sperelakis N., ed. *Physiology and Pathophysiology of the Heart,* 3rd Edition. Boston: Kluwer Academic, 1995:413–430.

Lyons D, Roy S, O'Byrne S et al. ACE Inhibition. Postsynaptic adrenergic sympatholytic action in men. *Circulation* 1997; 96:911–915.

Moncada S and Higgs A. The L-Arginine-Nitric oxide pathway. *N Engl J Med* 1993; 329:2002–2012.

Neubig RR. Membrane organization in G-protein mechanisms. *FASEB* 1994; 8:939–946.

Nicoll DA, Longoni S and Philipson KD. Molecular cloning and functional expression of the cardiac sarcolemmal Na^+-Ca^{2+} exchanger. *Science* 1990; 250:562–565.

Opie LH. Mechanisms of cardiac contraction and relaxation. In: Braunwald E., ed. *Heart Disease*, 5th Edition. Philadelphia: W B Saunders, 1997:360–393.

Pappano AJ and Mubagwa K. Actions of muscarinic agents and adenosine on the heart. In: HA Fozzard et al, ed. The Heart and Cardiovascular System, 2nd Edition. Vol. 2. New York: *Raven Press,* 1992:1765–1776.

Raymond JR, Hnatowich M, Lefkowitz RJ et al. Adrenergic receptors. Models for regulation of signal transduction processes. *Hypertension* 1990; 15:119–131.

Santana LF, Cheng H, Gomez AM et al. Relation between sarcolemmal Ca^{2+} current and Ca^{2+} sparks and local theories for cardiac excitation-contraction coupling. *Circ Res* 1996; 78:166–171.

Sicouri S and Antzelevitch C. A subpopulation of cells with unique electrophysical properties in the deep subepicardium of the canine ventricle. The M cell. *Circ Res* 1991; 68:1729–1741.

Stiles GL. Adenosine receptors. *J Biol Chem* 1992; 267:6451–6454.

Tracey WR, Magee W, Masamune H et al. Selective adenosine A_3 receptor stimulation reduces ischemic myocardial injury in the rabbit heart. *Cardiovasc Res* 1997; 33:410–415.

Wier WG, ter Keurs HE, Marban E et al. Ca^{2+} 'Sparks' and waves in intact ventricular muscle resolved by confocal imaging. *Circ Res* 1997; 81:462–469.

REVIEWS

Opie L.H. Vascular Smooth Muscle and Endothelium, In: Opie, L.H. *The Heart. Physiology, from Cell to Circulation,* Third Edition. Lippincott-Raven, Philadelphia, 1998: 233–264

Opie, L.H. Mechanisms of cardiac contraction and relaxation. In: Braunwald E, ed. *Heart Disease*, 5th Edition. Philadelphia: W.B. Saunders, 1997: 360–393.

CHAPTER 2

Effects of Anesthetic Agents on the Heart and Circulation

Hans-Joachim Priebe

All anesthetics used in clinical practice modify cardiovascular performance (Table 2-1). Such modification may be the result of either direct effects on the heart and the vasculature, or of indirect effects mediated by primary actions on neurohumoral control mechanisms of the circulation (Fig 2-1). Such interactions between direct and indirect effects render the interpretation of hemodynamic changes in response to drug administration difficult in vivo. For example, a change in blood pressure may be caused by a direct effect on the myocardium (thereby modifying contractility) and/or the vasculature (thereby modifying cardiac loading conditions), or by a primary effect on the autonomic nervous system (which, in turn, modifies myocardial contractility and loading conditions). Even for a given anesthetic agent, the relative contribution of the direct and indirect effects to the changes in hemodynamics may vary considerably with baseline conditions. For example, in patients whose cardiovascular performance is critically dependent on elevated sympathetic tone the hemodynamic consequences of anesthesia-mediated central depression of

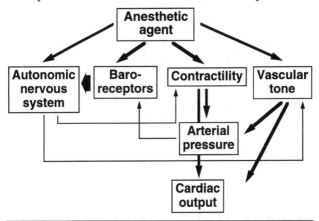

Fig 2-1. *Anesthetic agents and circulation. They exert both direct and indirect effects on the heart and the circulation resulting in changes in arterial pressure and cardiac output.*

Table 2-1: Hemodynamic Effects of Anesthetic Agents

FUNCTION	HALO	ENFL	ISO	DES	SEVO	N_2O	THIO	PRO	ETOM	KET	COMMENTS
Sympathetic nervous system	↓	↓	↓↑*	↓↑*	↓	↑	↓	↓	–	↑	↑* with rapid increase in concentration
Baroceptor response	↓	↓	↓	↓	↓	–/↓	↓	↓	–		iso < halo, enfl
Myocardial function	↓	↓	↓	↓	↓	↓/↑*	↓	↓	–	↓*	halo > iso, sevo, des, thio > pro *when sympathetic blocked
Lusitropic effects	↓	↓	↓	↓	↓	↓		–		↓	halo > sevo > des, iso
Coronary vasodilation	–	↑	↑*	↑	↑	–	–	↑/–	–	–	iso > des > sevo > halo, enfl * coronary steal, if steal – prone anatomy
Heart rate	↓	↓	↑*	↑*	–	–	–/↑	–/↓	–	↑	* with rapid ↑ conc des > iso
Systemic vascular resistance	↓	↓	↓	↓	↓	–/↑	↓	↓	–	↓*	* When sympathetic effect blocked or deficient

HALO = halothane; ENFL = enflurane; ISO = isoflurane; DES = desflurane; SEVO = sevoflurane; N_2O = nitrous oxide; THIO = thiopentone; PRO = propofol; ETOM = etomidate; KET = ketamine ↓ = reduction; – = little or no change; ↑ = increase sympathetic neural activity may be more pronounced than those of anesthetic-induced direct myocardial depression or vasodilation. Regardless of the relative contributions of centrally-mediated and direct drug-induced alterations of cardiovascular performance, it is well recognized that basically all anesthetics cause centrally-mediated cardiovascular depression. This short review will, therefore, start with some comments on the effects of anesthetics on the sympathetic nervous system.

ANESTHETICS AND THE AUTONOMIC NERVOUS SYSTEM

As the autonomic nervous system modifies heart rate, myocardial contractility, vascular resistance and venous capacitance, some knowledge of the effects of anesthetic agents on the autonomic nervous system is necessary for the correct interpretation of cardiovascular findings. Such knowledge is derived from recordings of sympathetic nerve activity via the peroneal nerve (Ebert and Kampine, 1989), from measurements of plasma catecholamines, and from evaluation of baroreceptor function.

Effects on the Sympathetic Nervous System

Induction of anesthesia with thiopental, propofol, or isoflurane inhibits skeletal muscle sympathetic nerve activity (Ebert et al, 1992; Sellgren et al, 1992; Selgren et al, 1990; Ebert et al, 1990). In contrast, etomidate has no significant effect on sympathetic tone (Ebert et al, 1992). The decrease in sympathetic nerve activity following propofol seems to be more pronounced in unpremedicated than in patients premedicated with benzodiazepines (Ebert et al, 1992; Sellgren et al, 1990). This underlines the importance of baseline sympathetic tone in determining the subsequent effects of anesthetic agents on sympathetic neural activity and, in turn, on hemodynamics. This would also explain why propofol may provoke pronounced hypotension in patients whose cardiovascular performance is presumably dependent on an elevated baseline sympathetic tone (i.e. patients with hypovolemia or compensated cardiac insufficiency). In contrast to other anesthetics, nitrous oxide (N_2O) increases sympathetic outflow (Ebert and Kampine, 1989; Sellgren et al, 1990). In healthy human volunteers, 40% N_2O produced a 60% increase in baseline efferent sympathetic nerve activity directed to skeletal muscle blood vessels (Ebert, 1990). Rapid and large increases in inspired concentrations of isoflurane and desflurane result in transient sympathetic hyperactivity (Ebert and Muzi, 1993; Yli-Hankala et al, 1993). The effects of some of the most commonly used anesthetics are summarized in Figure 2-2.

Effects on Plasma Catecholamines

Various studies have determined plasma catecholamine levels during anesthesia (Griffiths, 1993). In general, nor-

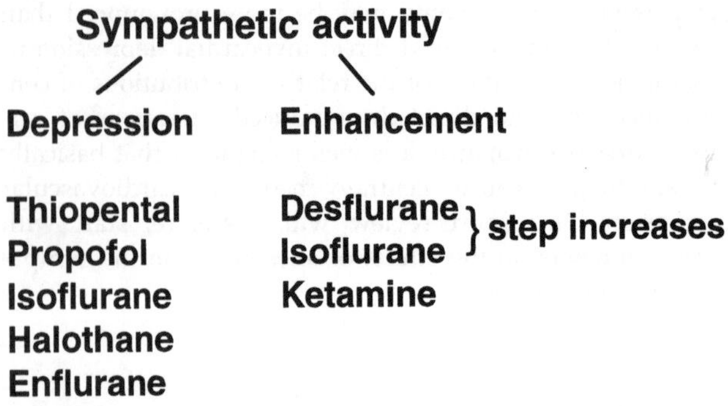

Sympathetic activity

/ \\

Depression   **Enhancement**

Thiopental   **Desflurane** } **step increases**
Propofol   **Isoflurane**
Isoflurane   **Ketamine**
Halothane
Enflurane

Fig 2-2. Effects of anesthetic agents on sympathetic activity

adrenaline levels correlate reasonably well with skeletal muscle sympathetic nerve activity in healthy volunteers. Various anesthetics have been shown to decrease plasma catecholamine levels (Pocock and Richards, 1991). However, in parallel with the increase in sympathetic nerve activity, catecholamine plasma levels increase markedly during the initial phase of the rapid increase in the inspired concentration of desflurane (Weiskopf et al, 1994).

Effects on Baroreceptor Function

Arterial baroflex control of heart rate can be studied in conscious and anesthetized individuals by injecting vasopressors (pressor test) and vasodilators (depressor test), and subsequently determining the slope derived from the change in the R-R interval of the ECG divided by the change in blood pressure. Thiopental and propofol in clinically relevant doses inhibit baroreflex control by up to 75% (Ebert et al, 1990 & 1992). In contrast, etomidate has only little effect on baroreceptor function (Ebert et al, 1992). Inhalational anesthetics also inhibit the baroreflex control of heart rate in both humans and animals (Kotrly et al, 1984 & 1986). Isoflurane seems to depress the barostatic reflexes less than halothane or enflurane (Kotrly et al, 1984). In human volunteers, 40% N_2O does not impair the hypotension-induced reflex augmentation of sympathetic nerve activity but decreases the baroreflex-mediated tachycardia (Ebert, 1990). Maintained ability of the baroreceptor reflex to augment sympathetic nerve activity may be partially responsible for the relatively stable hemodynamics during N_2O administration. Impairment of baroreceptor function may be of considerable clinical relevance as it blunts, or even prevents the reflexly mediated increase in heart rate following sleep- and drug-induced hypotension. Such reflex increase in heart rate is a physiological means of counteracting the adverse effects of hypotension.

Summary of Effects on Autonomic Nervous System

In summary, most anesthetics induce a centrally-mediated depression of cardiovascular performance as reflected by inhibition of sympathetic nerve activity, decreased plasma catecholamine levels, and impaired baroreflex control.

These indirect effects of anesthetics on hemodynamics occur independently of, and in addition to, the direct cardiovascular effects, and they are likely to vary with pre-existing sympathetic tone. They have to be taken into account when attempting to define the direct cardiovascular effects in vivo. Relative cardiovascular stability following etomidate, and at times profound hypotension following thiopental and propofol administration in patients dependent on elevated sympathetic tone can be explained, in part, by different effects on sympathetic outflow. N_2O is an exception in that it increases sympathetic nerve activity. In vivo, this characteristic may counteract direct negative inotropic effects associated with N_2O or other anesthetics.

TECHNIQUES USED TO ASSESS CARDIOVASCULAR PERFORMANCE

Assessment of the cardiovascular effects of anesthetics is complex. Not surprisingly, a wide variety of methods have been employed for this purpose. At times, findings appear contradictory. Seemingly contradictory results may, however, be the result of different techniques used in the evaluation of cardiovascular performance. A few general comments on advantages as well as limitations associated with the various techniques are, therefore, necessary in order to put study results in proper perspective.

As mentioned earlier, it is almost impossible to differentiate in vivo between the direct and the indirect centrally-mediated cardiovascular effects of anesthetics. Correct characterization of the direct cardiovascular effects requires stable heart rate, preload, and afterload during drug administration because changes in each of these parameters modify cardiac performance independent of the intervention. Such conditions are virtually impossible to achieve in vivo. Numerous techniques have been used to circumvent this problem. Possible solutions include the use of isolated in vitro preparations (cultured myocytes, papillary muscles, vascular rings, isolated working heart), and reliance on so-called "load-independent" indices of myocardial contractility in vivo.

In general, the more isolated the preparation the more artificial the functional environment. Obviously, cultured myocytes or skinned muscle fibers are far from reflecting physiological conditions. Papillary muscle and vascular ring preparations lack blood supply, and studies are frequently performed at room temperature to decrease basal metabolic rate. Isolated working heart preparations lack basal neuronal activity, and myocardial O_2 delivery is often unphysiologically low due to the use of crystalloid perfusion. It is, therefore, difficult to transfer findings obtained in isolated preparations to the clinical setting. On the other hand, preload, afterload and heart rate can be controlled in such preparations, and the modifying influences of the autonomic nervous system are eliminated.

As loading conditions and heart rate are virtually impossible to control in vivo, assessment of myocardial contractility in the intact organism requires considerable methodologic effort. Changes in blood pressure, left ventricular pressure, maximal velocity of rise in left ventricular pressure (dP/dt_{max}), stroke volume and stroke work in response to the administration of an anesthetic do not necessarily reflect changes in myocardial contractility. A change in blood pressure or stroke volume may reflect a true change in myocardial performance or merely altered loading conditions. Thus, for in vivo evaluation of cardiovascular performance load-independent indices of contractility are required.

The *end-systolic pressure/volume relationship* termed end-systolic elastance index (E_{es}) is considered to be relatively load-independent (Sagawa, 1978). End-systolic elastance is derived from instantaneous pressure-volume loops recorded during changes in preload and afterload (Fig 2-3). The slope of the regression line through the end-systolic pressure-volume points E_{es} is considered to reflect myocardial contractility. This approach to evaluating myocardial contractility has been extensively used in the intact experimental animal. Preload is usually varied by vena cava occlusion. Frequently, the autonomic nervous system is pharmacologically blocked (using β-adrenoceptor blockade, atropine, ganglionic blockade) to prevent baroreceptor reflex activation. In the experimental animal, left ventricular dimensions are usually determined by sonomicrometry.

The concept of end-systolic elastance has also been applied to humans (Mulier et al, 1991). Changes in loading conditions can be induced by bolus injections of nitroglycerin or phenylephrine, and left ventricular volume is determined by echocardiography. Since instantaneous measurement of end-systolic left ventricular pressure requires the introduction of a catheter-tip manometer into the left ventricle, it is reasonable to substitute peak aortic systolic pressure for end-systolic left ventricular pressure under clinical conditions.

The *preload recruitable stroke work* (PRSW) is considered to be even less load-dependent than end-systolic elastance

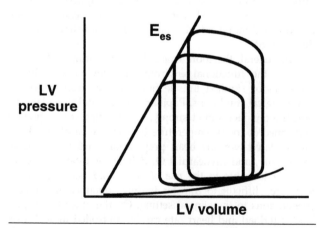

Fig 2-3. Effect of response to changes in preload or afterload on pressure-volume loop. At end-systole (top left corner of each loop), the pressure/volume points form a straight line, the slope of which is termed maximum elastance and designed as E_{es}. LV = left ventricular.

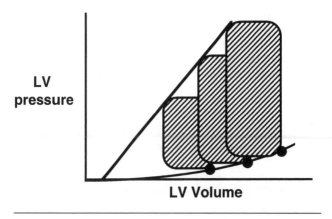

Fig 2-4. External work. The area of successive pressure/volume loops represents the external work (stroke work), and the bottom right corner of each loop represents its end-diastolic volume.

(Glower, 1985). Loading conditions are similarly varied by pharmacologic or mechanical means in order to obtain pressure-volume loops (Fig 2-4). Subsequently, stroke work (i.e. the area under the pressure-volume loop) is plotted against the end-diastolic dimensions of the left ventricle (i.e. end-diastolic volume or segment length determined by sonomicrometry). The slopes of the respective regression lines are considered to reflect myocardial contractility (Fig 2-5). It is obvious from the methodological requirements, that very few clinical studies have investigated the effects of anesthetics on myocardial contractility based on end-systolic elastance or PRSW. This might change with the more frequent use of transesophageal echocardiography. We have to be aware that it is difficult, if not impossible, to draw conclusions from studies that have not employed load-insensitive measures of cardiac performance.

In summary, a wide variety of techniques has been employed in the evaluation of the cardiovascular effects of anesthetics. Methods differ widely between studies. It is only to be expected that, at times, results will vary with the methodology employed (e.g. in vitro vs in vivo investigations; experimental animal vs human; awake, chronically instrumented vs anesthetized, acutely instrumented ani-

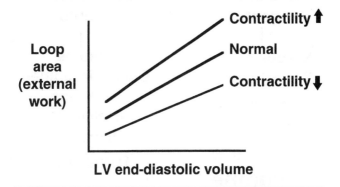

Fig 2-5. Slope of contractility. If the external work (loop area) is plotted against the corresponding end-diastolic volume, the values form straight lines, the slope of which quantify contractility.

mals; absence vs presence of blockade of autonomic nervous system; use of load-independent vs load-sensitive indices of myocardial contractility in vivo). Such differences in methodology have to be taken into account when interpreting results and defining their clinical implication.

Volatile Anesthetics and Cardiovascular Performance

Effects on Myocardial Function

Most anesthetic agents cause some depression of contractile performance (Fig 2-6). All volatile anesthetics depress myocardial contractility in a dose-dependent fashion in isolated preparations and in vivo. Using the slope (E_{es}) of the end-systolic pressure-mid-axis diameter relation as a relatively load-independent index of contractility in chronically instrumented dogs, equi-anesthetic concentrations of halothane and enflurane have been shown to depress myocardial contractility to similar degrees (Van Trigt et al, 1984).

Several studies had suggested different degrees of myocardial depression between halothane and isoflurane in experimental animals and humans. This suspected difference was quantified using the slope of regional PRSW relation and a stroke work analog of the end-systolic pressure-segment length relationship (ESPLR area) in chronically instrumented dogs with pharmacologic blockade of the autonomic nervous system (Pagel et al, 1990a). Isoflurane maintained contractile state an average of 22% higher than equi-anesthetic concentrations of halothane. The differential effects of halothane and isoflurane on myocardial contractility were maintained during pharmacologically-induced depression or enhancement of contractility (Hysing et al, 1990; Pagel et al, 1994).

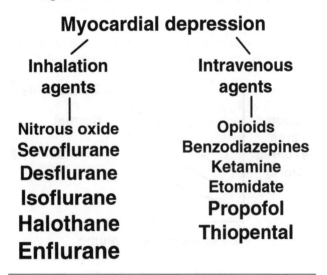

Myocardial depression

Inhalation agents	**Intravenous agents**

Inhalation agents

Nitrous oxide
Sevoflurane
Desflurane
Isoflurane
Halothane
Enflurane

Intravenous agents

Opioids
Benzodiazepines
Ketamine
Etomidate
Propofol
Thiopental

Fig 2-6. Most anesthetics decrease contractility. The size of the lettering indicates the relative magnitude of myocardial depression.

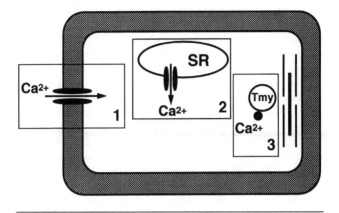

Fig 2-7. Depression of contractility may result from: (1) reduced sarcolemmal entry of calcium; (2) altered uptake and release of calcium by the sarcoplasmic reticulum (SR); or (3) altered interaction of calcium with tropomyosin (Tmy).

Depression of contractility results from alterations of calcium fluxes in the myocytes (Fig 2-7). The difference in myocardial depression between halothane and isoflurane may be due to differential modulation of intracellular Ca^{2+} kinetics at several subcellular sites within the cardiac myocyte (Rusy and Komai, 1987). Isoflurane and halothane inhibit the transsarcolemmal Ca^{2+} influx (resulting from membrane depolarization and responsible for initiating mechanical systole) to a different extent (Rusy and Komai, 1987). Such inhibition results in decreased availability of Ca^{2+} for contractile activation, reduced Ca^{2+}-dependent Ca^{2+}release from the sarcoplasmic reticulum, and a smaller amount of Ca^{2+} stored in the sarcoplasmic reticulum (Rusy and Komai, 1987). In addition, halothane may cause a greater leak of Ca^{2+} from the sarcoplasmic reticulum than isoflurane possibly related to a differential activation at the sarcoplasmic reticulum Ca^{2+} release channel (Connelly and Coronado, 1991).

The hemodynamic profile of *desflurane* is very similar to that of isoflurane during steady-state conditions. Using the slope of the PRSW relation in chronically instrumented dogs, desflurane and isoflurane have been shown to depress myocardial contractility equally in the absence (Pagel et al, 1993) and presence (Pagel et al, 1991a) of autonomic nervous system reflexes.

Sevoflurane also causes myocardial depression. Indeed, in healthy spontaneously breathing volunteers decreases in cardiac index, systemic vascular resistance (SVR), and systolic wall stress in the presence of unchanged cardiac filling pressures, heart rate, and echocardiographic ejection-phase indices of left ventricular function and preload, clearly indicate that sevoflurane anesthesia causes myocardial depression (Malan et al, 1995). The degree of myocardial depression is similar to that of isoflurane (Malan et al, 1995; Bernard et al, 1990). When employing the slope of PRSW vs end-diastolic length as a sensitive index of contractility, experimental work supports the finding of myocardial depression by sevoflurane (Harkin et al, 1994). The degree

of myocardial depression appears to be less during sevoflurane than during halothane (Lerman et al, 1990) or
enflurane anesthesia (Kikura and Ikeda, 1993). Indirect evidence would suggest that the magnitude of myocardial
depression is comparable between isoflurane, desflurane,
and sevoflurane (Pagel et al, 1991a; Pagel et al, 1993; Harkin et al, 1994).

All volatile anesthetics, including desflurane and sevoflurane, produce dose-related prolongation of isovolumic
relaxation (Harkin et al, 1994; Humphrey et al, 1990; Doyle
et al, 1989; Pagel et al, 1991b) and impairment of early ventricular filling (Pagel et al, 1994; Harkin et al, 1994). However, it seems unlikely that these anesthetics, with the
possible exception of halothane (Goldberg and Phear, 1970),
affect overall ventricular compliance in vivo (Harkin et al,
1994; Pagel et al, 1991b). Sevoflurane may produce a relatively greater negative lusitropic effect than desflurane or
isoflurane. At 1.5 MAC, the time constants of isovolumic
relaxation in animals with blocked autonomic nervous system were 51 ms (Harkin et al, 1994), 45 ms and 47 ms
(Pagel et al, 1991b) for sevoflurane, desflurane and isoflurane, respectively.

Whereas left ventricular-arterial coupling and myocardial efficiency seem to be preserved at low concentrations
of volatile anesthetics, they are impaired at higher concentrations (Hettrick, 1996). These alterations may contribute to
the overall reduction in cardiac performance observed during desflurane, sevoflurane and isoflurane.

*The mechanisms responsible for the negative lusitropic
effects of volatile anesthetics* are not entirely clear. It is, however, likely that the abnormal intracellular Ca^{2+} kinetics
acutely produced by the volatile anesthetics are not only
responsible for the depression of myocardial contractility,
but also for the prolongation of isovolumic relaxation, and
the delay in early ventricular filling.

In vitro, 50% N_2O causes a 5-15% depression of myocardial contractility (Lawson et al, 1990). The in vivo effects
of N_2O are complex. N_2O increases sympathetic nerve
activity, and increases blood pressure in some patients
(Ebert and Kampine 1989; Stellgren et al, 1990; Ebert et al,
1990). However, available evidence would suggest that
N_2O is a myocardial depressant when used as supplemental anesthetic. In chronically instrumented dogs with pharmacologic blockade of the autonomic nervous system,
myocardial contractility decreased when N_2O was added to
isoflurane and sufentanil (Pagel et al, 1990b). In addition to
its negative inotropic effect, N_2O impairs diastolic myocardial function in the experimental animal (Marsch, 1996).
Overall, N_2O seems to have a mild cardiodepressant effect
which is counteracted in the intact animal and the healthy
human by an increase in sympathetic tone.

Effects on the Coronary Circulation

In the experimental animal, halothane has little effect on
coronary vasomotor tone or autoregulation (Hickey et al,
1988). In the in situ canine heart, enflurane has a coronary

vasodilating effect similar to that of halothane, but less than that of isoflurane (Gurevicius, 1996).

Studies in acutely or chronically instrumented dogs indicate that enflurane is a mild coronary vasodilator (Hickey et al, 1988). In rat coronary microvessels, halothane attenuates endothelial-dependent vasodilation via interference at the endothelial receptor level (Park, 1997).

Numerous studies have shown that isoflurane is a coronary vasodilator that interferes with coronary autoregulation (Hickey et al, 1988; Priebe, 1989). In this regard, isoflurane is more potent than enflurane but less than adenosine (Hickey et al, 1988). Since isoflurane is an arteriolar-type coronary vasodilator it carries the potential of inducing coronary steal (Becker, 1978). This, however, requires underlying steal-prone coronary anatomy. In animals or humans with normal coronary arteries there is no evidence of isoflurane-induced coronary flow maldistribution. Isoflurane-induced coronary vasodilation is dose-dependent, and is mediated by the vascular endothelium (Blaise et al, 1987).

There is strong experimental evidence that sevoflurane is a less potent coronary vasodilator than isoflurane. In the isolated, quiescent perfused rat heart, the concentration-dependent decreases in coronary vascular resistance and flow reserve were significantly less during sevoflurane than during isoflurane anesthesia (Larach and Schuler, 1991). In the isolated, beating, perfused guinea pig heart, both sevoflurane and isoflurane increased coronary blood flow in a concentration-dependent fashion (Graf et al, 1995). However, at the higher concentration the increase was less prominent during sevoflurane administration.

In acute canine experiments, sevoflurane and isoflurane caused comparable decreases in myocardial O_2 consumption ($M\dot{V}O_2$) (Hirano, 1995). Despite these comparable decreases in $M\dot{V}O_2$, sevoflurane did not affect coronary vascular resistance, and it decreased coronary blood flow, whereas isoflurane decreased coronary vascular resistance with no change in coronary blood flow. Nevertheless, myocardial O_2 extraction decreased at 1.5 MAC sevoflurane. When coronary autoregulation is preserved, myocardial O_2 extraction will remain constant independent of metabolic needs as supply (coronary blood flow) and demand ($M\dot{V}O_2$) are closely coupled. The fact that myocardial O_2 extraction decreased indicates that sevoflurane interferes with coronary autoregulation. However, during isoflurane, (1) myocardial O_2 extraction decreased at lower concentrations (0.75 vs 1.5 MAC), and (2) the decrease at 1.5 MAC was much larger (39% vs 18%) during isoflurane than during sevoflurane anesthesia. Neither sevoflurane nor isoflurane had any direct effect on large coronary artery diameter, and on the endocardial/epicardial perfusion ratio. These data strongly suggest that sevoflurane is a considerably less potent arteriolar coronary vasodilator than isoflurane.

As sevoflurane is most likely to be an arteriolar coronary vasodilator, it has the potential for causing coronary steal. This potential was investigated in a canine model of multivessel coronary artery obstruction (Kersten et al, 1994).

When arterial pressure and heart rate were maintained at control values, 1.5 MAC sevoflurane actually increased blood flow to collateral-dependent myocardium. This would suggest preferential dilatation of coronary collateral vessels. In contrast, using an identical canine multivessel model, isoflurane (Hartman et al, 1991) and desflurane (Hartman et al, 1991) did not increase blood flow to collateral-dependent myocardium. Overall, evidence would suggest that sevoflurane is a rather weak coronary arteriolar vasodilator that lacks sufficient coronary vasodilating property to cause coronary steal. Unlike desflurane and isoflurane, it may preferentially increase collateral flow in the presence of maintained systemic perfusion pressure.

On the basis of calculated coronary vascular resistance and coronary blood flow, desflurane appears to be a coronary vasodilator with comparable (Merin et al, 1991) or somewhat less coronary vasodilator property (Pagel et al, 1991c) than isoflurane. Definitive statements regarding the direct effects of desflurane on coronary vasomotor tone are, however, not possible because there is a lack of data on the behavior of coronary sinus PO_2 or O_2 saturation in the presence of desflurane. In a canine model of multivessel coronary artery disease, desflurane did not redistribute blood flow away from collateral-dependent myocardium via a coronary steal mechanism (Hartman et al, 1991). The overall evidence would suggest that desflurane is a coronary vasodilator of similar, or perhaps slightly less potency than isoflurane.

Since N_2O has mostly been added to volatile or opioid anesthetics, there is hardly any data on the effects of N_2O per se on the coronary circulation. In dogs, N_2O decreased the diameter of epicardial coronary arteries with no effect on coronary resistance vessels (Wilkowski et al, 1987). In the isolated working guinea pig heart, N_2O had no direct effect on overall arteriolar coronary vasomotor tone (Stowe et al, 1990).

Effects on Heart Rate

An almost consistent finding of experimental and clinical studies is an increase in heart rate during the administration of desflurane (Merin et al, 1991; Pagel et al, 1991c; Kersten et al, 1993; Weiskopf et al, 1991). When compared to isoflurane, the increase in heart rate tends to be greater. The finding that blockade of the autonomic nervous system or administration of an $_2$-adrenoceptor agonist eliminates the differential effects of desflurane and isoflurane on heart rate, resulting in comparable decreases (Pagel et al, 1991c) or increases in heart rate (Kersten et al, 1993) would suggest that the greater increase in heart rate during desflurane anesthesia might be related to a lesser depression of sympathetic tone and autonomic reflexes. However, rapid increases in the inspired concentration of desflurane to above 1 MAC result in tachycardia and hypertension in healthy volunteers (Ebert and Muzi, 1993). This hyperdynamic circulatory response is associated with increased sympathetic nerve activity (Ebert and Muzi, 1993) and elevated plasma levels of epinephrine, norepinephrine, and vasopressin (Weiskopf et al, 1994). These responses are less pronounced during isoflurane anesthesia. Overall, the increase in heart rate during desflurane seems to be more pronounced than during isoflurane administration.

Although a couple of human studies suggest that sevoflurane may also cause an increase in heart rate (Frinkel et al, 1993; Lerman et al, 1994), the only clear evidence for sevoflurane-induced tachycardia during steady-state periods of anesthesia comes from chronically instrumented dogs (Bernard et al, 1990; Harkin et al, 1994). In one of these studies, the increase in heart rate during 1.2 MAC sevoflurane exceeded that during 1.2 MAC isoflurane (Bernard et al, 1990).

However, such data must be interpreted cautiously because, at times, the effects of volatile anesthetics on the autonomic nervous system differ widely between species. For example, several studies in dogs did not reveal any effect of desflurane on the autonomic nervous system (Pagel et al, 1993; Merin et al, 1991). In contrast, in humans the administration of desflurane has been associated consistently with large increases in sympathetic outflow, plasma catecholamines, heart rate and blood pressure (Weiskopf et al, 1994; Ebert and Muzi, 1993; Moore et al, 1994).

Recent work indicates that sevoflurane, in contrast to isoflurane and desflurane, does not increase heart rate in humans. Whereas heart rate increased during 1.5 and 2.0 MAC isoflurane in spontaneously breathing volunteers, it remained unchanged during equi-anesthetic concentrations of sevoflurane (Malan et al, 1995). Similarly, whereas heart rate increased at 1.24 MAC desflurane in ventilated volunteers, it remained unchanged during sevoflurane (Ebert et al, 1995). Overall, evidence would suggest that compared to isoflurane and desflurane, sevoflurane has the least potential for inducing an increase in heart rate. In this context it is worth noting that following blockade of the autonomic nervous system, sevoflurane decreases heart rate (Harkin et al, 1994).

Cardiac Arrhythmias

Cardiac arrhythmias during inhalational anesthesia are well documented (Atlee, 1995). They may, in part, involve depression of the fast inward Na^+ current during the action potential upstroke (Weight, 1997).

However, in general terms, contemporary anesthetic drugs are, per se, not arrhythmogenic, but are only so in the presence of other predisposing conditions and circumstances, e.g. excessive autonomic stimulation, electrolyte imbalance, hypoxia, hypercarbia, ischemic heart disease, congestive cardiac failure, to mention only the most common (Atlee, 1996).

Effects on the Peripheral Circulation

Anesthetics have direct and indirect effects on the peripheral circulation. As in the case of myocardial performance it is difficult to differentiate in vivo between direct and indirect effects. The centrally-mediated decrease in sympathetic outflow associated with induction of anesthesia with almost any anesthetic will, per se, modify peripheral vascular tone irrespective of the direct effect of the anesthetic on vascular smooth muscle. Alteration of peripheral vascular resistance is likely to affect regional flow and blood volume distribution. The effect on vascular smooth muscle may be direct or secondary by modifying the response to factors that modulate vasomotor tone.

Volatile anesthetics cause mild to moderate peripheral vasodilation. This is possibly caused by both reduced responsiveness of vascular smooth muscle to circulating catecholamines, and reduced vasomotor tone (Larach et al, 1987; Kenny et al, 1990). Interference with Ca^{2+} entry through vascular smooth muscle membranes (Larach et al, 1987), or attenuation of α_1-adrenoceptor-mediated vasoconstriction (Kenny et al, 1990) have been postulated. In addition, nitric oxide (NO) may play a significant role in cardiovascular control during both halothane and isoflurane anesthesia (Greenblatt et al, 1992). NO-mediated vasorelaxation appears to be more prominent during isoflurane anesthesia. This could be a mechanism for the prominent vasodilator effects of isoflurane.

In healthy, normocarbic human volunteers, desflurane causes a dose-dependent reduction in SVR (Weiskopf et al, 1991). Findings in experimental animals are inconclusive. Identical decreases in SVR during desflurane and isoflurane (Weiskopf et al, 1988), a decrease in SVR which tended to be larger than during isoflurane (Merin et al, 1991), as well as no change in SVR (compared to a decrease during isoflurane) have been reported (Pagel et al, 1991c; Kersten et al, 1993). Consistent with those findings, mean arterial pressure was reduced either to the same extent (Greenblatt et al, 1992) or to a lesser extent during desflurane than during isoflurane anesthesia (Pagel et al, 1991c, Kersten et al, 1993). However, the differences in responses to desflurane and isoflurane were eliminated following blockade of the autonomic nervous system. The decreases in mean arterial pressure were now comparable, and neither agent affected SVR (Pagel et al, 1991c). In view of comparable myocardial depression by desflurane and isoflurane, independent of autonomic nervous system activity (Pagel et al, 1991a & 1993), these results suggest that a lesser depression of sympathetic nerve activity and autonomic reflexes during desflurane anesthesia may explain the lesser reductions of mean arterial pressure and peripheral vascular tone during desflurane as compared to isoflurane anesthesia.

The role of the autonomic nervous system is confirmed by observations of the administration of the α_2-adrenoceptor agonist *dexmedetomidine*. Pretreatment with dexmedetomidine eliminated the differential effects of desflurane and isoflurane on mean arterial pressure and SVR (Kersten et al, 1993). The desflurane-induced decrease in SVR observed only in the presence of dexmedetomidine is suggestive of a direct peripheral vasodilator effect of desflurane. However, even during α_2-agonist administration, the decrease in SVR following isoflurane was more pronounced, unmasking its greater peripheral vasodilator property. Overall, evidence suggests that desflurane and isoflurane have similar peripheral vasodilatory properties. In vivo, there might be a tendency towards less peripheral vasodilation during desflurane related to less depression of sympathetic nerve activity and autonomic reflexes.

The effects of sevoflurane on SVR are somewhat controversial. In healthy, spontaneously breathing volunteers, the decreases in SVR and mean arterial pressure at 1.0, 1.5 and 2.0 MAC of sevoflurane were found to be quantitatively similar to those of isoflurane (Malan et al, 1995). Comparable decreases in SVR and mean arterial pressure during sevoflurane and isoflurane have also been observed in surgical patients (Frink et al, 1992), and in chronically instrumented dogs (Bernard et al, 1990; Merin et al, 1991). There is, however, experimental evidence that sevoflurane may be a somewhat less potent systemic vasodilator than isoflurane. In chronically instrumented animals, in which isoflurane usually causes a decrease in SVR (Pagel et al, 1991c, Kersten et al, 1993), sevoflurane did not affect SVR, neither during intact nor during blockade of the autonomic nervous system (Harkin et al, 1994).

There are hardly any studies that directly compare sevoflurane and desflurane with each other. In healthy, mechanically ventilated volunteers, both anesthetics produced similar progressive decreases in blood pressure (Ebert et al, 1995). In contrast, in pediatric patients blood pressure was maintained better during sevoflurane than during desflurane (Lerman et al, 1994). Overall, sevoflurane like isoflurane and desflurane causes systemic vasodilation. It is possible that the degree of systemic vasodilation is somewhat less than during isoflurane and desflurane.

INTRAVENOUS ANESTHETICS AND CARDIOVASCULAR PERFORMANCE

Barbiturates

Thiopental decreases ventricular dP/dt_{max} in a dose-dependent fashion in the isolated heart (Stowe et al, 1992), and depresses tension development and force-velocity relationships of atrial (Azari and Cork, 1993) and ventricular muscle (Frankle and Poole-Wilson, 1981) in vitro. These effects have been attributed to interference with transsarcolemmal Ca^{2+} flux which results in reduced levels of intracellular Ca^{2+} necessary for activation of myocardial fiber contraction (Azari and Cork, 1993; Frankl and Poole-Wilson, 1981). In isolated cat papillary muscle, the negative inotropic actions of small doses of thiopental depended on the presence of an intact endocardial endothelium (Bettens, 1996). The negative inotropic effects appeared to be mediated, in part, by the nitric oxide pathway.

Barbiturates decrease indirect indices of myocardial contractility in vivo (Conway and Ellis, 1969). Studies employing relatively load-independent indices of myocardial contractility such as invasively derived E_{es} or PRSW

would be required to assess quantitative changes in myocardial contractility in vivo. Such studies are not available.
When using several simplifying assumptions to noninva-
sively derive an approximation of E_{es}, barbiturates have
been shown to decrease myocardial contractility in humans
(Mulier, 1991). The combination of negative inotropy,
increase in venous capacitance (Eckstein et al, 1961), and
transient decrease in central sympathetic neural activity
(Sellgren et al, 1992), causes the decreases in blood pressure
and cardiac output typically observed during administration of barbiturates.

Etomidate

In vitro studies of isolated normal (Eckstein et al, 1961) and
cardiomyopathic (Riou et al, 1990) rat papillary muscle suggest that etomidate exerts little negative inotropic effect.
This may be related to maintained availability of intracellular Ca^{2+} for the excitation-contraction coupling (Komai et
al, 1985). The in vivo effects of etomidate on load-independent indices of myocardial contractility are unknown. Studies in isolated hearts (Stowe et al, 1992) and in dogs using
indirect, more load-dependent indices of myocardial contractility (De Hert et al, 1990) support the clinical impres-
sion of little or no cardiovascular depression in healthy
humans (Gooding and Corssen, 1977) and in patients with
cardiac disease (Gooding et al, 1979). Preserved sympathetic
nerve activity and autonomic reflexes contribute to the
hemodynamic stability observed during etomidate.

Propofol

In isolated guinea pig ventricular muscle, propofol
depresses voltage-dependent transsarcolemmal Ca^{2+} entry
and late Ca^{2+} release from the sarcoplasmic reticulum
resulting in mild myocardial depression (Park and Lynch,
1992). Despite reduced uptake of Ca^{2+} by the sarcoplasmic
reticulum, the rate constant of exponential decay of iso-
metric force does not change in vitro (Riou et al, 1992). In
patients, propofol decreased myocardial contractility at
least as much as thiopental (Mulier et al, 1991). It is likely,
however, that part of the negative inotropic effect was due
to the marked decrease in sympathetic outflow observed
during propofol anesthesia (Ebert et al, 1992).

   Evidence derived from in vitro (Park and Lynch, 1992)
as well as from in vivo studies in the experimental animal
(De Hert et al, 1990) and in humans (Mulier et al, 1991)
suggests that propofol causes less myocardial depression
than equipotent doses of thiopental and methohexital. In
the blood-perfused isolated rabbit heart, propofol (in contrast to thiopental) did not depress myocardial contractility
(Ismail et al, 1992). In the in situ canine heart, selective
intracoronary infusion of propofol did not cause myocardial
depression (Pagel et al, 1992b). Findings of unchanged isovolumic relaxation and regional chamber stiffness during
propofol administration in chronically instrumented dogs
indicate that propofol does not impair diastolic function
(Pagel et al, 1992b). The decrease in blood pressure follow-

ing induction of anesthesia with propofol is the result of a combination of a decrease in sympathetic nerve activity (Ebert et al, 1992; Sellgren et al, 1990), venous and arterial vasodilation (Muzi et al, 1992; Rouby et al, 1991), and a mild direct negative inotropy (Coetzee et al, 1989; Pagel and Warltier, 1993).

Propofol produces dose-related decreases in arterial blood pressure attributable to simultaneous reductions in myocardial contractility (Hettrick, 1997), left ventricular afterload (via decreases in peripheral resistance and increases in arterial compliance) (Lowe, 1996), and left ventricular mechanical efficiency (i.e. ratio of stroke work to left ventricular pressure-volume area) (Hettrick, 1997). The impairment of LV-arterial coupling and efficiency begin to plateau at higher dosages because they are compensated for by reductions in afterload (Hettrick, 1997). In humans, the peripheral vasodilatory effects of propofol appear to be due primarily to an inhibition of sympathetic vasoconstrictor nerve activity, rather than to direct vascular relaxation (Robinson, 1997). Propofol exhibits a direct negative inotropic effect in humans (Mulier, 1996).

The effects of propofol on the coronary vasculature are somewhat controversial. In vitro, propofol has been shown to possess coronary vasodilator properties, and to attenuate the effects of vasoconstrictors (White et al, 1982). However, in the blood-perfused isolated rabbit heart, propofol had no significant effect on coronary vasomotor tone (Ismail et al, 1992).

Propofol exhibits age-related effects on the cardiac conduction system, slowing conduction through atrial tissue, atrio-ventricular node and His-Purkinje system, as well as slowing spontaneous heart rate (Wu, 1997).

Ketamine

In most patients, ketamine markedly increases heart rate and blood pressure (White et al, 1982) because of its central and peripheral sympathomimetic effects. It is of clinical relevance that ketamine does not increase sympathetic tone by a direct effect, but indirectly by inhibiting neuronal and extraneuronal reuptake of catecholamines (Lundy et al, 1985). Consequently, when normal adrenergic nerve transmission is impaired ketamine causes myocardial depression in vitro (Cook et al, 1991; Kongsayreepong et al, 1993; Rusy et al, 1990). The negative inotropic effect is probably the result of inhibition of transsarcolemmal Ca^{2+} influx and subsequent decrease in available intracellular Ca^{2+} (Kongsayreepong et al, 1993; Rusy et al, 1990). It is to be expected that depletion of catecholamines will unmask the direct vasodilator and myocardial depressant effects of ketamine. Such mechanism would explain the hemodynamic collapse in some critically ill patients receiving ketamine (Waxman et al, 1980).

Because of the simultaneous increase in sympathetic tone, the direct effects of ketamine on myocardial performance in vivo are difficult to evaluate. In dogs with pharmacological blockade of the autonomic nervous system, ketamine reduces the regional PRSW slope indicating direct myocardial depression (Pagel et al, 1992a). In addition, ketamine prolongs isovolumic relaxation and increases regional chamber stiffness consistent with a negative lusitropic effect (Muzi et al, 1992). Ketamine has no direct effect on the tone of large or small canine coronary arteries at concentrations seen in routine clinical practice (Coughlan et al, 1992).

Benzodiazepines

There are surprisingly few data on the direct cardiovascular effects of benzodiazepines using load-independent indices of myocardial performance. Diazepam and midazolam depress indirect indices of contractility in the experimental animal (Messina et al, 1995). Using systolic function indices derived from transesophageal echocardiography in humans with coronary artery disease, there is evidence that midazolam has a mild negative inotropic effect that appears to be offset by a concomitant reduction in afterload resulting in maintained cardiac pump function (Strauer, 1972).

Opioids

Isolated heart or papillary muscle studies have shown that opioids can cause dose-dependent myocardial depression (Strauer 1972; Zhang et al, 1990). However, in these studies opioid concentrations by far exceeded those observed in clinical practice. Opioids seem to produce peripheral vasodilation by a direct action on vascular smooth muscle (Kawar et al, 1985).

ANESTHETICS AND BLOOD VOLUME DISTRIBUTION

As sympathetic tone influences central venous pressure via changes in effective compliance (Bonica et al, 1972), the decrease in sympathetic activity associated with induction of anesthesia should not only be expected to depress cardiac performance but also to redistribute blood volume from the intrathoracic to the extrathoracic compartment. This may contribute to the decrease in blood pressure during induction of anesthesia. Surprisingly, no systematic studies on the effects of anesthesia and different anesthetics on blood volume distribution are available. A decrease in intrathoracic blood volume has been observed during halothane anesthesia (Hedenstierna et al, 1985).

SUMMARY

1. *Anesthetic agents modify cardiovascular performance* by a variety of mechanisms. They interfere with intracellular Ca^{2+} kinetics, local regulation of vasomotor tone, autonomic nervous system activity and reflexes, and/ or myocardial contractility. In general, the direct effects

of anesthetic agents on the circulation result in cardio-vascular depression. In vivo, numerous hemodynamic control mechanisms interfere with and subsequently modify each other.

2.   *Direct vs indirect effects of anesthetic agents.* Direct effects on specific components of the circulation can, there-fore, only be determined under controlled in-vitro con-ditions. It is to be expected that results obtained in vitro will, at times, differ from those obtained in vivo. In the intact organism, the hemodynamic alteration in response to the anesthetic is the net result of direct ef-fects on central and peripheral neurohumoral control mechanism, and on the heart and the vasculature, and of indirect effects elicited by the primary alteration (e.g. secondary changes in cardiac loading conditions, reflexly mediated increases in sympathetic tone, initia-tion of autonomic reflexes). The in vivo response to the administration of an anesthetic will, therefore, de-pend to a large degree on the magnitude of the sec-ondary effects. These, in turn, are dependent on preexisting sympathetic tone, intravascular volume, and reactivity of the autonomic nervous system. Since these factors vary widely between patients, it is not surprising that the hemodynamic response to a given anesthetic cannot reliably be predicted for the indivi-dual patient.

3.   *Differences in preexisting hemodynamic status* explain why in certain patients induction of anesthesia with in-travenous anesthetics causes profound hypotension, whereas some patients with impaired myocardial func-tion seem to tolerate the myocardial depressant effects of inhalational anesthetics quite well. Although the di-rect effects of most anesthetics on the cardiovascular system and its control mechanisms have been well de-fined in vitro, the in vivo effects remain less predict-able.

REFERENCES

Atlee JL III. Cardiac electrophysiology. In: *Cardiovascular Physiology.* Priebe H-J, Skarvan K (Eds). BMJ Publishing Group 1995, 62–96.

Atlee JL. Arrhythmias: Causes and associations. In: *Arrhythmias and Pacemakers.* WB Saunders Co, Philadelphia, 1996, 59–104.

Azari DM and Cork RC. Comparative myocardial depressive ef-fects of propofol and thiopental. *Anesth Analg* 1993; 77: 324–329.

Becker LC. Conditions for vasodilator-induced coronary steal in ex-perimental myocardial ischemia. *Circulation* 1978; 57:1103–1110.

Bernard J-M, Wouters PF, Doursout MF, et al. Effects of sevoflur-ane and isoflurane on cardiac and coronary dynamics in chronically instrumented dogs. *Anesthesiology* 1990; 72: 659–662.

Bettens KM, De Hert SG, Sys SU, Brutsaert DL. Role of the endo-cardial endothelium in the negative inotropic effects of thiopental. *Anesthesiology* 1996; 85:1100–1110.

Blaise G, Sill JC, Nugent M, et al. Isoflurane causes endothelium-dependent inhibition of contractile responses of canine coronary arteries. *Anesthesiology* 1987; 67: 513–517.

Bonica JJ, Kennedy WF, Nakamatsu TJ and Gerberrshagen HU. Circulatory effects of peridural block: III. Effects of acute blood loss. *Anesthesiology* 1972; 36: 219–227.

Coetzee A, Fourie P, Coetzee J, et al. Effect of various propofol plasma concentrations on regional myocardial contractility and left ventricular afterload. *Anesthesiology* 1991; 75: 32–42.

Connelly TJ and Coronade R. Activation of the Ca^{2+} release channel of cardiac sarcoplasmic reticulum by volatile anesthetics. *Anesthesiology* 1994; 81:459–469.

Conway CM and Ellis DB. The haemodynamic effects of short-acting barbiturates. Br J Anaesth 1969; 41: 534–542.

Cook DJ, Carton EG, Housmans PR. Mechanism of the positive inotropic effect of ketamine in isolated ferret ventricular papillary muscle. *Anesthesiology* 1991; 74: 880–888.

Coughlan MG, Flynn NM, Kenny D, et al. Differential relaxant effect of high concentrations of intravenous anesthetics on endothelin-constricted proximal and distal canine coronary arteries. *Anesth Analg* 1992; 74: 378–383.

De Hert SG, Vermeyen KM and Adriaensen HF. Influence of thiopental, etomidate, and propofol on regional myocardial function in the normal and acute ischemic heart segment in dogs. *Anesth Analg* 1990; 70: 600–607.

Doyle RL, Foex P, Ryder WA and Jones LA. Effects of halothane on left ventricular relaxation and early diastolic coronary blood flow in the dog. *Anesthesiology* 1989; 70: 660–666.

Ebert TJ, Kampine JP. Nitrous oxide augments sympathetic outflow: Direct evidence from human peroneal nerve recordings. *Anesth Analg* 1989; 69: 444–449.

Ebert TJ, Kanitz DD, Kampine JP. Inhibition of sympathetic neural outflow during thiopental anesthesia in humans. *Anesth Analg* 1990; 71: 319–326.

Ebert TJ, Muzi M, Berens R et al. Sympathetic responses to induction of anaesthesia in humans with propofol or etomidate. *Anesthesiology* 1992; 76: 725–733.

Ebert TJ, Muzi M and Lopatka CW. Neurocirculatory responses to sevoflurane in humans. A comparison to desflurane. *Anesthesiology* 1995; 83: 88–95.

Ebert TJ and Muzi M. Sympathetic hyperactivity during desflurane anesthesia in healthy volunteers. *Anesthesiology* 1993; 79: 444–453.

Ebert TJ. Differential effects of nitrous oxide on baroreflex control of heart rate and peripheral sympathetic nerve activity in humans. *Anesthesiology* 1990; 72: 16–22.

Eckstein JW, Hamilton WK and McCammond JM. The effect of thiopental induction on peripheral venous tone. *Anesthesiology* 1990; 72: 330–340.

Frankl WS and Poole-Wilson PA. Effects of thiopental on tension development, action potential, and exchange of calcium and potassium in rabbit ventricular myocardium. *J Cardiovasc Pharmacol* 1981; 3: 554–565.

Frink EJ, Malan TP, Atlas M, et al. Clinical comparison of sevoflurane and isoflurane in healthy patients. *Anesth Analg* 1992; 74:241–245.

Glower DD, Spratt JA, Snow ND, et al. Linearity of the Frank-Starling relationship in the intact heart: the concept of preload recruitable stroke work. *Circulation* 1985; 71: 994–1009.

Goldberg AH and Phear WPC. Halothane and paired stimulation: Effects on myocardial compliance and contractility. *J Appl Physiol* 1970; 28: 391–396.

Gooding JM and Corssen G: Effect of etomidate on the cardiovascular system. *Anesth Analg* 1977; 56:717–719.

Gooding JM, Weng JT, Smith RA, et al. Cardiovascular and pulmonary responses following etomidate induction of anesthesia in patients with demonstrated cardiac disease. *Anesth Analg* 1979; 58: 40–41.

Graf BM, Viceenzi MN, Bosnjak ZJ, Stowe DF. The comparative effects of equimolar sevoflurane and isoflurane in isolated hearts. *Anesth Analg* 1995; 81:1026–1032.

Griffiths R and Norman RI. Effects of anesthetics on uptake, synthesis and release of transmitters. *Br J Anaesth* 1993; 71: 96–107.

Greenblatt EP, Loeb AL, and Longnecker DE. Endothelium-dependent circulatory control — a mechanism for the differing peripheral vascular effects of isoflurane versus halothane. *Anesthesiology* 1992; 77:1178–1185.

Gurevicius J, Holmes CB, Salem R, et al. The direct effects of enflurane on coronary blood flow, myocardial oxygen consumption, and myocardial segmental shortening in in situ canine hearts. *Anesth Analg* 1996; 83: 68–74.

Harkin CP, Pagel PS, Kersten JR, et al. Direct negative inotropic and lusitropic effects of sevoflurane. *Anesthesiology* 1994; 81:156–167.

Hartman JC, Kampine JP, Schmeling WT and Warltier DC. Alterations in collateral blood flow produced by isoflurane in a chronically instrumented canine model of multivessel coronary artery disease. *Anesthesiology* 1991; 74:120–133.

Hartman JC, Pagel PS, Kampine JP, et al. Influence of desflurane on regional distribution of coronary blood flow in a chronically instrumented canine model of multivessel coronary artery obstruction. *Anesth Analg* 1991; 72: 289–299.

Hedenstierna G, Strandberg A, Brismar B, et al. Functional residual capacity, thoracoabdominal dimensions and central blood volume during general anesthesia with muscle paralysis and mechanical ventilation. *Anesthesiology* 1985; 62: 247–254.

Hettrick DA, Pagel PS and Warltier DC. Alterations in canine left ventricular-arterial coupling and mechanical efficiency produced by propofol. *Anesthesiology* 1997; 86:1088–1093.

Hettrick DA, Pagel PS and Warltier DC. Desflurane, sevoflurane, and isoflurane impair canine left ventricular-arterial coupling and mechanical efficiency. *Anesthesiology* 1996; 85: 403–413.

Hickey RF, Sybert PE, Verrier ED and Cason BA. Effects of halothane, enflurane, and isoflurane on coronary blood flow autoregulation and coronary vascular reserve in the canine heart. *Anesthesiology* 1988; 68: 21–30.

Hirano M, Fujigaki T, Shibata O and Sumikawa K. A comparison of coronary hemodynamics during isoflurane and sevoflurane anesthesia in dogs. *Anesth Analg* 1995; 80: 651–656.

Humphrey LS, Stinson DC, Humphrey MJ, et al. Volatile anesthetic effects on left ventricular relaxation in swine. *Anesthesiology* 1990; 73: 731–738.

Hysing ES, Chelly JE, Jacobson L, et al. Cardiovascular effects of acute changes in extracellular ionized calcium concentration induced by citrate and CaCl$_2$ infusion in chronically instrumented dogs, conscious and during enflurane, halothane, and isoflurane anesthesia. *Anesthesiology* 1990; 72: 100–104.

Ismail EF, Kim S-J, Salem R and Crystal GJ. Direct effects of propofol on myocardial contractility in in situ canine hearts. *Anesthesiology* 1992; 77:964–972.

Jones DJ, Stehling LC and Zander HL. Cardiovascular responses to diazepam and midazolam maleate in the dog. *Anesthesiology* 1979; 51: 430–434.

Kawar P, Carson IW, Clarke RSJ, et al. Haemodynamic changes during induction of anesthesia with midazolam and diazepam (Valium) in patients undergoing coronary artery bypass surgery. *Anesthesia* 1985; 40: 767–771.

Kenny D, Pelch LR, Brooks HL, et al. Calcium channel modulation of α_1 and α_2 adrenergic pressor responses in conscious and anesthetized dogs. *Anesthesiology* 1990; 72: 874–881.

Kersten JR, Brayer AP, Pagel PS, et al. Perfusion of ischemic myocardium during anesthesia with sevoflurane. *Anesthesiology* 1994; 81: 995–1004.

Kersten J, Pagel PS, Tessmer JP, et al. Dexmedetomidine alters the hemodynamic effects of desflurane and isoflurane in chronically instrumented dogs. *Anesthesiology* 1993; 79:1022–1032.

Kikura M and Ikeda K. Comparison of effects of sevoflurane-nitrous oxide and enflurane-nitrous oxide on myocardial contractility in humans. Load-independent and noninvasive assessment with transesophageal echocardiography. *Anesthesiology* 1993; 79: 235–243.

Komai H, DeWitt DE and Rusy BF. Negative inotropic effects of etomidate in rabbit papillary muscle. *Anesth Analg* 1985; 64: 400–404.

Kongsayreepons S, Cook DJ and Housmans PR. Mechanism of the direct, negative inotropic effect of ketamine in isolated ferret and frog ventricular myocardium. *Anesthesiology* 1993; 79: 313–322.

Kotrly KJ, Ebert TJ, Vucins E, et al. Baroreceptor reflex control of the heart rate during isoflurane anesthesia in humans. *Anesthesiology* 1984; 60: 173–179.

Kotrly KJ, Ebert TJ, Vucins EJ, et al. Effects of fentanyl-diazepam-nitrous oxide anesthesia on arterial baroreflex control of heart rate in man. *Br J Anaesth* 1986; 58: 406–414.

Larach DR, Schuler HG, Derr JA, et al. Halothane selectively attenuates $_2$-adrenoreceptor mediated vasoconstriction, in vivo and in vitro. *Anesthesiology* 1987; 66: 781–791.

Larach DR and Schuler HG. Direct vasodilation by sevoflurane, isoflurane, and halothane alters coronary flow reserve in the isolated rat heart. *Anesthesiology* 1991; 75: 268–278.

Lawson D, Frazer MJ and Lynch C III. Nitrous oxide effects on isolated myocardium: a reexamination in vitro. *Anesthesiology* 1990; 73: 930–943.

Lerman J, Oyston JP, Gallagher TM, et al. The minimum alveolar concentration (MAC) and hemodynamic effects of halothane, isoflurane, and sevoflurane in newborn swine. *Anesthesiology* 1990; 73:717–721.

Lerman J, Sikich N, Kleinmans S and Yentis S. The pharmacology of sevoflurane in infants and children. *Anesthesiology* 1994; 80: 814–824.

Lowe D, Hettrick DA, Pagel PS and Warltier DC. Propofol alters left ventricular afterload as evaluated by aortic input impedance in dogs. *Anesthesiology* 1996; 84: 368–376.

Lundy PM, Gverzdys S and Frew R. Ketamine: Evidence of tissue specific inhibition of neuronal and extraneuronal catecholamine uptake processes. *Can J Physiol Pharmacol* 1985; 63:298–303.

Malan TP, DiNardo JA, Isner J, et al. Cardiovascular effects of sevoflurane compared with those of isoflurane in volunteers. *Anesthesiology* 1995; 83: 918–928.

Marsch SCU, Dalmas S, Philbin DM, et al. Effects and interactions of nitrous oxide, myocardial ischemia, and reperfusion on left ventricular diastolic function. *Anesth Analg* 1997; 84:39–45.

Merin RG, Bernard J, Doursout M, et al. Comparison of the effects of isoflurane and desflurane on cardiovascular dynamics and regional blood flow in the chronically instrumented dog. *Anesthesiology* 1991; 74: 568–574.

Messina AG, Paranicas M, Yao F-S, et al. The effect of midazolam on left ventricular pump performance and contractility in anesthetized patients with coronary artery disease: effect of preoperative ejection fraction. *Anesth Analg* 1995; 81:793–799.

Moore MA, Weiskopf RB, Eger EI II, et al. Rapid 1% increases of end-tidal desflurane concentration to greater than 5% transiently increase heart rate and blood pressure in humans. *Anesthesiology* 1994; 81: 94–98.

Mouren S, Baron J-F, Albo C, et al. Effects of propofol and thiopental on coronary blood flow and myocardial performance in an isolated rabbit heart. *Anesthesiology* 1994; 80:634–641.

Mulier JP and Van Aken H. Comparison of eltanolone and propofol on a pressure-volume analysis of the heart. *Anesth Analg* 1996; 83:233–237.

Mulier JP, Wouters P, Van Aken H, et al. Cardiodynamic effects of propofol in comparison with thiopental: Assessment with a transoesophaegeal echocardiographic approach. *Anesth Analg* 1991; 72:28–35.

Muzi M, Berens RA, Kampine JP and Ebert TJ. Ventilation contributes to propofol-mediated hypotension in humans. *Anesth Analg* 1992; 74: 877–883.

Pagel PS, Hettrick DA and Warltier DC. Left ventricular mechanical consequences of dihydropyridine calcium channel modulation in conscious and anesthetized chronically instrumented dogs. *Anesthesiology* 1994; 81:190–208.

Pagel PS, Kampine JP, Schmeling WT and Warltier DC. Comparison of end-systolic pressure-length relations and preload recruitable stroke work as indices of myocardial contractility in the conscious and anesthetized, chronically instrumented dog. *Anesthesiology* 1990a; 73: 278–290.

Pagel PS, Kampine JP, Schmeling WT and Warltier DC. Effects of nitrous oxide on myocardial contractility as evaluated by the preload recruitable stroke work relationship in chronically instrumented dogs. *Anesthesiology* 1990b; 73:1148–1157.

Pagel PS, Kampine JP, Schmeling WT and Warltier DC. Influence of volatile anesthetics on myocardial contractility in vivo: Desflurane versus isoflurane. *Anesthesiology* 1991a; 74: 900–907.

Pagel PS, Kampine JP, Schmeling WT and Warltier DC. Alteration of left ventricular diastolic function by desflurane, isoflurane and halothane in the chronically instrumented dog with autonomic nervous system blockade. *Anesthesiology* 1991b; 74: 1103–1114.

Pagel PS, Kampine JP, Schmeling WT and Warltier DC. Comparison of the systemic and coronary hemodynamic actions of desflurane, isoflurane, halothane and enflurane in the chronically instrumented dog. *Anesthesiology* 1991c; 74: 539–551.

Pagel PS, Kampine JP, Schmeling WT and Warltier DC. Ketamine depresses myocardial contractility as evaluated by the preload recruitable stroke work relationship in chronically instrumented dogs with autonomic nervous system blockade. *Anesthesiology* 1992a; 76: 564–572.

Pagel PS, Kampine JP, Schmeling WT and Warltier DC. Evaluation of myocardial contractility in the chronically instrumented dog with intact autonomic nervous system function: Effects of desflurane and isoflurane. *Acta Anaesthesiol Scand* 1993; 37: 203–210.

Pagel PS, Schmeling WT, Kampine JP and Warltier DC. Alteration of canine left ventricular diastolic function by intravenous anesthetics in vivo: Ketamine and propofol. *Anesthesiology* 1992b; 76: 419–425.

Pagel PS and Warltier DC. Negative inotropic effects of propofol as evaluated by the regional preload recruitable stroke work relationship in chronically instrumented dogs. *Anesthesiology* 1983; 78: 100–108.

Park KW, Dai HB, Lowenstein E, et al. Isoflurane and halothane attenuate endothelium-dependent vasodilation in rat coronary microvessels. *Anesth Analg* 1997; 84: 278–28.

Park WK and Lynch C III. Propofol and thiopental depression of myocardial contractility: A comparative study of mechanical and electrophysiologic effects in isolated guinea pig ventricular muscle. *Anesth Analg* 1992; 74: 395–405.

Pocock G and Richards CD. Cellular mechanisms in general anaesthesia. *Br J Anaesth* 1991; 66:116–128.

Priebe H-J. Isoflurane and coronary hemodynamics (Review Article). *Anesthesiology* 1989; 71: 960–976.

Riou B, Besse S, Lecarpentier Y and Viars P. In vivo effects of propofol on rat myocardium. *Anesthesiology* 1992; 76: 609–616.

Riou B, Lecarpentier Y, Chemla D and Viars P: In vitro effects of etomidate on intrinsic myocardial contractility in the rat. *Anesthesiology* 1990; 72: 330–340.

Riou B, Lecarpentier Y and Viars P. Effects of etomidate on the cardiac papillary muscle of normal hamsters and those with cardiomyopathy. *Anesthesiology* 1993; 78:83–90.

Robinson BJ, Ebert TJ, O'Brien TJ, et al. Mechanisms whereby propofol mediates peripheral vasodilation in humans. Sympathoinhibition or direct vascular relaxation? *Anesthesiology* 1997; 86: 64–72.

Rouby JJ, Andreev A, Léger P, et al. Peripheral vascular effects of thiopental and propofol in humans with artificial hearts. *Anesthesiology* 1991; 75: 32–42.

Rusy BF, Amuzu JK, Bosscher HA, et al. Negative inotropic effect of ketamine in rabbit ventricular muscle. *Anesth Analg* 1990; 71: 275–278.

Rusy BF and Komai H: Anesthetic depression of myocardial contractility: A review of possible mechanisms. *Anesthesiology* 1987; 67: 745–766.

Sagawa K. The ventricular pressure-volume diagram revisited. *Circ Res* 1978; 46: 677–687.

Sellgren J, Ponten J and Wallin BG. Characteristics of muscle sympathetic nerve activity during general anaesthesia in humans. *Acta*

Anaesthesiol Scand 1992; 36: 336–345.

Sellgren J, Ponten J and Wallin G. Percutaneous recordings of muscle nerve sympathetic nerve activity during propofol, nitrous oxide, and isoflurane anesthesia in humans. *Anesthesiology* 1990; 73: 20–27.

Stowe DF, Bosnjak ZJ and Kampine JP. Comparison of etomidate, ketamine, midazolam, propofol, and thiopental on function and metabolism of isolated hearts. *Anesth Analg* 1992; 74: 547–558.

Stowe DF, Monroe SM, Marijic J, et al. Effects of nitrous oxide on contractile function and metabolism of the isolated heart. *Anesthesiology* 1990; 73: 1220–1226.

Strauer BE. Contractile responses to morphine, piritramide, meperidine, and fentanyl: a comparative study of effects on the isolated ventricular myocardium. *Anesthesiology* 1972; 37:304–310.

Van Trigt P, Christian CC, Fagraeus L, et al. Myocardial depression by anesthetic agents (halothane, enflurane and nitrous oxide): Quantitation based on end-systolic pressure-dimension relations. *Am J Cardiol* 1984; 53: 243–247.

Waxman K, Shoemaker WC and Lippmann M. Cardiovascular effects of anesthetic induction with ketamine. *Anesth Analg* 1980; 59: 355–358.

Weight HU, Kwok W-M, Rehmert GC, et al. Voltage-dependent effects of volatile anesthetics on cardiac sodium current. *Anesth Analg* 1997; 84:285–293.

Weiskopf RB, Cahalan MK, Eger EI II, et al. Cardiovascular actions of desflurane in normocarbic volunteers. *Anesth Analg* 1991; 73: 143–156.

Weiskopf RB, Holmes MA, Eger EI II, et al. Cardiovascular effects of I 653 in swine. *Anesthesiology* 1988; 69: 303–309.

Weiskopf RB, Moore MA, Eger EI II, et al. Rapid increase in desflurane concentration is associated with greater transient cardiovascular stimulation than with rapid increase in isoflurane concentration in humans. *Anesthesiology* 1994; 80: 1035–1045.

White PF, Way WL and Trevor AJ. Ketamine - its pharmacology and therapeutic uses. *Anesthesiology* 1982; 56: 119–136.

Wilkowski DAW, Sill JC, Bonta W, et al. Nitrous oxide constricts epicardial coronary arteries without effect on coronary arterioles. *Anesthesiology* 1987; 66: 659–665.

Wu M-H, Su M-J and Sun S S-M Age-related propofol effects on electrophysiological properties of isolated hearts. *Anesth Analg* 1997; 84: 964–971.

Yamanoue T, Brum JM and Estafanous FG. Vasodilation and mechanism of propofol in porcine coronary artery. *Anesthesiology* 1994; 81: 443–451.

Yli-Hankala A, Randell T, Seppälä Tand Lindgren L. Increases in hemodynamic variables and catecholamine levels after rapid increase in isoflurane concentration. *Anesthesiology* 1993; 78:266–271.

Zhang C-C, Su JY and Calkins D. Effects of alfentanil on isolated cardiac tissues of the rabbit. *Anesth Analg* 1990; 71: 268–274.

CHAPTER 3

Adrenergic Receptor Agonists in Anesthetic Practice

Michael G. Mythen and Debra A. Schwinn

Adrenergic receptor (AR) agonists have a relevance to 4 aspects of anesthetic practice:

i Manipulation of Pathologically Deranged Cardio-respiratory Variables

The primary goal of the cardio-respiratory system is delivery of oxygen to the body's cells. Cardio-respiratory monitoring is used during anesthetic practice to allow the detection and correction of cardio-respiratory derangements with the aim of improving patient outcome. AR agonists are commonly used to manipulate pathologically deranged cardio-respiratory variables with the aim of improving cellular oxygenation and thus patient outcome.

ii Adjuncts to the Use of Other Drugs

AR agonists are used during routine clinical practice as adjuncts to the use of other drugs. For example epinephrine is often added to local anesthetics that are injected into tissues with the aim of prolonging their action by producing local vasoconstriction. Vasoconstrictors, such as ephedrine, are sometimes given systemically at the same time as a spinal local anesthetic block is produced with the aim of avoiding the cardiovascular instability that may result from sympathetic blockade.

iii As a Part of Organ-protective Regimens

There is some evidence to suggest that the prophylactic administration of a combination of intravenous fluids and AR agonists with the aim of increasing oxygen delivery to cells prior to the trauma of surgery may result in an improved outcome. Similarly many administer drugs such as dopamine or dopexamine as they are believed to be protective of renal and/or splanchnic perfusion, and thus function.

iv Adrenergic Agonists May Adversely Interact With Other Drugs

Many commonly prescribed drugs have effects on adrenergic receptors. It is therefore important for the anaesthetist to have a clear understanding of the effects of AR agonists with the aim of avoiding adverse effects of co-administration.

PHARMACODYNAMICS AND MECHANISMS OF ACTION OF ADRENERGIC RECEPTOR AGONISTS

Adrenergic receptor agonists mediate their action via adrenergic receptors (ARs). ARs were first described and divided into α and β by Ahlquist in his landmark manuscript in the Journal of Physiology in 1948 (Ahlquist, 1948). By 1967 Lands had subdivided βARs into β_1 and β_2 subtypes (Lands et al, 1967a; Lands et al, 1967b) and by the mid 1970s αARs had been subdivided into α_1 and α_2 (Fig 3-1). It is important to note that ARs mediate physiologic responses in many tissues, however only the predominant cardiovascular properties of ARs will be presented in this chapter. To delve further into other properties of AR subtypes (including gluconeogenesis, glycogenolysis, sedation, etc.) the reader is referred to a relatively recent textbook about ARs (Bergowitz and Schwinn, 1994). Classically, ARs have the following locations and properties (Figs 3-2 and 3): α_1ARs are located postsynaptically and mediate vasoconstriction (Fig 1-9, page 11); α_2ARs when located presynaptically inhibit norepinephrine release, and when located postsynaptically mediate vaso- and venoconstriction; β_1ARs are located predominantly in the heart and mediate increased myocardial chronotropy and inotropy (Fig 3-2); and β_2ARs are located predominantly in the lungs and

Adrenergic Receptor Subtypes

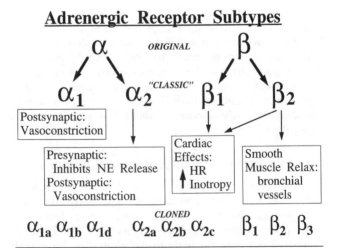

Fig 3-1. Adrenergic receptor (AR) subtypes. Individual AR subtypes are listed historically along with associated cardiovascular responses to activation. See text for details. NE = norepinephrine; HR = heart rate.

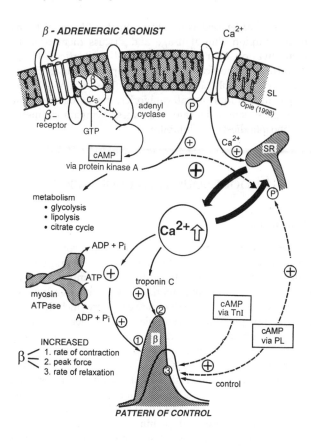

Fig 3-2. β-adrenergic signal systems leading to an increased rate of contraction, increased peak force of contraction, and increase rate of relaxation. SL = sarcolemma; SR = sarcoplasmic reticulum. (Fig. copyright © L.H. Opie, 1998)

vessels and mediate bronchodilation and vasodilation, respectively. Recent evidence suggests that β_2ARs are clearly located in the human myocardium as well and also mediate myocardial inotropy. These properties of AR subtypes conveniently explain most of the clinical cardiovascular actions of drugs acting on ARs. However, most AR agonists and antagonists available today are not very subtype selective. For example, dopamine alone can activate dopamine receptors (of which nine have now been cloned) as well as all AR subtypes (depending on the dose used). In addition, there has been an explosion recently in the number of AR subtypes identified and cloned using genetic techniques. By the late 1980s and early 1990s, at least nine AR subtypes had been discovered, described, and cloned (Fig 3-1). The ability to express an individual cloned receptor gene in a cell previously not containing the receptor enables a researcher to study individual receptor subtypes and analyze their signal transduction properties. Since multiple ARs are usually expressed simultaneously in various tissues, the ability to study individual subtypes greatly enhances the understanding of molecular pharmacology of ARs. This should lead eventually to more selective compounds for use in the peri-operative period.

This chapter will concentrate on the AR agonists that are in common clinical usage and discuss them from the perspective of their pharmacological properties, dosage, administration, indications for peri-operative use, interactions and possible adverse effects. The commonly used agents fall into four overall catagories: the endogenous catecholamines; synthetic catecholamines, sympathomometics, and phosphodiesterase inhibitors.

ENDOGENOUS CATECHOLAMINES

Dopamine

Dopamine is the immediate metabolic precursor of norepinephrine and epinephrine (Fig 3-3) and is a central nervous system neurotransmitter. In addition to stimulating dopamine receptors, dopamine binds to and activates adrenergic receptors (both α and βARs). Indirect effects include inhibition of norepinephrine reuptake at the nerve terminal, release of norepinephrine at the nerve terminal, and metabolism by hydroxylation of the a carbon to form norepinephrine (Weiner 1985; Ghosh et al, 1991). Although increases in renal blood flow and sodium excretion both occur with dopamine administration, it is not clear that increases in renal blood flow are the sole cause of enhanced diuresis and natriuresis; dopamine may also inhibit tubular solute reabsorption directly (Hiberman et al. 1984; Miller, 1984). Dopamine receptors exist in the central nervous system, however dopamine administration does not result in CNS effects since intravenous dopamine cannot cross the blood brain barrier.

Administration and dosage of dopamine. Dopamine is a substrate for both catechol-o-methyl transferase (COMT)

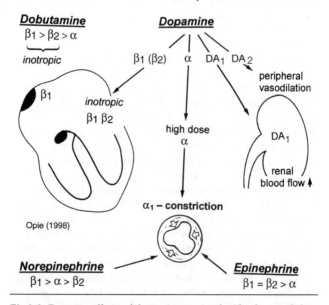

Fig 3-3. Receptor effects of dopamine compared with other catecholamines. (Fig. copyright © L.H. Opie, 1998)

and mondamine oxidase (MAO), therefore it is ineffective when administered orally and is rapidly metabolized by the liver and other tissues when administered intravenously. Therefore, dopamine is most commonly given as an intravenous infusion. The primary effects of dopamine are dose dependent (see table). At relatively low intravenous doses (1–5 μg/kg/min), dopamine stimulates predominantly dopamine receptors which mediate renal and mesenteric arterial relaxation (Szerlip, 1991). At moderate intravenous doses (5–10 μg/kg/min), dopamine is classically thought to directly stimulate predominantly ARs, thus accounting for its positive inotropic effects. Recent evidence suggests that the exact mechanism of dopamine-mediated positive inotropic responses in this dose range actually depends on conversion of dopamine to norepinephrine in noradrenergic nerves, and secondary release in the myocardium (Brown, 1990). At high intravenous dose (10–15 μg/kg/min), αAR stimulation becomes apparent and vasoconstriction results, reversing potential renal perfusion benefits seen at lower doses.

Using dopamine peri-operatively. Dopamine is often used peri-operatively for its effects on renal artery blood flow and as a positive inotrope. It can been used effectively in heart failure and various hypotensive states including septic shock. Probably the most common peri-operative use of dopamine is as a low dose infusion primarily for its effects on renal and splanchnic blood flow. Many believe the prophylactic infusion of "renal dose dopamine" (typically 2.5 μg/kg/min) confers protection on the kidneys and or splanchnic organs. This remains highly controversial because, although numerous animal experiments support such practices, more than 20 years of clinical trials have failed to demonstrate a significant clinical effect (Miller, 1984; Szerlip, 1991; Flancbaum et al, 1994; Vincent 1994). Indeed some argue that a low dose dopamine infusion may have a deleterious effect as it can increase myocardial oxygen demand and maintain the sytemic blood pressure and urine output in the face of occult hypovolemia. Interestingly, one study has recently compared the effects of low dose infusions of both dopamine and dobutamine in critically ill patients and found that although dopamine increased urine flow, only dobutamine increased creatinine clearance (Duke et al, 1994). Another study of patients undergoing cardiac surgery found that peri-operative administration of low dose dopamine only produced natriuresis if the patients had first been adequately fluid loaded (Bryan et al, 1995) re-emphasising the key role of good fluid balance in the maintenance of renal perfusion. Despite lack of evidence to support its prophylactic low dose administration, dopamine is undoubtedly a clinically useful AR agonist.

Interactions and adverse effects of dopamine. Since dopamine is a substrate for both COMT and MAO it should be used with extreme caution in patients on MAO inhibitor medication for symptoms of depression. Dopamine can cause or exacerbate tachyarrythmias. Since much of dopamine's effect is mediated by increasing levels of norepinephrine, co-administration of dopamine with norepine-phrine in an attempt to offset any reductions in splanchnic or renal blood flow that may occur is illogical and may actually have deleterious effects.

Epinephrine

Epinephrine is a potent α and βAR agonist, with β effects predominating at lower doses. In the heart, epinephrine is a potent stimulant of myocardial inotropy, has significant arrhythmogenic potential, and increases stroke volume, coronary blood flow, and heart rate. Intravenous injection of epinephrine results in vasoconstriction, particularly in the skin and kidneys, while vessels to skeletal muscles dilate. Increases in blood pressure mediated by intravenous administration of epinephrine are mediated predominantly by constriction of small arterioles and precapillary sphincters (although some constriction occurs on large arteries and veins); a characteristically higher systolic blood pressure than diastolic blood pressure is produced, hence widening the pulse pressure (Weiner, 1985). Since epinephrine acts directly on adrenergic receptors (instead of indirectly by releasing norepinephrine from the nerve terminal), repeated bolus doses of epinephrine mediate continued increases in blood pressure. Epinephrine also causes relaxation of bronchial smooth muscle and increases in cAMP in mast cells, which then stabilizes these cells and prevents degranulation.

Administration and dosage of epinephrine. As can be seen in Table 3–1, the route of administration and dose of epinephrine depend on the condition being treated. Epinephrine is rapidly conjugated and oxidized in gastrointestinal mucosa and liver by the enzymes COMT and MAO; thus oral administration of epinephrine does not provide therapeutic drug levels. Epinephrine can be administered either via subcutaneous, intravenous or pulmonary routes. Subcutaneous administration of epinephrine slows absorption significantly, enabling beneficial effects to last longer and potential side-effects to be minimized; this route has proved useful in the out-of-hospital emergency treatment of anaphylaxis and asthma. Patients with known life threatening allergies will often carry a pre-loaded subcutaneous injector on a chain around their neck and hope to have time to self inject on exposure to their known allergen. Subcutaneous injection of epinephrine is occasionally recommended for the in-hospital treatment of anaphylaxis or asthma. However, if the patient is already in shock the subcutaneous administration of any drug is illogical, as there will be reduced skin perfusion and thus poor systemic drug delivery. For any emergency situation the drug should ideally be given intravenously. For a collapsed patient who has an endotracheal tube *in-situ*, but no access to a great vein or the heart, epinephrine can effectively be administered into the pulmonary circulation via the endotracheal tube. This route of administration remains controversial and can only be recommended if central venous access is unavailable. Nebulized epinephrine can be an effective treatment for swelling of the upper airway or severe bronchospasm. In

Table 3–1. Adrenergic receptor agonists and related inotropic drugs.

Drug	Catecholamine Receptor Activation					Non-catecholamine Mechanism	Drug Doses and Suggested Intravenous Infusion Schemes
	α1	α2	β1	β2	Dopamine		
Endogenous Catecholamines:							
Epinephrine	+++ (high dose)	+++	++ (low dose)	++	–	No	Drip: 1 mg/250 ml. Start 2–4 μg/min or 0.03–0.06 μg/kg/min or 0.3–0.5 mg s.c.; 1 μg/kg/min IV CPR: 0.5–5 mg IV or ETT Asthma: 0.3–0.5 mg s.c.; 1 μg/kg/min IV
Norepinephrine	+++	+++	+ (low dose)	little	–	No	Drip: 1 mg/250 ml. Start 2–4 μg/min or 0.03–0.06 μg/kg/min
Dopamine	++ (high dose)	+	++ (low dose)	+	+++	No*,**	Drip: 200 mg/250 ml (800 μg/ml) or 400 mg/250 ml (1600 μg/ml) 2–5 μg/kg/min → ↑ renal blood flow (dopamine effects, some β) 5–10 μg/kg/min → ↑ HR & contractility, β effects 10–20 μg/kg/min → vasoconstriction
	Direct and indirect actions: 1) NE 2° metabolism via hydroxylation of α carbon, 2) inhibition of NE reuptake, 3) promotion of NE release						
Synthetic Catecholamines:							
Isoproterenol	–	–	+++	+++	–	No	Drip: 1 mg/250 ml (4 μg/ml), 0.01–0.1 μg/kg/min (keep HR < 120) Arrhythmogenic. Use in status asthmaticus, complete heart block.
Dobutamine	little	little	+++	++	–	No*	Drip: 250 mg/250 ml (1000 μg/ml), 2–15 μg/kg/min 5–40 μg/kg/min for stress echocardiography
			Direct and minimal indirect effects				
Arbutamine	++	–	+++	+++	–	No	Drip: 0.2–0.8 μg/kg/min for stress echocardiography
Dopexamine	–	–	little	+++	++	No*	Drip: 1–10 μg/kg/min
			Both direct and indirect effects				
Sympathomimetic Agents:							
Denopamine	antag	–	++	–	–	No	Oral administration
Ephedrine	+	+	+	+	–	No**	Bolus: 50 mg/10 ml (5 mg/ml), 10–25 mg IV boluses effect lasts 10–15 min, ↑CO ↑SVR ↑HR
			Both direct and indirect effects				
Phosphodiesterase Inhibitors:							
Amrinone	–	–	–	–	–	Yes	Loading Dose: 0.75 mg/kg IV (maximum up to 3 mg/kg in CHF) Drip: 2–10 μg/kg/min IV (higher infusion rates have been used in CHF)
	Peripheral vasodilator, ↑inotropy (additive to other types), ↑cAMP in heart						
Milrinone	–	–	–	–	–	Yes	Loading Dose: 50–75 μg/kg IV bolus Drip: 0.35–0.85 μg/kg/min (usually 0.5 μg/kg/min)
	Similar to amrinone, but more potent inotropy, less vasodilation						
Enoximone	–	–	–	–	–	Yes	Not available

Notes: Do not give inotropes in same IV line as HCO₃– or alkaline solutions since these drugs will be inactivated (by auto–oxidation). Doses should always be checked on individual package inserts before administering drug. *Blocks reuptake of norepinephrine from the nerve terminal. **Promotes the release of norepinephrine from the nerve terminal.

Abbreviations: α1, α2, β1, β2=adrenergic receptor subtypes (catecholamine receptors), antag=antagonist, – =no effect, + =positive effect, 2°=secondary to, cAMP=cyclic adenosine monophosphate, CHF=congestive heart failure, CPR=cardiopulmonary resuscitation, ETT=endotracheal tube, gm=gram, HR=heart rate, IV=intravenous, kg=kilogram, max=maximum, mg=milligram, μg=microgram, min=minute, ml=milliliter, NE=norepinephrine, sc=subcutaneous cardiopulmonary resuscitation, 1mg bolus doses are given intravenously or directly into the ventricle (1mg = 1ml of 1:1,000 or 10ml of 1:10,000 epinephrine). For the treatment of myocardial failure, intravenous infusions are more commonly used. Doses ranging from $0.01-0.03$ $\mu g/kg/min$ provide low dose epinephrine effects in which βAR agonist effects predominate. However, at higher dose range (maximum 0.1 $\mu g/kg/min$), vasoconstrictive αAR effects predominate. This is potentially useful in the setting of hypotensive cardiac failure where both positive inotropic and some vasoconstrictive effects are desired.

Epinephrine peri-operatively. The most common perioperative uses of epinephrine are in the treatment of anaphylactic shock and during cardiopulmonary resuscitation. In the treatment of anaphylactic shock, the early administration of fluids and epinephrine are thought to be the most important interventions for a favourable outcome. In the treatment of acute cardiac failure, although the use of epinephrine infusions have become less fashionable, there is no evidence to demonstrate that the alternative use of the synthetic catecholamines or phosphodiesterase inhibitors (with their added expense) is associated improved outcome beyond epinephrine.

Interactions and potential adverse effects of epinephrine. Epinephrine has been shown to mediate renal artery constriction, suggesting that it should be avoided in patients with renal failure. However, since severe hypotension may be more detrimental to renal function in the long term than acute therapy with epinephrine (in which renal perfusion pressure is re-established), renal failure should not neccessarily be regarded as a contraindication. Epinephrine administration may result in serious side-effects, including cerebral hemorrhage (from an acute elevation of blood pressure) and cardiac arrhythmias (usually ventricular arrhythmias including ventricular fibrillation). For this reason epinephrine should be used with extreme caution in patients on MAO inhibitor medication for symptoms of depression, since metabolism of epinephrine is reduced in this scenario, potentially leading to severe hypertension. In the presence of inhalational anesthetics, cardiac arrhythmias may occur at a lower epinephrine dose (Sumikawa et al, 1983). However, when used properly, epinephrine can be a safe and life saving drug.

Norepinephrine

Norepinephrine, structurally similar to epinephrine, is the endogenous postganglionic neurotransmitter for the sympathetic nervous system. In addition, norepinephrine constitutes 10–20% of the catecholamine content of the adrenal medulla, and is secreted in >95% of pheochromocytomas (Weiner, 1985). Norepinephrine stimulates predominantly $\alpha_1 ARs$ but there is also some stimulation of βARs (β_1 to a far greater extent than $\beta_2 AR$) (see table). From this information, most of the cardiovascular effects of norepinephrine can be derived. Blood pressure increases with intravenous administration of norepinephrine primarily based on significant increases in systemic vascular resistance (SVR) ($\alpha_1 AR$

stimulation without opposing β_2AR stimulation). Because of the rise in SVR, heart rate tends to decrease with norepinephrine administration due to reflex activation of vagal pathways which overcome direct stimulation of myocardial β_1ARs. Norepinephrine stimulation of myocardial β_1ARs mediating increases in contractility does occur, so norepinephrine is a positive inotropic agent, particularly at low doses where αAR effects are minimised. In contrast to low dose norepinephrine, the cardiac effects of moderate dose norepinephrine in the intact animal or patient include increases in stroke volume and coronary blood flow (in the absence of coronary vasospasm), significant arrhythmogenic potential (although less than epinephrine or isoproterenol), little overall change in cardiac output, and potential decreases in heart rate. Compared to epinephrine, where increases in blood pressure result predominantly from increases in heart rate and cardiac output with a mild concurrent decrease in SVR (due to vascular β_2AR stimulation), moderate dose infusion of norepinephrine increases blood pressure predominantly via vasoconstriction. Under normal circumstances norepinephrine will decrease renal artery blood flow (with little to no change in glomerular filtration rate), in addition to mesenteric, splanchnic, and hepatic blood flow in man (see below).

Administration and dosage of norepinephrine. Like epinephrine, norepinephrine is easily oxidized and is metabolized by enzyme systems such as COMT and MAO. Therefore it is not effective when administered orally. Because of its predominant vasoconstrictive properties, it should only be administered centrally (or very proximally in a large peripheral vein) in order to avoid severe tissue necrosis and sloughing resulting from potential extravasation of the drug at the site of administration. Although small intravenous boluses can be given, it is most commonly used as an infusion. As listed in the table, the usual clinical dose range for intravenous norepinephrine ranges from 0.01 to 0.1 $\mu g/kg/min$.

Norepinephrine peri-operatively. Norepinephrine can be used for its inotropic (low dose) and vasoconstrictive properties (moderate-high dose), and titrated to effect. It is important that cardiac output be monitored when norepinephrine is used, since blood pressure increases predominantly due to increased SVR, can be detrimental to forward blood flow from the heart and in some circumstances contribute to myocardial failure. Moderate dose norepinephrine may have a detrimental effect on end organ perfusion and, as a result, has developed a poor reputation in the treatment of shock. However, in situations where peripheral vascular failure is the predominant cause of a low perfusion pressure and the cardiac output is in fact elevated, such as in septic shock, the use of norepinephrine has been shown to improve renal and splanchnic blood flow (by increasing blood pressure) provided the patient has been adequately volume resuscitated.

Interactions and potential adverse effects of norepinephrine. Like epinephrine, norepinephrine should be used with extreme caution in patients on MAO inhibitor medication.

Extravasation may result in severe tissue necrosis. The treatment of hypovolemic shock with norepinephrine will result in end organ hypoperfusion. If such treatment is sustained it may be a significant factor in the patient's demise. The use of norepinephrine for the treatment of low output, low volume, shocked states justifiably earned it the nick-name "embalming fluid".

SYNTHETIC CATHECHOLAMINES

Isoproterenol/isoprenaline

Isoproterenol is a synthetic catecholamine derivative. It is the only clinically available drug with pure βAR agonist activity. Hence, isoproterenol causes a decrease in peripheral vascular resistance (via activation of β_2ARs) concurrent with increases in heart rate and myocardial contractility (and hence cardiac output via both β_1 and β_2ARs). Isoproterenol is also an excellent bronchodilator and causes an increase in pulmonary blood flow associated with a decrease in pulmonary vascular resistance. However, isoproterenol is very pro-arrythmogenic. Interestingly, isoproterenol stimulates secretion of atrial natriuretic peptide from atria (Schiebinger et al, 1987), a process which is dependent on calcium influx through voltage-sensitive calcium channels as well as calcium release from the sarcoplasmic reticulum (Schiebinger, 1989); this process is inhibited by calcium channel antagonists. Since atrial natriuretic peptide mediates vasodilation, this may add to the vasodilation already seen with isoproterenol from direct β_2AR agonist activity in vascular beds.

Administration and dosage of isoproterenol. As with other catecholamines, isoproterenol is rapidly metabolized in the liver and other tissues by the enzyme COMT and thus is unsuitable for oral administration. Intravenous administration of isoproterenol is usually by infusion beginning with 2–4 μg/min and titrated to effect (Table 3-1). Optimal titration of intravascular volume is essential with isoproterenol administration, to maintain myocardial preload secondary to the vasodilatory properties of this drug.

Isoproterenol peri-operatively. Because of its direct effects on stimulation of heart rate, isoproterenol is useful in the treatment of heart block and conduction abnormalities resulting in life-threatening bradycardia. Isoproterenol is also useful, but less commonly used, in the treatment of low cardiac output states that are not associated with tachycardia since it stimulates increases in both myocardial inotropy and chronotropy. Despite being such a good bronchodilator its cardiovascular effects (particularly arrhythmogenicity) restrict its use in asthma: more selective β_2AR agonists (such as terbutaline and salbutamol) tend to be used instead. Isoproterenol has combined effects on pulmonary blood flow and bronchial muscle tone, that can be used to good effect in conditions associated with pulmonary hypertension and right heart dysfunction secondary to lung pathology. Similarly isoproterenol can be used during congenital heart surgery or lung transplantation surgery specifically for pulmonary vasodilatory effects.

Interactions and possible adverse effects of isoproterenol. Isoproterenol is not well metabolised by MAO and is not taken up by sympathetic neurons to the same extent as epinephrine and norepinephrine. Therefore, its use is less of a concern in patients taking MAO inhibitor medications. Of all the AR agonists, isoproterenol seems to have the most significant arrhythmogenic potential.

Dobutamine

Dobutamine is similar in structure to dopamine except for the addition of a bulky aromatic group. Dobutamine is primarily a direct acting βAR agonist, relatively selective for the β_1AR subtype. Minimal indirect effects of preventing reuptake of norepinephrine at the nerve terminal are also seen. Dobutamine is more effective in providing positive inotropic effects than increases in heart rate (although some increase in sinus node automaticity are apparent with dobutamine). Dobutamine does not bind to dopamine receptors and therefore does not provide the selective increases in renal blood flow seen with dopamine (see above). In typical clinical concentrations of dobutamine (2-15 μg/kg/min), positive inotropic responses are seen with modest increases in heart rate and little change in SVR (in spite of some αAR agonist properties of the drug). However, in patients receiving βAR antagonists, cardiac output may not change and SVR can increase with dobutamine administration. In contrast to other catecholamines, higher doses of dobutamine in general do not cause large increases in blood pressure due to increasing vasoconstriction. In patients with pure myocardial pump failure, this may be an advantage. However, in patients with combined myocardial failure and vasodilation, an additional vasopressor may be required in conjunction with dobutamine. Although both isoproterenol and dobutamine are agonists at the β_1AR subtype, increases in heart rate tend to be higher with isoproterenol than dobutamine, even when reflex tachycardia secondary to isoproterenol induced vasodilation is taken into account. In some patients dobutamine may increase heart rate profoundly, although this side-effect can be minimized by optimizing intravascular volume.

Administration and dosage of dobutamine. Dobutamine is rapidly metabolised in the liver (see below) and cannot be effectively administered orally. It is usually given as an intravenous infusion at 2–15 μg/kg/min guided by its effects on pre-load, after load and cardiac output, and titrated to effect (see table).

Dobutamine peri-operatively. Dobutamine is used almost exclusively as an inotrope. There is some evidence to suggest that it can be used to increase both splanchnic and renal perfusion (Price et al, 1992; Silverman and Tuma, 1992; Shoemaker et al, 1988). However, its effects on splanchnic perfusion remain controversial. Some clinicians use combinations such as dopamine and dobutamine simultaneously to achieve clinical benefits while minimizing side-effects such as tachycardia for any one single agent

(Richard et al, 1983). The chemical structure of dobutamine (which is missing the hydroxyl group thought to confer selectivity for β_1ARs) may have some effect in this regard (Weiner, 1985). Others would choose to use epinephrine rather than the dopamine/dobutamine combination as the same pharmacological effect can be produced but with a single agent and at a far lower cost. As mentioned above, the idea of the combined inotropic effects of dobutamine and splanchno-reno-protective effects of low dose dopamine remain fanciful. In one study of high risk surgical patients, the use of dobutamine as part of a therapeutic regimen aimed at prophylactically increasing oxygen delivery variables to predetermined supranormal levels, resulted in a significant reduction in post operative mortality. It is not known from this study if the use of dobutamine, rather than an alternative inotrope, was a significant component in the final outcome (Shoemaker et al, 1988). However, one other similar study demonstrated equal efficacy with dopexamine (see below) in achieving similar goals of oxygen delivery (Boyd et al, 1993). In the treatment of septic shock there is some evidence from animal models that the use of dobutamine may have a destructive effect on tissue morphology when compared to other synthetic catecholamines such as dopexamine (Webb et al, 1991). In one human study of critically ill patients, the use of dobutamine to achieve supra-normal oxygen flow variables, sometimes in extraordinarily high doses (up to 200 μg/kg/min), was associated with an excess mortality when compared to control patients (Hayes et al, 1994).

Interactions and possible adverse effects of dobutamine. Dobutamine is metabolized somewhat differently from other catecholamines in that while it is rapidly metabolized in the liver, different enzyme systems (glucuronic acid and not COMT or MAO) are involved. Because the chemical structure of dobutamine is similar to both epinephrine and isoproterenol, dobutamine is also capable of inducing ventricular arrhythmias, but to a lesser extent than the other two agents.

Dopexamine

Dopexamine, a synthetic analog of dopamine, has potent β_2AR, dopamine agonist properties, little to no β_1 or αAR activity, and inhibits reuptake of catecholamines at the nerve terminal (Ghosh et al, 1991; Gray et al, 1990; Foulds, 1988). Because of its potent β_2AR agonist properties, dopexamine causes vasodilation (similar to isoproterenol); dopexamine has no demonstrable venous effects. This can be beneficial in unloading the heart by reducing after load and thus enhancing forward flow of blood, particularly in congestive heart failure. Effects of dopexamine on the heart include direct β_2AR stimulation of heart rate and positive inotropy, indirect increases in heart rate from β_2AR-mediated vasodilation, and effects of norepinephrine release at the nerve terminal which include β_1 and β_2AR increases in heart rate and inotropy (Foulds, 1988). In heart failure, β_1ARs are desensitised and decreased in numbers compared with β_2AR — hence dopexamine has theoretical advantages in heart failure. In spite of these theoretical advantages, dopexamine appears to have more marked direct positive inotropic effects in healthy myocardium and less vasodilatory effects; most inotropic effects in patients with heart failure appear to be manifest from effects of decreased afterload (from decreased SVR) and heart rate increases, and not direct increases in myocardial inotropy. Because of the combined DA_1, DA_2 and β_2AR receptor agonism dopexamine causes an increase in both splanchnic and renal blood flow. Some dispute exists whether increases in mesenteric and renal artery blood flow actually occur secondary to regional arterial dilatation or simply secondary to increases in cardiac output (Sinclair et al, 1997). In one human study of patients undergoing cardiopulmonary bypass for cardiac surgery, a dopexamine infusion had no effect on indirect measures of splanchnic perfusion but did result in significantly greater maintenance of gut barrier function (Tighe et al, 1994). This may have significant benefits in the prevention of the translocation of bacteria and endotoxins from the GI tract that is thought to occur during many types of major surgery. There are no outcome trials to support either this hypothesis nor the notion that dopexamine might be reno-protective if infused prophylactically. However, as mentioned there is one prospective randomized placebo controlled trial which demonstrated a reduction in mortality following major surgery when dopexamine was used to prophylactically increase oxygen delivery. Again, as there was no positive control group, it is not known if the use of dopexamine was a significant component in the success of the therapeutic regimen (Boyd et al, 1993).

Administration and dosage of dopexamine. Dopexamine is given by continuous intravenous infusion at a recommended dose of 1–10 μg/kg/min guided by measurement of indices of pre-load, after load and cardiac output, and titrated to effect (Table 3-1). Rather like dopamine, it is believed that low dose infusion (1–2 μg/kg/min) will result in selective renal and splanchnic effects with minimal global cardiovascular effects. Although this seems to be the case in animal models (including models of septic shock) the human data is highly conflicting (Ghosh et al, 1991; Foulds, 1988; Sinclair et al, 1997; Tighe et al, 1994; Trinder et al, 1995; Uusara et al, 1995; Smithies et al. 1994).

Dopexamine peri-operatively. Dopexamine has been most often used in the treatment of myocardial failure during cardiac surgery. Its product license in the UK is restricted to this use, and to exacerbations of chronic heart failure. It is not licensed in the USA. Dopexamine has a very favorable pharmacological profile in the treatment of the failing heart, causing both inotropy and after load reduction, provided that the reduction in systemic blood pressure is not so great as to compromise both myocardial and end organ perfusion. As with all inotropes, but particularly with the inodilators, it is essential to optimize intravascular volume before and during administration.

Interactions and potential adverse effects of dopexamine. Dopexamine is metabolized in the liver (methylation and sulphation) and taken up into the tissues via extraneuronal catecholamine uptake mechanisms (Ghosh, 1991). Although dopexamine produces atrial tachycardia (mostly from reflex tachycardia secondary to vasodilation or increases in dose directly), it shows no propensity for development of ventricular arrhythmias either with halothane administration or ischemia. There have even been some suggestions that dopexamine may have a class 1-like antiarrhythmic effect (Boachie-Ansa 1989). Many of the early reports of dopexamine administration being associated severe tachycardia seem to have been as a result of sub-optimal fluid loading and titration of intravascular volume (Friedel et al. 1992). Subsequent studies have demonstrated that with careful monitoring these reflex HR changes can be avoided (Boyd et al, 1993).

Arbutamine

Arbutamine is a novel synthetic catecholamine with β_1, β_2 and β_1AR activity. In vitro experiments demonstrate a 25 to 30-fold selectivity for βAR activity. *In vivo* experiments demonstrate that arbutamine exhibits similar degrees of inotropic and chronotropic activity while eliciting less peripheral vasodilatation than isoproterenol and less inotropy than dobutamine. Once infusion of arbutamine has been stopped, there is rapid and predictable resolution of tachycardia (Young et al, 1994). Arbutamine has been specifically developed as a pharmacological stress agent to aid in the diagnosis of coronary artery disease and myocardial ischaemia. Early results from both animal and human studies suggest that administration of arbutamine may be more effective than dobutamine in the detection of regional heart wall motion abnormalities, particularly during stress echocardiography (Young et al 1994). However, it is unlikely that this agent will become useful to the anesthetist in the peri-operative period.

Clonidine

Clonidine is an α_2AR agonist (Kamibayashi et al, 1997). Presynaptic α_2ARs mediate feedback inhibition by norepinephrine of further neurotransmitter release (Fig 3-1). Clonidine was developed as an anti-hypertensive agent and has both peripheral and central actions. Initial blood pressure reduction is secondary to a central reduction in sympathetic outflow and increased vagal tone. Clinically there may be reduced venous return, bradycardia and thus a reduced cardiac output without any direct negative inotropic effects. Clonidine also reduces renovascular resistance without altering renal blood flow or glomerular filtration rate. There has been an increased interest in the peri-operative use of clonidine as α_2AR agonists can blunt the adrenergic response to the stresses of surgery without the penalty of respiratory depression associated with opiates. However, there is little "hard" evidence to suggest any meaningful benefits in terms of outcome from its peri-operative use. Clonidine administered peri-operatively is known to reduce anesthetic requirements, it produces drowsiness and has analgesic properties particularly when used as an adjunct to opiates. The potential role for new α_2AR agonists in pain management is increased by the recent identification of receptor sub-types present in human spinal cord (Stafford-Smith et al, 1996). Unwanted side effects of clonidine include dry mouth and postural hypotension. Sudden withdrawal may be associated with rebound hypertension that can be life threatening.

SYMPATHOMIMETIC AMINES

Sympathomimetics have many of the same properties as catecholamines, but do not contain the catecholamine ring moiety as part of their chemical structure. Phenylisopropylamines are such a class of compounds which stimulate α and βARs and are powerful CNS stimulants, but have divergent chemical structures compared with catecholamines. Amphetamines, methamphetamine, ephedrine, denopamine, mephentermine, metaraminol, hydroxyamphetamine, phenylephrine, and methoxamine are all phenylisopropylamines. These clinically used agents are discussed below.

Ephedrine

Pharmacological actions of ephedrine. While catecholamine and phosphodiesterase inhibitors provide rapid changes in cardiac output, they are all administered via an infusion and usually used in critically ill patients. Most patients with and without cardiovascular disease coming to the operating room, however, do not require inotropic support for long periods. Hence, ephedrine has become a common drug (administered by intravenous bolus) in the perioperative period, used specifically to increase blood pressure predominantly by increasing cardiac output. Ephedrine is a naturally occurring compound found in several plants. It was used in China for over 2000 years before being introduced into western medicine in 1924 (Weiner et al, 1985). Ephedrine has both direct effects (stimulation of myocardial βARs) and indirect effects (release of norepinephrine from the nerve terminal); it therefore has a mixture of properties. Since both ephedrine and norepinephrine stimulate βARs, the primary effect of ephedrine is to increase cardiac output, and hence blood pressure, by stimulation of myocardial βARs. However, since norepinephrine also activates αARs, some vasoconstriction can be seen with ephedrine predominantly due to its secondary effect of release of norepinephrine at the nerve terminal. Taking into account both mechanisms of action, the overall effect of ephedrine administration is to increase cardiac output, increase heart rate, and increase SVR. These effects are most striking when parasympatholytic agents have been administered, effectively preventing reflex HR responses in the heart.

Administration and dosage of ephedrine. Ephedrine is administered as an intravenous bolus of 5–10 mg (see table), and its clinical effect lasts for approximately 10–15 minutes. One unique feature of phenylisopropylamines in general is that they are effective when administered orally. Ephedrine is not a substrate for metabolism by the enzyme COMT, and only a small amount is oxidatively deaminated in humans; the vast majority of ephedrine is excreted unchanged. Two asymmetric carbon atoms exist in the ephedrine molecule, creating the possibility of several isomers; only l-ephedrine and racemic forms are used clinically.

Ephedrine peri-operatively. Because ephedrine increases blood pressure primarily by increasing heart rate and cardiac output, it is considered the drug of choice in clinical situations where blood pressure increases are required but vasoconstriction is not desired, for example during pregnancy and Caesarean section surgery. There is now preliminary data to suggest that using only an ephedrine infusion, rather than fluid pre-loading, may be just as effective at maintaining both maternal and fetal blood supply during epidural anaesthesia for Caesarean section. However, no study has been done to date with adequate power to justify such practices.

Potential adverse effects of ephedrine. Ephedrine is not metabolised by MAO and is therefore a suitable agent to be given to patients receiving MAO inhibitor therapy for depression. As with any drug that increases myocardial inotropy, myocardial oxygen consumption is increased, and therefore ephedrine can precipitate myocardial ischemia in patients with coronary artery disease. Hence, like all catecholamines and positive inotropic agents, it should be used with extreme caution in patients with cardiovascular disease. The injudicious use of ephedrine peri-operatively to maintain blood pressure in the face of hypovolemia will result in reduced end organ perfusion and a worse patient outcome. The administration of anything other than a small dose of ephedrine to counteract a predictable effect of another pharmacological agent (eg. vasodilatation associated with spinal anesthesia) should be discouraged without the measurement of cardiac output.

Denopamine

Denopamine is unique in having selective β_1AR agonist and α_1AR antagonist properties (Aikawa et al, 1991). It is used clinically as an oral positive inotropic agent, particularly in patients with congestive heart failure. Denopamine mediates direct positive inotropic effects via myocardial β_1AR stimulation and also decreases SVR via α_1AR antagonist properties, providing afterload reduction and effective forward flow from the heart. The net cardiovascular effects are positive inotropic effects with little change in blood pressure. Denopamine also causes concentration dependent relaxation in canine coronary, mesenteric, and renal arteries. Although not yet clinically available, denopamine promises to provide effective therapy for patients in congestive heart failure. Therefore in the future, anesthesiologists may encounter patients maintained on chronic oral denopamine therapy coming to the operating room for heart surgery and various other non-cardiac surgeries.

Phenylephrine

Pharmacological actions of phenylephrine. Phenylephrine has a chemical structure virtually identical to epinephrine, only lacking a hydroxyl group at position 4 on the benzene ring. However, agonist binding properties of phenylephrine are significantly different from epinephrine. Phenylephrine is a pure α_1AR agonist at clinical concentrations; it binds α_2ARs only at extremely high concentrations and βARs in concentrations approximately ten times the clinical concentration. Hence phenylephrine is the most selective α_1AR agonist clinically available to date. Increases in SVR secondary to α_1AR stimulation are the primary effects of phenylephrine, although in the absence of parasympatholytic agents such as atropine, reflex bradycardia may be seen. Vasoconstriction occurs in most vascular beds (renal, splanchnic, cutaneous, and limbs) at the level of the arteriole, but coronary artery perfusion is increased. This may be due to increased diastolic perfusion pressure generated by phenylephrine providing improved coronary artery driving pressure. Large epicardial coronary arteries have relatively high concentrations of α_1ARs, with less present in distal coronary branches; the opposite is true of α_2ARs (Feigl, 1987); therefore, phenylephrine stimulation of α_1ARs results in epicardial coronary artery constriction with less constriction of normal distal coronary vascular beds. This increases perfusion pressure across concentric coronary stenoses, potentially providing an anti-steal effect (Feigl, 1987). However, phenylephrine does constrict coronary vessels with eccentric stenoses, potentially eliciting myocardial ischemia in this setting (Shoemaker et al, 1988). In general, increases in diastolic perfusion pressure provide increased coronary artery blood flow even in the presence of occlusive lesions. In addition to acute therapy in patients with cardiovascular disease, phenylephrine is available in several other formulations, most notably as an integral ingredient in nasal and ophthalmic decongestants. It is also useful as a vasoconstricting agent in combination with local anesthetic administration.

Administration and dosage of phenylephrine. Phenylephrine is frequently administered in bolus form (50–100 µg) intravenously (see table); clinical effects are apparent within one minute and may last from 5–20 minutes. When continued administration of vasopressors is required, phenylephrine can be administered as a continuous intravenous infusion at rates of 20–40 µg/min (0.5–1.0 µg/kg/min). The ℓ-form is the active isomer.

Potential adverse effects of phenylephrine. As with the use of any vasoconstrictor, careful monitoring of fluid balance and cardiac output is required in order to ensure that vasoconstriction is not used to treat hypotension when more appropriate therapies such as fluid resuscitation or inotropic support are indicated.

Methoxamine

Methoxamine is an isopropylamine type compound with potent α_1AR agonist and mild α_2AR agonist properties.

Methoxamine has many of the same properties as phenylephrine (increases in SVR, increases in blood pressure, no myocardial βAR activation, potential for reflex bradycardia, and vasoconstriction of many vascular beds), but has one important difference. Once bolus methoxamine is administered (2–10 mg) intravenously, the clinical effect is rapidly apparent and lasts significantly longer than phenylephrine (60–90 minutes). This is advantageous in some settings (such as after removal of a pheochromocytoma surgically), but may last too long to be clinically useful in other settings. Methoxamine does have slightly more propensity to induce bradycardia compared to phenylephrine and in contrast to epinephrine, slows A-V conduction in the heart and does not provoke cardiac arrhythmias. Although not used frequently in the perioperative period any longer, methoxamine is still a useful drug and an important part in an anesthesiologist's and intensivist's range of options for vasoconstrictors.

Mephenteramine

Mephentermine acts directly as an α_1AR agonist and has secondary effects of releasing norepinephrine at the nerve terminal, lasting several hours. The pressor response is mediated predominantly by increases in SVR, but also some increases in cardiac output. Administration is accomplished via intramuscular injection.

Meteraminol

Metaraminol is essentially identical to mephenteramine but can also be given intravenously. Meteraminol has one additional interesting characteristic. It can replace norepinephrine in storage vesicles in the nerve terminal where it acts as a false transmitter (1/10 as effective at α_1ARs compared to norepinephrine). Hence after approximately 5 hours, hypotension may result from metaraminol therapy.

PHOSPHODIESTERASE INHIBITORS

Phosphodiesterase inhibitor drugs provide myocardial inotropy via a different mechanism than catecholamines and sympathomimetics. Although stimulation of βARs results in the production of cAMP, this product is rapidly inactivated by metabolism by phosphodiesterases in the cell. Phosphodiesterase inhibitors act by preventing the breakdown of cAMP, prolonging its effectiveness, and augmenting its physiologic response. Since endogenous circulating catecholamines provide a basal level of cAMP production, via tonic stimulation of βARs, phosphodiesterase inhibitors are effective in producing increases in myocardial inotropy when given alone. However, when βARs are stimulated with βAR agonists such as isoproterenol, epinephrine, dopamine, or norepinephrine, the addition of a phosphodiesterase inhibitor (which inhibits the breakdown of cAMP) will have synergistic effects. In addition to positive inotropic properties, phosphodiesterase inhibitors cause vasodilation. Hence, they are "inodilators," inotropic agents which also reduce afterload (see dopamine above). They are also arrhythmogenic. Three phosphodiesterase inhibitors have been used clinically, namely amrinone, milrinone, and enoximone. These agents are described in more detail below.

Amrinone

The phosphodiesterase inhibitor amrinone is a commonly used clinical positive inotropic agent (Goenen, 1989; Rutman et al, 1987). In addition to positive inotropy, amrinone has potent vasodilatory (potentially profound decreases in SVR) effects. In fact, when administered clinically, the vasodilatory effects of amrinone are immediately apparent while approximately 10–15 minutes are required before positive inotropic effects become appreciable. Because amrinone acts via phosphodiesterase inhibition, its inotropic and vasodilator effects are not reversed by βAR blocking drugs or by norepinephrine depletion from the nerve terminal.

Administration and dosage of amrinone. Amrinone is administered as a bolus loading dose (0.75 mg/kg over 2–3 minutes), followed by continuous intravenous infusion at 2–10 μg/kg/min (see table) (Bailey et al. 1991). The maximum suggested daily dose of amrinone should not exceed 10 mg/kg. In the presence of congestive heart failure, however, up to 3 mg/kg is considered an acceptable loading dose (Hayes et al,. 1994); recent limited experience suggests that short term infusion rates can be increased to 20 μg/kg/min in patients with congestive heart failure (Bailey et al, 1991). Monitoring of central venous pressure and cardiac output is essential when amrinone therapy is contemplated.

Amrinone peri-operatively. This combination of vasodilation and positive inotropy is useful in heart failure where combined afterload reduction and inotropic support provide more effective forward flow of blood from the heart. Interestingly, administration of amrinone to patients with severe congestive heart failure has been shown to improve myocardial performance while decreasing myocardial oxygen consumption by 30% (Baim, 1989). Hence short term amrinone may be beneficial in patients with congestive heart failure or conditions such as mitral regurgitation where combined inotropy and vasodilatation is advantageous.

Interactions and possible adverse effects of amrinone. Although bolus doses of amrinone can be injected directly into an infusion line containing glucose, a slow reaction with glucose occurs over 24 hours; therefore long term intravenous infusions of amrinone should not be mixed in glucose containing solutions. Amrinone ampules should be protected from light and stored at room temperature. Furosemide precipitates with amrinone and therefore should not be administered in the same intravenous line. Positive inotropic drugs in general increase myocardial oxygen consumption, and since vasodilation can decrease diastolic blood pressure and hence decrease coronary blood flow, amrinone has the potential for exacerbating myocardial ischemia in the presence of coronary artery disease. This potential side-effect can be minimized or avoided with careful fluid management and vasopressor therapy when required, in order to increase diastolic blood pressure and improve coronary perfusion. Other potential side-effects of amrinone therapy (in addition to hypotension), include thrombocytopenia in 2–3% of patients, and to a far lesser degree gastrointestinal upset, myalgia, fever, hepatic dysfunction, and ventricular irritability. Since amrinone solution contain metabisulfite, it is contraindicated in patients with allergy to sulfonamides.

Milrinone

Milrinone is a 2-methyl, 5-carbonitrile derivative of amrinone (Makela and Kapu, 1988). Milrinone has nearly twenty times the inotropic potency of amrinone and does not cause fever or thrombocytopenia (Baim et al, 1983; Colucci, 1989). As with amrinone, milrinone has vasodilator properties (Colucci, 1989) although severe vasodilation is less frequently seen clinically with milrinone compared to amrinone. Vasodilation also occurs in the coronary artery bed, resulting in increased coronary blood flow. When administered to patients with congestive heart failure, milrinone reduced ventricular filling pressures by 30–40% (Packer et al, 1991).

Administration and dosage of milrinone. Milrinone is most commonly administered intravenously as a bolus loading dose (50 µg/kg over 10 minutes), followed by continuous intravenous infusion at 0.375–0.75 µg/kg/min (see table). Milrinone can also be administered orally long-term (see table) and therefore can be administered to patients with congestive heart failure on an outpatient basis (see below).

Milrinone peri-operatively. The indications for the peri-operative use of milrinone are the same as amrinone above (i.e. predominantly as an adjunct to a direct βAR agonist). However, milrinone has fewer serious side effects and therefore may be a more suitable choice, particularly for more prolonged usage.

Interactions and possible adverse effects of milrinone. Milrinone forms a precipitate with frusemide. Dose adjustment is recommended according to the patients baseline renal function as judged by creatinine clearance. As mentioned above milrinone can be administered orally and thus has potential for the treatment of chronic heart failure. However, a recent multicentre study has found that in spite of its beneficial hemodynamic actions, long-term therapy with oral milrinone increases morbidity (hypotension, syncope) and mortality (28% increase in overall mortality, 34% increase in cardiovascular mortality) compared with other agents in patients with severe congestive heart failure (Packer et al, 1991; Curfman, 1991); the mechanism for these severe effects is not known. Increased myocardial levels of arrhythmogenic cyclic AMP is a possibility (Lubbe et al, 1992).

Enoximone

Enoximone is an imidazole derivative that is also a phosphodiesterase inhibitor (Baim et al, 1983). While enoximone has positive inotropic properties, it is has more vasodilator effects than either amrinone or milrinone. Since enoximone is a relatively new phosphodiesterase inhibitor drug, many more studies are needed before its role among other vasoactive agents is firmly established. As a vasodilator it seems to add nothing to the established pharmacopeia (Squara et al, 1994). When used acutely as an inotrope following cardiopulmonary by-pass there is no evidence to suggest that enoximone is any more efficacious than established agents such as dobutamine. However, in the setting of acute myocardial infarction results are more encouraging as enoximone has been shown to have a similar inotropic effect to dobutamine but with fewer adverse effects (such as arrhythmias) (Caldicott et al, 1993). Similarly, oral enoximone has been shown in a small group of patients with refractory heart failure, secondary to cardiomyopathy, to provide symptomatic relief (Dee et al, 1993). Presently, there are no outcome data available from any large study prospective randomised clinical trial to determine the efficacy of oral enoximone in this setting.

Summary

1. *Adrenergic receptor agonists* have a relevance to 4 aspects of anesthetic practice: i) manipulation of pathologically deranged cardiovascular variables; ii) as adjuncts to the use of other drugs; iii) as a part of organo-protective regimens; and iv) because adrenergic agonists may adversely react with other drugs.

2. *Adrenergic receptors* mediate the actions of adrenergic receptor agonists. There has been an explosion recently in the number of adrenergic receptor subtypes identified and cloned using genetic techniques. Since multiple adrenergic receptors are usually expressed simultaneously in various tissues, the ability to study individual subtypes greatly enhances the understanding of their molecular pharmacology. This process should eventually lead to more selective compounds for use in the peri-operative period.

3. *The clinical usage of adrenergic receptor agonists* is discussed from the perspective of their pharmacological properties, dosage, administration, indications for peri-operative use, interactions and possible adverse effects.

References

Ahlquist RP. A study of adrenotropic receptors. *Am J Physiol* 1948; 153:586–600.

Aikawa J, Koike K and Takayanagi I. Vascular smooth muscle relaxation by $_1$-adrenoceptor blocking action of denopamine in isolated rabbit aorta. *J. Cardiovasc Pharm* 1991; 17:440–444.

Bailey JM, Levy JH, Rogers HG, et al. Pharmacokinetics of amrinone during cardiac surgery. *Anesthesiology* 1991; 75:961–968.

Baim DS. Effect of phosphodiesterase inhibition on myocardial oxygen consumption and coronary blood flow. *Am J Cardiol* 1989; 63:23A–26A.

Baim DS, McDowell AV, Cherniles J, et al. Evaluation of a new bipyridine inotropic agent, milrinone, in patients with severe congestive heart failure. *N Engl J Med* 1983; 309:748–756.

Berkowitz DE and Schwinn DA. Basic pharmacology of α and β-adrenergic receptors. In: *The Pharmacological Basis of Anesthesiology.* Bowdle A, Kharasch E, Horita A (eds). Churchill Livingstone, New York, 1994, 581–668.

Boachie-Ansa G, Kane KA and Parratt JR. The cardiac electrophysiologic effects of dopexamine under normal and simulated ischaemic conditions. *J Mol Cell Cardiol* 1989; 21:S23.

Boyd O, Grounds RM and Bennett ED. A randomized clinical trial of the effect of deliberate perioperative increase of oxygen delivery on mortality in high risk surgical patients. *JAMA* 1993; 270:2699–2707.

Boyd O, Grounds RM and Bennett ED. The use of dopexamine hydrochloride to increase oxygen delivery perioperatively. *Anesth Analg* 1993; 76:372–376.

Brown L. Pharmacological responses to dopamine in isolated guinea-pig cardiovascular tissues: mechanisms of action. *Arch Int Pharmacodyn* 1990; 308:47–62.

Bryan AG, Bolsin SN, Fianna PT and Haloush H. Modification of the diuretic and natriuretic effects of a dopamine infusion by fluid loading in preoperative cardiac surgical patients. *J Card Vasc Anesth* 1995; 9:158–163.

Caldicott LD, Hawley K, Heppell R, et al. Intravenous enoximone or dobutamine for severe heart failure after acute myocardial infarction: a randomized double-blind trial. *Eur Heart J* 1993; 14:696–700.

Colucci WS. Myocardial and vascular actions of milrinone. *Eur Heart J* 1989; 10:32–38.

Curfman GD. Inotropic therapy for heart failure, an unfulfilled promise. *N Engl J Med* 1991; 325:509–1510.

Dec GW, Fifer MA, Herrman HC, et al. Long-term outcome of enoximone therapy in patients with refractory heart failure. *Am Heart J* 1993; 125:423–9.

Duke GJ, Briedis JH and Weaver RA. Renal support in critically ill patients: low-dose dopamine or low-dose dobutamine? *Crit Care Med* 1994; 22:1919–25.

Feigl EO. The paradox of adrenergic coronary vasoconstriction. *Circulation* 1987; 76:737–745.

Flancbaum L, Choban PS and Dasta JF. Quantitative effects of low dose dopamine on urine output in oliguric surgical intensive care unit patient patients. *Crit Care Med* 1994; 22:61–66.

Foulds RA. Clinical development of dopexamine hydrochloride and an overview of its hemodynamic effects *Am J Cardiol* 1988; 62:41C–45C.

Friedel N, Wenzel R, Matheis G, et al. Haemodynamic effects of different doses of dopamine hydrochloride in low cardiac output states following cardiac surgery. *Eur Heart J* 1992; 13:1271–1276.

Ghosh S, Gray B, Oduro A and Latimer RD. Dopexamine hydrochloride: pharmacology and use in low cardiac output states. *J Cardiovasc Vasc Anesth* 1991; 5:382–389.

Goenen M. Historical perspectives and update of amrinone. *J Cardiovasc Anesth* 1989; 3:15–23.

Gray PA, Bodenham AR and Park GR. The pharmacokinetics of dopexamine hydrochloride in patients undergoing orthotopic liver transplantation. *Intensive Care Med* 1990; 16:A143.

Hayes MA, Timmins AG, Yau E, et al. Elevation of systemic oxygen delivery in the treatment of critically ill patients. *N Engl J Med* 1994; 330:1717–1722.

Hilberman M, Maseda J, Stinson EB , et al. The diuretic properties of dopamine in patients after open-heart operation. *Anesthesiology* 1984; 61:489–494.

Kambiyashi T and Harasawa K, Maze M. α_2-adrenergic agonists. *Can J Anaesth* 1997; 44:R13–22.

Lands AM, Arnold A, McAuliff JP, et al. Differentiation of receptor systems activated by sympathomimetic amines. *Nature* 1967; 214: 597–598.

Lands AM, Luduena FP and Bruzzo HJ. Differentiation of receptors responsive to isoprenaline. *Life Sci* 1967; 6:2241–2249.

Lubbe WH, Podzuweit T and Opie LH. Potential arrhythmogenic role of cyclic adenosine monophosphate (AMP) and cytosolic calcium overload: Implications for prophylactic effects of beta-blockers in myocardial infarction and proarrhythmic effects of phospodiesterase inhibitors. *J Am Coll Cardiol* 1992; 19:1622–1633.

Makela VHM, Kapur PA. New drugs for the treatment of heart failure: amrinone and milrinone. *Seminars Anes* 1988; 7:92–99.

Miller ED, Jr. Renal effects of dopamine. *Anesthesiology* 1984; 61:487–488.

Packer M, Carver JR, Rodeheffer RJ, et al. Effect of oral milrinone on mortality in severe chronic heart failure. *N Engl J Med* 1991; 325:1468–1475.

Price K, Clark C and Guttierrez G. Intravenous dobutamine improves gastric intramucosal pH in septic patients. *Am Rev Resp Dis* 1992; 145:A316.

Richard C, Ricome JL, Rimailho A, et al. Combined hemodynamic effects of dopamine and dobutamine in cardiogenic shock. *Circulation* 1983; 67:620–626.

Rutman HI, LeJemtel TH and Sonnenblick EH. Newer cardiotonic agents: implications for patients with heart failure and ischemic heart disease. *J Cardiothor Anesth* 1987; 1:59–70.

Schiebinger RJ. Calcium, its role in isoproterenol-stimulated atrial natriuretic peptide secretion by superfused rat atria. *Circ Res* 1989; 65:600–606.

Schiebinger RJ, Baker MZ and Linden J. The effect of adrenergic and muscarinic cholinergic agonists on atrial natriuretic peptide secretion by isolated rat atria: a potential role of the autonomic nervous system in modulating atrial natriuretic peptide secretion. *J Clin Invest* 1987; 80:1687–1691.

Shoemaker WC, Appel PL, Kram HB, et al. Prospective trial of supranormal values of survivors as therapeutic goals in high-risk surgical patients. *Chest* 1988; 94:1176–1186.

Silverman HJ and Tuma P. Gastric tonometry inpatients with sepsis: effects of dobutamine infusions and packed red blood cell transfusions. *Chest* 1992; 102:184–188.

Sinclair DG, Houldsworth, Keogh B, et al. Gastrointestinal permeability following cardiopulmonary bypass: a randomised study comparing the effects of dopamine and dopexamine. *Intensive Care Med* 1997; 23:510–516.

Smithies M, Yee TH, Jackson L, et al. Protecting the gut and the liver in the critically ill: effects of dopexamine. *Crit Care Med* 1994; 22:789–95.

Squara P, Denjean D, Godard P, et al. Enoximone vs nicardipine during the early postoperative course of patinets undergoing cardiac surgery. A prospective study of two therapeutic strategies. *Chest* 1994; 106: 52–58.

Stafford-Smith M, Schambra UB, Wilson KH, et al. α_2 receptors in human spinal cord: specific localized expression of mRNA encoding α_2-adrenergic receptor subtypes at four distinct levels. *Mol Brain Res* 1996; 34:109–117.

Sumikawa K, Ishizaka N and Suzaki M. Arrhythmogenic plasma levels of epinephrine during halothane, enflurane, and pentobarbital anesthesia in the dog. *Anesthesiology* 1983; 58:322–325.

Szerlip HM. Renal-dose dopamine: fact and fiction. *Ann Int Med* 1991; 115:153–154.

Tighe D, Moss R, Webb A et al. Post-treatment with dopexamine provides hepatic protection when compared to dobutamine hydrochloride in porcine septic shock. *Clin Intensive Care* 1994; 5:99.

Trinder TJ, Lavery GG, Fee JP and Lowry KG. Correction of splanchnic oxygen deficit in the intensive care unit: dopexamine and colloid versus placebo. *Anaesth Intensive Care* 1995; 23:178–82.

Uusara A, Ruokonen E and Takala J. Gastric mucosal pH does not reflect changes in splanchnic blood flow after cardiac surgery. *Brit J Anaesth* 1995; 74:149–54.

Vincent J-L. Renal effects of dopamine: can our dream ever come true? *Crit Care Med* 1994; 22: 5–6.

Webb AR, Moss RF, Tighe D, et al. The effects of dobutamine on hepatic histological responses to porcine fecal peritonitis. *Intensive Care Med* 1991; 17:487–493.

Weiner N. E pinephrine and the sympathomimetic amines. In: *The Pharmacological Basis of Therapeutics*. Gilman AG, Goodman LS, Rall TW, Murad F (Eds) MacMillan Publishing Co. New York 1985; 145–180.

Young M, Pan W, Bullough D, et al. Characterization of arbutamine: A novel catecholamine stress agent for diagnosis of coronary artery disease. *Drug Develop Res* 1994; 32:19–28.

CHAPTER 4

Adrenergic Inhibitors

D. Joseph Meyer, Jr. and Noel W. Lawson

The autonomic nervous system (ANS), as implied by its name, performs an ubiquitous role as "self-regulator" of bodily functions. Pharmacological uncoupling of a single component of the ANS will affect numerous physiological systems, inhibiting some while stimulating others. This chapter focuses on antagonists of the sympathetic (adrenergic) division of the ANS. The reader will be provided with a discussion of the topic organized to encompass pre-operative patient evaluation and perioperative usage of adrenergic antagonists.

Adrenergic antagonists may be divided into five categories based on their mechanism of blockade: 1) peripheral adrenergic receptor antagonists, 2) autonomic ganglion antagonists, 3) drugs which form false sympathetic neurotransmitters, 4) drugs which deplete stores of sympathetic neurotransmitter and 5) drugs which inhibit presynaptic release of sympathetic neurotransmitter. Several of these drugs satisfy the criterion for more than one category.

PERIPHERAL ADRENERGIC RECEPTOR ANTAGONISTS

Traditionally, the catecholamines epinephrine (EPI) and norepinephrine (NE) were considered the exclusive mediators of peripheral sympathetic nervous system activity. Epinephrine release from the adrenal medulla into the vasculature acts as the circulating (hormonal) sympathetic mediator. Release of NE from postganglionic sympathetic terminals acts as the peripheral sympathetic neurotransmitter. Catecholamine receptors may be subdivided into three principal groups: alpha- and beta-adrenergic receptors and dopaminergic receptors. The locations and physiological actions of the alpha- and beta-adrenergic receptors (and their subtypes) are listed in Table 4-1. Dopamine (DA) is a precursor in the synthetic cascade forming NE and EPI in adrenergic neurons. DA acts as a neurotransmitter in the central nervous system. Receptors specific for DA are found both in the CNS and in tissues such as renal, mesenteric and coronary vessels. They are also found on post-ganglionic sympathetic nerve terminals where their activity is simi-

Table 4-1. Alpha- and beta-adrenergic receptors: locations, antagonists and effects of inhibition

Receptor	Location	Effects of Antagonists	Antagonists
Alpha$_1$	Smooth muscle (vascular, iris, pilomotor, uterus, ureter, trigone, and bladder sphincters)	Relaxation Vasodilation Altered neuro-transmission	Phenoxyben-zamine Phentolamine Prazosin
	Brain	Contraction	Doxazosin
	Smooth muscle (gastrointestinal)	↓ force ↓ glycolysis	Terazosin Tolazosin
	Myocardium	↓ secretion (K^+, H_2O)	Labetalol
	Salivary glands		
	Adipose tissue	↓ glycogenolysis	
	Sweat glands	↓ secretion	
	Kidney (proximal tubule)	↓ Na^+ reabsorption ↓ gluconeogenesis	
Alpha$_2$	Adrenergic nerve endings (presynaptic)	↑NE release vasodilation	Yohimbine Piperoxan
	Vascular smooth muscle	↓ aggregation	Phentolamine
	Platelets	↓ granule release	Phenoxybenza-mine
	Adipose tissue	↑ lipolysis	Tolazoline
	Endocrine Pancreas	↑ insulin release	
	Kidney	↑ renin release	
	Brain	Altered neuro-transmission	
Beta$_1$	Heart	↓ rate ↓ contractility	Acebutolol Practolol
	Adipose tissue	↓ conduction velocity	Propranolol Alprenolol Metoprolol
		↓ Lipolysis	Esmolol Labetalol Carvedilol
Beta$_2$	Liver	↓ glycogenolysis ↓ gluconeogenesis	Propranolol Butoxamine
	Skeletal muscle	↓ glycogenolysis ↓ lactate release	Alprenolol Nadolol
	Smooth muscle (bronchi, uterus, vascular, gastrointestinal, detrusor, spleen)	Contraction Vasoconstriction ↓ insulin secretion (minimal)	Timolol Labetalol Carvedilol
	Endocrine pancreas	↓ amylase secretion	
	Salivary glands		

lar to other adrenergic receptors (Kuchel and Kuchel, 1991; Goldberg, 1989).

Evidence accumulated over the past few decades, suggests a role for compounds such as ATP and neuropeptide Y as sympathetic neurotransmitters (Burnstock, 1993). These substances are either co-released with NE or differentially released from the postganglionic sympathetic nerve terminal. The roles of these additional transmitters are under active investigation and promise to further understanding of the workings of the sympathetic nervous system. For example, ATP is co-transmitted with NE at vascular nerve terminals, apparently acting synergistically in its post-synaptic smooth muscle effects. Thus, while the peripheral effects of the adrenergic system are mediated largely by activation of the receptors to NE and EPI, our understanding of this system is evolving and future pharmacologic agonists and antagonists may be directed at "newer" transmitters.

This section will devote itself to discussion of pharmacological antagonists to beta-adrenergic, alpha-adrenergic and dopaminergic receptors.

BETA-ADRENOCEPTOR ANTAGONISTS

Beta-adrenoceptors stimulate activation of adenylate cyclase through a G protein-mediated pathway. Subsequent formation of cyclic AMP triggers responses of considerable variability between tissues (Fig 4-1).

Beta-adrenoreceptor antagonists (also known as beta-blockers) are amongst the most common cardiovascular drugs in clinical use today. They enjoy front-line status in the management of cardiovascular disorders such as hypertension, coronary artery disease and arrhythmias. Many of these drugs are marketed on the basis of their relative selectivity for blockade of beta$_1$- versus beta$_2$-adrenoceptor function. However, the selectivity of these drugs is only relative. Larger doses will inhibit the activity of both receptor subtypes (Fig 4-2). For example, the use of a beta$_1$-selective blocker in a patient with reactive airway disease may result in clinically significant bronchoconstriction; and by no means should it be considered a "safe drug" in this patient population. When used in these patients, beta$_2$-agonist therapy is often co-administered.

Table 4-2 lists pharmaco-kinetic and -dynamic properties of several beta-blockers. The dynamic effects of adrenergic receptor blockade depend on circulating catecholamine levels. When sympathetic tone is low (resting or basal conditions), the corresponding effect of receptor

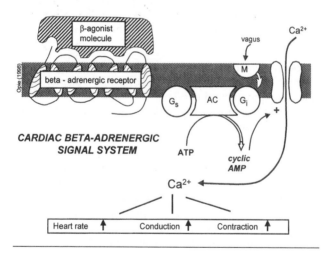

Fig 4-1. *The cardiac beta-adrenoreceptor and signalling system.*
The beta-antagonist molecule interacts with the beta-receptor, whose molecular structure has recently been revealed and the amino-acid sequence characterized. In the presence of the stimulatory form of the G-protein (G$_s$), adenylate cyclase (AC) converts ATP to cyclic AMP which, acting via a protein kinase, enhances phosphorylation of the calcium channel and permits more calcium to enter through the calcium channel during voltage-induced depolarization. Such calcium releases much more from the sarcoplasmic reticulum (calcium-induced calcium release) to increase cytosolic calcium, heart rate, conduction and contraction, as well as the rate of relaxation (the latter via phosphorylation of the protein phospholamban in the sarcoplasmic reticulum). G$_i$ = inhibitory G-protein, part of signalling system for vagal muscarinic stimulation. (Fig. copyright © L.H. Opie, 1998)

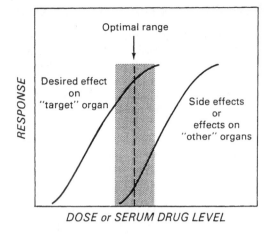

Fig 4-2. *Relative drug selectivity is illustrated by showing the relationship between two dose-response curves.* The curves on the left and right represent the desired and undesired responses to a given drug. For example, consider the case of a beta$_1$-selective adrenergic antagonist. The left curve represents the desired effects of beta$_1$-adrenoceptor blockade while the curve on the right represents the nonspecific effects of this drug due to blockade of beta$_2$-adrenoceptors. Thus, it can be seen that deleterious effects such as bronchoconstriction may occur with higher doses of the drug (reflecting beta$_2$-blockade). The optimal range is the concentration of drug that will give the maximal desired response with minimal effects on other receptors. The size of the optimal range is dependent on the therapeutic index, or distance between the two curves.

blockade is modest. When sympathetic tone is high (during exercise or stress, for example), adrenergic receptor blockade has a pronounced effect.

In the absence of catecholamines, a few beta-blockers (including pindolol and acebutolol) act as partial (weak) beta-agonists. They are said to have *intrinsic sympathomimetic activity*. The remainder of the beta-adrenoceptor antagonists have no intrinsic receptor activity; they simply prevent beta-adrenoceptor activation. In the absence of sympathetic tone, use of a beta-blocker with intrinsic sympathomimetic activity may cause less bradycardia and negative inotropy than its counterparts.

Several of the beta-blockers in Table 4-2 exhibit Class 1 (quinidine-like) *membrane stabilizing effects* which are independent of their effects on beta-receptors. The slope of phase 0 of the cardiac action potential is reduced, slowing conduction. This activity is specific to the *d*-isomer of the drug, which is devoid of beta-adrenoceptor blocking properties. The *d*-isomer of sotolol exhibits Class 3 antiarrhythmic properties (via potassium channel inhibition) and no significant beta-adrenoceptor antagonism. Most beta-adrenoceptor antagonists are supplied as racemic mixtures (containing both *d*- and *l*-isomers). While no clinically untoward effects have been demonstrated with the use of racemic mixtures (Stoschitzky and Linder, 1997), the use of the optically pure isomer *d*-sotolol increased mortality by 65% compared with placebo in patients with left ventricular

Table 4-2. Beta adrenoceptor antagonists: properties and pharmacokinetics

Drug	Trade Name	Relative Beta₁ Selectivity	Anti-arrhythmic Properties△	ISA	Predominant Route of Elimination	Preparations	Usual Dose (mg)◇	Usual Frequency (hr)	Time to Peak Effect	Plasma Half-life (hr)
Noncardioselective										
Propranolol	Inderal	0	Class I & II	0	hepatic and renal	oral, iv	10-80, 1-3	8-12	1-1.5 hr, 1-2 min	3-5
Carteolol	Cartrol	0	Class II	+	hepatic and renal	oral	2.5-5	24	1-3 hr	6
Carvedilol*	Coreg	0	Class II	0	hepatic	oral	3.125-25	12		6-7
Labetalol*	Trandate Normodyne	0	Class II	+**	hepatic	oral, iv	100-400, 0.1-1 mg/kg	12, as needed	2-4 hr, 5 min	5-8, 5-6
Nadolol	Corgard	0	Class II	0	renal	oral	40-320	24	4 hr	14-24
Penbutolol	Levatol	0	Class II	+	hepatic ***	oral	10-40	24	1.5-3 hr	20-100
Pindolol	Visken	0	Class I & II	++	hepatic and renal	oral	5-30	24	1-2 hr	3-4
Sotalol	Betapace	0	Class II & III	0	renal	oral	80-160	12-24	2.5-4 hr	
Timolol	Blocadren	0	Class II	0	hepatic and renal	oral+	10-30	12	1-2 hr	4-5
Cardioselective										
Acebutolol	Sectral	+	Class I & II	+	hepatic ***	oral	200-600	12-24	2-4 hr	3-4
Atenolol	Tenormin	++	Class II	0	renal	oral, iv	50-100, 5-10	12-24	5 mins	6-9
Betaxolol	Kerlone	+++	Class I & II	0	hepatic ***	oral+	10-20	24	1.5-6 hr	14-22
Bisoprolol	Zebeta	+++	Class II	0	hepatic and renal	oral	2.5-20	24	2-4 hr	9-12
Esmolol	Brevibloc	++	Class II	0	RBC Esterase	iv	Bolus: 500 µg/kg Infusion: 50-300µg/kg/min	as needed++	6-10 min	0.13 (8 min)
Metoprolol	Lopressor	++	Class II	0	hepatic	oral, iv	50-450, 5-15	12-24	1-2 hr, 20 min	3-7

* Combined alpha-beta-blocker, see table 4-3
** Intrinsic sympathomimetic activity at the beta₂-adrenoceptor
*** Primarily hepatic, but active metabolites are formed that must be renally excreted

◇ Doses are in milligrams unless otherwise indicated. Oral doses are total daily doses.
+ Also as eye drops
ISA = intrinsic sympathomimetic activity
++ Esmolol is usually dosed as a bolus given over 1 minute and followed immediately by continuous infusion. To increase the dose, an additional bolus of 500 µg/kg must be administered prior to increasing the infusion rate.
△ Vaughan Williams classification scheme: Class I drugs are membrane stabilizers, Class II drugs are beta-adrenoceptor antagonists, Class III drugs prolong repolarization, Class IV drugs are calcium-channel antagonists.

dysfunction following myocardial infarction (Waldo et al, 1996).

Labetalol represents a relatively new category of beta-blocker. It is a non-selective beta-receptor antagonist, but also blocks alpha$_1$-adrenoceptor activity and exhibits intrinsic sympathomimetic activity (ISA) at the beta-receptor. These latter two properties are responsible for the *vasodilatory activity* of labetalol. Carvedilol is a newer drug which also exhibits alpha$_1$-adrenoceptor blocking activity in conjunction with non-selective beta-blocking activity. Unlike labetolol, carvedilol is only available in tablet form and is of limited utility in the perioperative setting.

Beta-Adrenoceptor Antagonists and Pre-Anesthetic Assessment

Pre-anesthetic evaluation of beta-blocker usage must include consideration of the effects of the drug on each of the principal organ systems.

Cardiovascular responses to beta-blockade

Antagonism of the beta$_1$-adrenoceptor in the myocardium reduces its chronotropic, dromotropic and inotropic effects (Fig 4-1). Thus, beta-blockade reduces the tachycardia, increased conduction velocity and elevated contractility observed during periods of high sympathetic tone. Cardiac output, though, is less affected secondary to an increase in stroke volume during blockade. At rest (low sympathetic tone), the effect of beta-blockade is much less pronounced.

By virtue of the reduction in inotropy, acute beta-blockade is best avoided in the presence of *congestive heart failure*. Nevertheless, it is noted that beta-blockade has been utilized under well-controlled circumstances in an attempt to upregulate myocardial beta$_1$-adrenoceptor numbers in refractory heart failure (Shanes, 1987; Waagstein et al, 1993). Recently, the CIBIS 2 trial was stopped because of the reduction in mortality achieved by bisoprolol.

Beta-adrenoceptor antagonists acutely increase *systemic vascular resistance* (SVR) due to blockade of pre-synaptic beta$_1$-receptors in the periphery. Blockade of the beta-receptor enhances NE release at presynaptic membranes, increasing NE-induced activation of postsynaptic alpha$_1$-receptors. A subsequent increase in vascular resistance and reduction in blood flow is observed in most organs. The notable exception is the brain, which possesses few alpha$_1$-receptors on the resistance vessels. SVR returns to pre-blockade levels with long term beta-blocker use. For reasons yet to be understood, long term use of beta-blockers in hypertensive patients is associated with a net reduction in SVR. This may be secondary to decreased renin release or, possibly, decreased central sympathetic outflow. This drop in SVR in conjunction with beta-blocker-induced myocardial depression is largely responsible for the observed drop in blood pressure in these patients (Hoffman and Lefkowitz, 1990).

In patients with coronary artery disease, beta-blockers will decrease *myocardial oxygen demand* by reducing heart rate and contractility, yet decrease flow through stenosed vessels by increasing end diastolic pressure. Overall, the balance between oxygen delivery and demand is improved, reducing anginal symptoms, and improving exercise tolerance. Further, beta-blockade has been shown to diminish platelet activity, which may confer additional myocardial protection (Frishman and Weksler, 1984). Use of beta-blockers in patients following myocardial infarction is one of the few regimens associated with reduced risk of reinfarction and improved longevity (Yusuf et al, 1988).

Beta-blockers are class II antiarrhythmic agents and are widely used in the treatment of *tachyarrhythmias*. Blockade of $beta_1$-receptors slows phase 4 depolarization, thereby decreasing sinus rate and automaticity of ectopic pacemakers and prolonging the effective refractory period of the atrioventricular (AV) node. Thus, beta-blockers may be used in the treatment of supraventricular and reentrant arrhythmias such as atrial fibrillation, atrial flutter or the AV-reciprocating tachycardia of Wolff-Parkinson-White syndrome. The goal of beta-blocker therapy in these cases is to slow the ventricular rate rather than abolish the arrhythmia. Beta-blockers are often used to control the tachycardia and dysrrhythmias observed with pheochromocytomas and hyperthyroidism. Administration of large doses of propranolol is occasionally effective in treatment of ventricular arrhythmias. This may reflect its quinidine-like membrane stabilizing effect at high doses. Lastly, beta-blocker therapy is occasionally used in the management of prolonged QT syndromes, which are thought to result from an imbalance in the distribution of sympathetic cardiac innervation (Jackman et al, 1984).

Pulmonary responses to beta-blockade

Blockade of pulmonary $beta_2$-receptors causes bronchoconstriction. This effect is clinically insignificant in normal individuals. However, $beta_2$-blockade in patients with asthma or chronic obstructive pulmonary disease may cause life-threatening increases in airway resistance.

Cerebrovascular responses to beta-blockade

Cerebral vascular resistance is generally unaffected by beta-blockade.

Metabolic responses to beta-blockade

$Beta_1$-adrenoceptor antagonism blocks catecholamine-induced glycogenolysis and glucose mobilization. Thus, beta-blockers reduce the ability to recover from hypoglycemia. This effect is particularly prominent in insulin-dependent diabetics, who risk potentially life-threatening hypoglycemic episodes during beta-blockade. Further, beta-blockers inhibit the tachycardia observed in response to hypoglycemia, masking an important warning sign. While insulin secretion is potentiated by $beta_1$-adrenoceptor stimulation, the effect of beta-blockade on insulin release is clinically insignificant. Beta-blockade is best avoided in insulin-dependent diabetics. Nevertheless, when clinical circumstances mandate their use, beta$_1$-selective blockers are preferable (Deacon et al, 1977).

Uterine and fetal response to beta-blockade

Beta$_2$-adrenoceptor blockade may interfere with tocolysis and, in theory, precipitate uterine contractions and reduce uterine perfusion. When necessary, beta$_1$-selective agents are preferable to nonspecific beta-blockers. Clinical experience has demonstrated the safety of beta$_1$-selective blockers such as atenolol and metoprolol in the treatment of maternal hypertension (Rubin, 1987). Labetalol, with its combined beta- and alpha-blocking activity, results in insignificant fetal adrenergic blockade and does not decrease uterine blood flow in pre-eclamptic patients (Jouppila et al, 1986; Pickles et al, 1989).

Esmolol is ultra short acting and may be useful for intra-operative blood pressure control. Caution should be exercised when using this drug: studies in sheep demonstrate persistent fetal bradycardia and hypoxemia (up to 30 minutes) following exposure to esmolol (Eisenbach and Castro, 1989). Similar controlled studies in gravid humans do not exist. The anesthesiologist, though, may encounter maternal pathology which mandates use of a short-acting drug such as esmolol. For example, esmolol has been used in conjunction with sodium nitroprusside to induce hypotension during resection of a cerebrovascular malformation in a pregnant patient (Larson et al, 1990). Fetal heart rate decreased during the esmolol infusion, but returned to pre-infusion values when the infusion was terminated three hours later. No adverse fetal sequelae were noted.

Glaucoma

Topical ophthalmic administration of beta-adrenergic antagonists is occasionally used to decrease aqueous humor formation in patients with open angle glaucoma. Systemic absorption of the beta-antagonist may place the patient at risk for enhanced cardiovascular suppression by anesthetic agents or other cardiovascular drugs administered by the anesthetist. For example, administration of verapamil or diltiazem may result in high grade AV nodal blockade due to the synergistic effects of beta-blockers and calcium channel-antagonism (Murad, 1990).

Beta-Adrenoceptor Antagonist Dosage and Pharmacokinetics

See Table 4-2.

Peri-Anesthetic Usage of Beta-Adrenoceptor Antagonists

Controlled hypotension

In attempt to reduce blood loss and transfusion requirements intraoperatively, controlled induction and maintenance of hypotension may be utilized. Mean arterial pressure (MAP) is reduced to a level which is safely tolerated by the patient. This level is determined by the anesthesiologist preoperatively and must be continuously reevaluated intraoperatively. A MAP one third less than the patient's baseline is usually well tolerated. Beta-blockade may be used as the primary hypotensive agent or as a means to control tachycardia during the use of direct-acting vasodilators. Labetalol and esmolol are two commonly used drugs for this purpose. *Labetalol* is a competitive antagonist at the $alpha_1$-receptor, in addition to its nonselective beta-blocking properties. As a result, it triggers vasodilation in addition to reducing cardiac contractility and rate. The onset of action of labetalol following intravenous (IV) administration is within 5-10 minutes and duration is 3-6 hours. It may be administered as intermittent boluses of 0.1-0.5 mg/kg or as a continuous infusion at rates up to a maximum of 2 mg/min. Advantages of labetalol include a limited effect on intracranial pressure and a lack of effect on hypoxic pulmonary vasoconstriction and intrapulmonary shunting. Disadvantages include prolonged hypotension following discontinuation of the infusion. As with all beta-blockers, it may cause heart block, congestive heart failure or bronchospasm.

Esmolol is a short-acting, $beta_1$-selective blocker. Its onset of action is 3 minutes following IV bolus administration of 500 μg/kg, with an elimination half-life of 9.2 minutes due to rapid hydrolysis by blood borne esterases. The hypotensive effect may be maintained by a continuous infusion of 50-300 μg/kg/min. A short half-life allows for quick reversal in the event of any adverse effect. Another advantage of esmolol may be its cardioselectivity. Its effect on pulmonary airway resistance is less than with a non-specific antagonist, making it a more suitable drug for patients with increased pulmonary reactivity. Lastly, its elimination is unaffected by renal or hepatic failure and it may be used safely in these patients.

Endotracheal intubation

Beta-adrenoceptor blockade is occasionally used to blunt the sympathetic cardiovascular response to placement of an endotracheal tube during anesthetic induction or during other noxious intraoperative stimuli. A short-acting drug such as esmolol may be administered as a bolus or infusion and then stopped as soon as the stimulus ceases (Helfman et al, 1991).

Pheochromocytoma

Beta-blockade is often necessary to reduce catecholamine-induced tachycardias and arrhythmias in patients with pheochromocytoma. Intraoperative catecholamine surges may be sporadic and a short acting beta-blocking drug, such as esmolol, may be preferred. The anesthetist must assure that adequate $alpha_1$-blockade is present prior to institution of beta-blockade in order to avoid potentially severe vasoconstriction. Blockade of $beta_2$-mediated vasodilation in these instances will leave $alpha_1$-mediated vasoconstriction unopposed. Labetalol has the advantage of acting as an alpha$_1$-blocker and beta-blocker simultaneously, thereby reducing the risk of beta-blockade-induced vasoconstriction. Potent direct vasodilators may still be required, but at reduced dosage.

Coronary artery disease

Episodes of chronic exertional angina may be reduced in severity and frequency by chronic beta-blockade. Beta-blockade reduces myocardial oxygen demand in these patients through its negative inotropic and chronotropic effects. Beta-blockade may be used alone or in conjunction with nitrate or calcium channel antagonist therapy. Caution must be exercised when instituting beta-blockade in the presence of a calcium channel blocker which antagonizes AV nodal conduction (i.e. verapamil or diltiazem). This combination risks the onset of high grade AV nodal blockade with subsequent hemodynamic compromise (Murad, 1990). Beta-blockade must be avoided in patients with vasospastic (also known as variant or Prinzmetals) angina. In these cases, blockade of beta-adrenoceptors may leave alpha-adrenoceptor-mediated   coronary   vasoconstriction unopposed.

Use of beta$_1$-selective antagonists during the course of an acute myocardial infarction may reduce morbidity and mortality by one or more mechanisms: 1) by decreasing myocardial oxygen demand, 2) redistribution of myocardial perfusion, 3) reduction of circulating free fatty acids, and 4) reduction of tachyarrhythmias. Chronic beta-blockade following a myocardial infarction is epidemiologically associated with reduced mortality (Yusuf et al, 1988).

Dissecting aortic aneurysm

The rate of propagation of dissecting aortic aneurysms is directly proportional to the rate of change of blood pressure (dP/dt) with each cardiac contraction. Thus, the goal of medical management is to simultaneously reduce blood pressure and myocardial contractility. This is most often accomplished with the use of beta-blockade in combination with a direct arterial vasodilator (such as sodium nitroprusside or alpha-adrenoceptor blockade). Arterial vasodilators must not be administered alone due to reflex increases in cardiac contractility and rate.

Hypertrophic cardiomyopathy

Historically, hypertrophic cardiomyopathy (HCM) has been referred to by several names including idiopathic hypertrophic subaortic stenosis (IHSS) and hypertrophic obstructive cardiomyopathy (HOCM). HCM is due to idiopathic myofibrillar disarray and asymmetric left ventricular hypertrophy. Symptoms result primarily from increased chamber stiffness resulting in diastolic dysfunction. In a small group of patients, left ventricular outflow obstruction is observed. By lengthening diastolic filling time and reducing myocardial oxygen demand, beta-blockers improve symptoms of angina and dyspnea, but have not been shown to improve long-term survival. The calcium channel blocker verapamil reduced diastolic dysfunction and improved survival in a retrospective study (Seiler et al, 1991).

Tetrology of Fallot

Beta-adrenoceptor antagonists are useful in the management of cyanotic episodes (tet spells) in patients with tetrology of Fallot. Right to left intracardiac shunting and cyanosis are observed under conditions of systemic vasodilation and/or increased pulmonary outflow (infundibular) obstruction. This most commonly occurs when the child is upset or agitated. Intravenous propranolol or esmolol will reduce cyanosis by slowing the heart rate, increasing diastolic filling and reducing myocardial contractility, all of which tend to reduce pulmonary infundibular obstruction. Concurrent intravenous administration of the alpha-adrenergic agonist phenylephrine, placement in a knee-chest position or external compression of the abdominal aorta will increase systemic vascular resistance and reduce intracardiac right to left shunting. Beta-blockade itself triggers vasoconstriction. The subsequent increase in systemic vascular resistance may contribute to the beneficial effects of beta-antagonists in these patients.

Tachyarrhythmias

Beta-blockers are widely used in the treatment of tachyarrhythmias (see earlier discussion).

Perioperative hypertension

Perioperative hypertension is frequently transient and multifactorial in etiology. Episodes may be fairly straightforward, representing continued manifestation of hypertensive disease; or they may be more complex, perhaps reflecting a combination of processes such as pain, hypoxemia, and hypercarbia. It is incumbent upon the anesthesiologist to define the nature of the episode prior to instituting therapy.

Beta-blockers may be used as antihypertensives. Short acting beta-blockers are preferable in the perioperative period due to the often transient nature of hypertensive episodes. Labetalol may be administered as intermittent boluses or infusion. Esmolol may be used diagnostically if the clinician believes beta-blockade is warranted, but is unsure of potential detrimental effects. A single bolus will produce a short-lived beta-blockade allowing assessment of the effects. Beta-blockade may be maintained by continuously infusing esmolol.

Hyperthyroidism and thyroid storm

Beta-antagonists are useful in the treatment of the cardiovascular symptoms of hyperthyroidism and thyroid storm, including tachycardia, arrhythmias, palpitations, and angina. They also appear to reduce tremors. Beta-blockers must be used with caution in patients with hyperthyroid-induced congestive heart failure.

ALPHA-ADRENOCEPTOR ANTAGONISTS

As shown in Fig 4-3, alpha$_1$-adrenoceptors stimulate phospholipase C (PLC), triggering formation of the cytoplasmic second messenger inositol 1,4,5-trisphosphate (IP$_3$) and the membrane-bound second messenger 1,2-diacylglycerol (DAG). Alpha$_2$-adrenoceptors, on the other hand, act through one or more G-protein-mediated mechanisms to 1) inhibit cyclic AMP formation, 2) increase potassium efflux (hyperpolarize the cell), and 3) decrease calcium influx (see Lawson and Meyer, 1996, 1997; Bockman, 1993; Dorn, 1997; Hohlfeld, 1990; Mironneau, 1995; Vanhoutte, 1989). These intermediary compounds and ion fluxes then trigger the diverse cellular responses to alpha-agonists (Table 4-1).

Alpha-adrenoceptor antagonists bind to and selectively inhibit alpha$_1$- and alpha$_2$-adrenoceptor activation. As with beta-adrenoceptor antagonists, the effect of alpha-blockers will depend upon the underlying level of sympathetic tone. The resulting effects of alpha-blockade may be ascribed to the unopposed activity of beta-adrenergic receptors. Indeed, alpha-blockers are classically defined as those drugs which convert the vascular response to epinephrine from constriction (alpha-mediated) to dilation (beta-mediated).

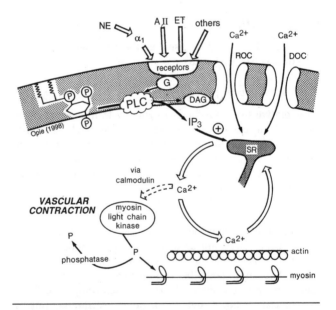

Fig 4.3 *Vasoconstrictory agonists.* These include post-synaptic alpha$_1$-receptor agonists and act by releasing calcium from the sarcoplasmic reticulum (SR). For example, stimulation of vascular receptors by alpha$_1$-agonists, endothelin (ET), angiotensin II (AII), leads to increased activity of phospholipase C, which splits phospatidyl inositol into two messengers: IP$_3$ (inositol triphosphate) and 1,2-DG (1,2 diacyglycerol). IP$_3$ promotes the release of calcium from the SR. Membrane-bound DAG activates PKC. The latter may act by a breakdown product on the contractile apparatus to promote a sustained contractile response. Vasoconstriction also occurs in response to enhanced activity of the calcium channels which are either receptor-operated channels (ROC) or depolarization-operated channels (DOC). NE = norepinephrine. (Fig. copyright © L.H. Opie, 1998)

Alpha-adrenoceptor antagonists may be classified according to 1) their selectivity for alpha$_1$- and alpha$_2$-receptors and 2) whether their receptor binding is reversible and competitive or irreversible and noncompetitive (Table 4-3).

Phenoxybenzamine binds covalently to alpha$_1$- and alpha$_2$-adrenoceptors, producing a noncompetitive, irreversible blockade. Reversal requires synthesis of new receptors, which may take days. The remaining alpha-blockers in Table 4-3 bind reversibly, producing a competitive antagonism of the alpha-adrenoceptor response. Phentolamine and tolazoline are relatively nonselective, antagonizing alpha$_1$- and alpha$_2$-adrenoceptor function equivalently. Prazosin and yohimbine are markedly specific. Prazosin antagonizes alpha$_1$-adrenoceptors while yohimbine antagonizes alpha$_2$ receptors. Phenoxybenzamine antagonizes both receptor subtypes with alpha$_1$-antagonism predominating. Terazosin, doxazosin and indoramin are similar to prazosin, demonstrating alpha$_1$-specificity.

Alpha-Adrenoceptor Antagonists and Preanesthetic Assessment

The anesthesiologist must consider the impact of alpha-adrenoceptor antagonists on each organ system prior to administration.

Cardiovascular response to alpha-blockade

Vascular. Alpha$_1$-adrenoceptors are found on vascular smooth muscle cells of the peripheral vasculature, including the coronary arterial, skin, uterine, intestinal, and splanchnic vasculatures (see Table 4-1). The alpha$_1$-receptor is located strictly post-synaptically at sympathetic nerve terminals on the peripheral vasculature. Alpha$_1$-receptors are also found post-synaptically on intestinal smooth muscle and endocrine glands (see below). The vascular response to alpha$_1$-stimulation is vasoconstriction, both in the resistance (arterial) and capacitance (venous) circulations. Thus, blockade of the alpha$_1$-receptor causes vasodilation, decreasing peripheral vascular resistance, cardiac afterload and cardiac preload. The magnitude of these responses will depend on underlying sympathetic tone.

In animal studies, epicardial vasodilation results with alpha$_1$-blockade, due to the predominance of alpha$_1$-receptors on these larger vessels. Alpha$_2$-adrenoceptors are the primary mediators of catecholamine-induced vasoconstriction of the smaller coronary vessels (Jones et al, 1993). Coronary vascular resistance is affected little by alpha$_1$-adrenoceptor activation or blockade since the epicardial vasculature accounts for only 5% of total coronary vascular resistance. Coronary flow, on the other hand, may be profoundly altered depending on the effects of alpha$_1$-blockade on peripheral vascular resistance (afterload) and capacitance (preload) with subsequent changes in coronary perfusion pressure.

Alpha$_2$-adrenoceptors are found on both pre- and post-synaptic membranes of the adrenergic neuroeffector junction. In the peripheral vasculature, post-synaptic alpha$_2$-

Table 4-3. Alpha-adrenoceptor antagonists

Drug	Trade Name	Type of Antagonism	Selectivity	Predominant Route of Elimination	Preparations	Usual Dose (mg)◇	Frequency (hr)	Peak Effect
Phenoxybenzamine	Dibenzyline	Noncompetitive	$\alpha_1 > \alpha_2$	hepatic and renal	oral	10-40	8-12	1-2 days
Phentolamine	Regitine	Competitive	$\alpha_1 = \alpha_2$	renal	iv	2.5-5	as needed	1-5 min
Tolazoline	Priscoline	Competitive	$\alpha_1 = \alpha_2$	renal	iv	1-2 mg/kg**	1	30 min
Prazosin	Minipress	Competitive	$\alpha_1 >> \alpha_2$	hepatic	oral	0.5-5	8-12	2-4 hr
Doxazosin	Cardura	Competitive	$\alpha_1 >> \alpha_2$	hepatic	oral	1-4	24	
Terazosin	Hytrin	Competitive	$\alpha_1 >> \alpha_2$	hepatic and renal	oral	1-5	12-24	2-3 hr
Labetalol*	Trandate	Competitive, also beta	α_1, also beta	hepatic	oral	100-400	12	2-4 hr
	Normodyne				iv	0.1-1 mg/kg	as needed	5 minutes
Carvedilol*	Coreg	Competitive, also beta	α_1, also beta	hepatic	oral	3.125-25	12	
Yohimbine	several trade names	Competitive	$\alpha_2 >> \alpha_1$	renal	oral	2.7-5.4	8	

◇ Doses are in milligrams unless otherwise indicated; oral doses are total daily doses.

iv = intravenous

* see Table 4-2

** In neonates, initial bolus administration of 1-2 mg/kg may be followed by a continuous infusion of 1-2 mg/kg/hr.

adrenoceptors mediate arterial and venous vasoconstriction (Faber, 1988; Vanhoutte, 1989). Alpha$_2$-post-synaptic activity predominates over alpha$_1$-activity in the arterioles (primary resistance vasculature) and in the veins (Faber, 1988). Pre-synaptic alpha$_2$-adrenoceptors inhibit the release of NE from the nerve terminal, thereby serving as a feedback inhibitory mechanism for peripheral sympathetic activity. Alpha$_2$-adrenoceptors located on vascular endothelium mediate vasodilation by releasing endothelium-derived nitric oxide in response to blood borne stimuli (Vanhoutte, 1989; Jones, 1993; Ohgushi, 1993). The alpha$_2$-D subtype is involved (Bockman et al, 1996). The net effect of peripheral alpha$_2$-blockade is the algebraic sum of blockade of endothelial, smooth muscle and presynaptic-neural alpha$_2$-adrenoceptors, acting through the various receptor subtypes (Bockman et al, 1993). In most vascular beds, alpha$_2$-adrenergic blockade causes a net vasodilatory response, due to the predominance of smooth muscle alpha$_2$-receptor activity over alpha$_2$-mediated endothelial nitric oxide release. Again, the magnitude of the vasodilatory effect also will depend on the prevailing sympathetic tone at the time of blockade.

The peripheral vasodilating properties of alpha-adrenoceptor antagonists have lead to their frequent use in the treatment of hypertensive disorders. A major side effect in patients taking alpha-blockers is postural hypotension, most often observed upon initiation of therapy. In these patients, a deficit in cerebral perfusion results from inadequate compensatory tachycardia possibly reflecting alpha-blockade-induced reduction of central sympathetic outflow.

Prazosin and its congeners terazosin, trimazosin and doxazosin are selective alpha$_1$-blockers which decrease peripheral vascular resistance and capacitance with little reflex increase in heart rate. Compensatory tachycardia is common to other primary vasodilators. The difference between these two groups may reflect one or more of the following:

1. preservation of alpha$_2$-activity reduces sympathetic output in the heart;

2. reduced preload from venodilation with alpha$_1$-blockade may trigger a Bainbridge-type reflex, thereby reducing heart rate (in contrast to primary arterial vasodilators); and

3. prazosin and its congeners may have a central nervous system effect reducing sympathetic outflow and, hence, baroreceptor function (Cubeddu, 1988).

Myocardial response. Recent studies have demonstrated the presence of alpha$_1$-adrenoceptors on the myocardium which exert a significant positive inotropic effect. In the healthy heart, myocardial post-synaptic alpha$_1$-receptors mediate perhaps as much as 30-50% of basal inotropic tone and 20-30% of total inotropy during exercise or stress (Schmitz et al 1989; Osnes et al, 1989). Thus, alpha$_1$-blockade directly contributes to a decrease in cardiac inotropy. In the normal individual, this negative inotropic effect is negligible due to reflex, beta$_1$-adrenoceptor-mediated changes in response to the drop in peripheral vascular resistance and increase in vascular capacitance.

Myocardial alpha$_1$-adrenoceptors play a more prominent role in the chronically failing heart due to the observed down-regulation in beta$_1$-adrenoceptor number. There is no evidence for down-regulation of the alpha$_1$-receptor number in myocardial failure and its contribution to total inotropy is consequently enhanced. Thus, alpha$_1$-blockade may cause significant reductions in inotropy in the failing heart. Nevertheless, alpha$_1$-antagonists such as prazosin have been used to reduce afterload in patients with congestive heart failure and cardiac valvular disorders such as mitral or aortic insufficiency (Stanaszek et al, 1983). Long-term prazosin therapy does not, however, improve mortality in chronic heart failure.

A similar relative enhancement in alpha$_1$-adrenoceptors is observed in ischemic myocardium. This may contribute to the positive inotropism observed during ischemia as well as to the malignant arrhythmias observed during reperfusion. Alpha$_1$-adrenoceptor antagonists such as prazosin and phentolamine possess significant antiarrhythmic activity but are often of limited utility due to their hypotensive effects. Reflex cardiac stimulation in response to the hypotension of alpha$_1$-blockade may lead to further ischemia and cardiac arrhythmias (Murdock et al, 1990).

Pulmonary response to alpha-blockade

Alpha-adrenoceptors located on bronchial smooth muscle may mediate contraction, though the clinical importance of this effect is minimal. Alpha-blockade is essentially ineffective in the treatment of bronchospastic disorders.

The pulmonary vascular response to alpha-adrenergic blockade mimics the peripheral vascular response. Tolazoline decreases pulmonary vascular resistance and has been used in neonates with respiratory distress syndrome and pulmonary hypertension in attempt to improve pulmonary blood flow. Its effectiveness is inconsistent and complications include hypotension, oliguria, thrombocytopenia, and hemorrhage of the gastrointestinal, renal and pulmonary systems (Goetzman et al, 1976).

Cerebrovascular response to alpha-blockade

There are relatively few alpha-adrenoceptors in the cerebral arterial vasculature. Thus, alpha-adrenoceptor activation or blockade cause little change in cerebrovascular resistance. Changes in cerebral perfusion during alpha-blockade reflect alterations in perfusion pressure, not cerebrovascular resistance.

Metabolic response to alpha-blockade

Alpha-adrenoceptors contribute to glucose mobilization by the liver. Alpha-blockade is less potent than beta-blockade in reducing catecholamine-induced glucose mobilization. This is due to the predominance of the beta$_2$-adrenoceptor in mediating this response. Alpha$_2$-blockade might facilitate insulin release from the islet cells of the pancreas.

Uterine and fetal response to alpha-blockade

Alpha$_1$-blockade and alpha$_2$-activation (with clonidine) have both been employed in the treatment of pre-eclampsia with good results. Alpha$_1$-blockade or alpha$_2$-activation will decrease uterine vascular resistance. As long as maternal blood pressure is maintained, uterine perfusion will be preserved or even enhanced.

Miscellaneous responses to alpha-blockade

Alpha-receptors of the trigone and sphincter muscles of the urinary bladder may be blocked in attempt to relieve urinary outflow obstruction. Direct intracavernous injection of phentolamine in combination with papaverine has been proposed for treatment of male sexual dysfunction. Orthostatic hypotension and priapism may result, necessitating treatment with an alpha-agonist such as phenylephrine.

Alpha$_2$-adrenoceptors facilitate platelet aggregation. The clinical effect of alpha-blockade on platelet function in not clear, though hemorrhagic complications have been reported with the use of alpha-blockers (Goetzman et al, 1976).

Alpha-Adrenoceptor Antagonist Dosage and Pharmacokinetics

See Table 4-3.

Peri-Anesthetic Usage of Alpha-Adrenoceptor Antagonists

Pheochromocytoma

Alpha-adrenergic blockade is a mainstay in the treatment of the adrenergic hyperactivity of pheochromocytoma. The goal of alpha-adrenergic-blockade in these patients is to control the episodes of severe hypertension and increase vascular capacitance to allow adequate hydration. Phenoxybenzamine is frequently used to treat the patient in preparation for surgery. It may be administered orally two or three times a day. Patients may require from 40 to 120 mg daily to control blood pressure. Total dosage may be limited by symptoms of postural hypotension. Phentolamine may be administered intravenously and is useful in the short term control of hypertension in these patients. The usual dose is 5 mg, administered slowly to avoid precipitous hypotension. Prazosin and other alpha$_1$-blockers are ineffective in the treatment of hypertension of pheochromocytoma due to persistent alpha$_2$-mediated vasoconstriction.

Autonomic hyperreflexia

Phenoxybenzamine has been used in the chronic treatment of spinal cord injured patients who exhibit hypertensive symptoms of autonomic hyperreflexia (Sizemore, 1970). Phentolamine may be administered intravenously during an acute vasospastic crisis in these patients.

Controlled hypotension

Labetalol may be used to induce intraoperative hypotension as discussed above.

Perioperative hypertension

Alpha-adrenergic blockers are often used in the treatment of primary hypertensive disorders. Perioperative use of most of these drugs is restricted by the inability to administer medications orally. The nonspecific alpha-blocker, phentolamine, and the combined $alpha_1$- and beta-blocker, labetalol, are available to the anesthetist for intravenous administration. The use of labetalol perioperatively is discussed above.

Phentolamine may be used to treat rebound hypertension following abrupt withdrawal of clonidine therapy or following ingestion of tyramine-containing foods by individuals taking monoamine oxidase inhibitors (see below). Phentolamine may be used to manage vasospastic hypertension in pheochromocytoma as discussed above.

Phenothiazines such as chlorpromazine and the butyrophenones haloperidol and droperidol exhibit significant alpha-adrenoceptor blocking properties. These drugs may cause perioperative hypotension particularly in the presence of other drugs such as inhalational anesthetics.

Miscellaneous

Local injection of phentolamine has been used to prevent dermal necrosis in cases of extravasation of alpha-adrenergic agonists.

Phentolamine may cause gastrointestinal stimulation and has been used to relieve catecholamine-induced pseudo-obstruction of the bowel in patients with pheochromocytoma. Phentolamine should be used with caution in patients with a history of peptic ulcers.

DOPAMINERGIC ADRENOCEPTOR ANTAGONISTS

Five ligand-specific dopaminergic receptors have been identified to date (Grandy and Civelli, 1992). The first two receptor types, D_1 and D_2, are the best studied. Peripheral D_1 receptors are post-synaptic and stimulate adenylate cyclase while D_2 receptors inhibit adenylate cyclase. The D_1 receptors are found on smooth muscle cells and act in a manner similar to beta-adrenergic receptors, triggering relaxation (e.g. vasodilation).

The role of the peripheral D_2 receptors is unclear; they may act like pre- and post-synaptic $alpha_2$-receptors, causing vasoconstriction and inhibiting NE release (Kuchel and Kuchel, 1991; Goldberg, 1989). The D_2 receptor antagonists metoclopramide and domperidone exhibit prokinetic effects on the upper gastrointestinal tract. They also exhibit antiemetic effects at the level of the chemoreceptor trigger zone

(CTZ). Clinically, they exhibit no peripheral vascular effects. Neuroleptic medications, phenothiazines (e.g. chlorpromazine) and butyrophenones (e.g. droperidol and haldol), exhibit potent antiemetic activity by antagonizing D_2 receptors in the CTZ. The peripheral vascular effects of the neuroleptics are complex and unpredictable, reflecting combined antidopaminergic, antihistaminic, antitryptaminergic and alpha$_1$-adrenergic inhibitory actions (see above).

AUTONOMIC GANGLION ANTAGONISTS

Hexamethonium, pentolinium, trimethaphan and mecamylamine constitute a group of drugs which selectively and competitively inhibit the nicotinic cholinergic receptors of the autonomic ganglia (Table 4-4). The physiological impact of these drugs depends on the prevailing level of sympathetic versus parasympathetic tone at the effector sites. As shown in table 4-5, for example, the normal (resting) predominant tone in the vasculature is sympathetic; thus, ganglionic blockade will decrease peripheral vascular resistance and increase venous capacitance. Postural hypotension is a major problem with the use of these drugs in ambulating patients. It reflects the inability of the autonomic nervous system to mount a reflex increase in sympathetic tone and cardiac output. Trimethaphan is the only ganglionic blocker which may be administered intravenously.

Table 4-4. Autonomic ganglion antagonists

Drug	Trade name
Nicotine (high concentrations)	
Hexamethonium	
Mecamylamine	Inversine
Trimethaphan	Arfonad
Pentolinium	

Table 4-5. Effector site predominance of autonomic tone

Site	Predominant Tone
Heart	Parasympathetic
Arterial vasculature	Sympathetic
Venous vasculature	Sympathetic
Bronchial tree	Parasympathetic
Gastrointestinal tract	Parasympathetic
Uterus	Parasympathetic
Eye muscles	Parasympathetic
Urinary bladder	Parasympathetic
Salivary glands	Parasympathetic
Sweat glands	Sympathetic (cholinergic)
Liver glycogenolysis	Sympathetic

Ganglionic antagonists may be used in the management of acute dissecting aortic aneurysms. In these patients, *trimethaphan* may be administered to reduce blood pressure and, more importantly, reduce the rate of rise of the pulse pressure at the level of the aortic tear. Trimethaphan may be infused intravenously at 0.3 to 3 mg per minute until the pain of aortic dissection abates or blood pressure is in the low-normal range.

Trimethaphan infusions may be used to induce controlled hypotension intraoperatively. It carries the advantages of rapid onset and offset, it is easily titrated, and it does not increase intracranial pressure. Unfortunately, rapid tachyphylaxis usually develops. It may result in significant histamine release and bronchospasm. Trimethaphan is metabolized by plasma cholinesterase. It may also inhibit this enzyme, potentially prolonging the effects of drugs such as succinylcholine and ester local anesthetics. Lastly, ganglionic blocking effects such as mydriasis, ileus, and urinary retention may complicate patient management.

Trimethaphan is also effective in the acute management of episodes of autonomic hyperreflexia.

Table 4-6. Indirect-acting adrenergic antagonists

Category	Drug	Trade name
Drugs which form false sympathetic neurotransmitters	Methyldopa	Aldomet
	Guanethidine	Ismelin
	Guanadrel	Hylorel
	Monoamine oxidase inhibitors:	
	Isocarboxazid	Marplan
	Pargyline	Eutonyl
	Phenelzine	Nardil
	Tranylcypromine	Parnate
Drugs which deplete stores of sympathetic neurotransmitters	Reserpine	Diupres, Hydropres*
	Guanethidine	Ismelin
	Metyrosine	Demser
Drugs which inhibit presynaptic release of sympathetic neurotransmitter	Clonidine	Catapres
	Dexmedetomidine	
	Guanabenz	Wytensin
	Guanfacine	Tenex
	Guanethidine	Ismelin
	Bretylium	Bretylol
	Muscarinic cholinergic agonists:	
	Acetylcholine	
	Methacholine	Provocholine
	Carbamylcholine	
	Bethanechol	Urecholine, Myotonachol
	Pilocarpine	Salagen

* Combined with diuretic

DRUGS WHICH FORM FALSE SYMPATHETIC NEUROTRANSMITTERS

Methyldopa

Methyldopa (alpha-methyldopa or Aldomet) exerts its antihypertensive effect by replacing NE in the central nervous system with methylnorepinephrine or methylepinephrine. One or both of these, in turn, reduces central sympathetic outflow, apparently by activation of central alpha$_2$-adrenoceptors.

Guanethidine and Guanadrel

The adrenergic blocking effect of guanethidine appears bimodal in nature. First, guanethidine binds to the presynaptic membrane of post-ganglionic sympathetic neurons. There, it inhibits release of NE from the neuron, producing a peripheral sympathetic blockade. Guanethidine does not cross the blood brain barrier and does not affect CNS function. Second, guanethidine is taken up by the neurons wherein it replaces NE in the storage vesicles. NE is depleted and guanethidine is released in its place when the nerve is depolarized by a stimulus. The released guanethidine then acts as a false neurotransmitter and the sympathetic blockade persists. Arterial and venous vasodilation occur with a concomitant reduction in cardiac inotropy and rate. Postural hypotension is a prominent side effect. Further, post-synaptic effector cell membranes become supersensitized to adrenergic agonists due to up-regulation of adrenergic receptors.

Guanadrel acts in essentially the same manner as guanethidine. It is more rapidly eliminated and therefore dosed twice daily instead of once a day.

Monoamine Oxidase Inhibitors

Monoamine oxidase inhibitors (MAOIs) block oxidative deamination of endogenous catecholamines by the enzyme monoamine oxidase. They do not inhibit catecholamine synthesis. Thus, the bioactive amines NE, epinephrine, dopamine, and serotonin accumulate in adrenergically active tissues. MAOIs are used to treat refractory cases of psychotic depression. Their antidepressant activity may reflect elevation of endogenous catecholamines in the brain. Their use in psychiatry has largely been supplanted by the tricyclic antidepressants, which have a larger margin of safety. Potential side effects of MAOI therapy may be severe and are discussed below.

MAOIs have an antihypertensive effect which is thought to result from formation of a false adrenergic neurotransmitter. Oxidative deamination of tyramine in the liver is blocked by MAOIs. Excess tyramine is taken up in adrenergic nerve terminals and transformed into the false neurotransmitter, octopamine, by the enzyme dopamine beta-hydroxylase. Octopamine is stored in adrenergic nerve varicosities, displacing NE. Upon stimulation, octopamine is released in place of NE. Octopamine is only a weak agonist at sympathetic receptors. A relative sympathectomy results and blood pressure drops. MAOIs are not used clinically as antihypertensives secondary to their low therapeutic index.

MAOI toxicity may manifest as agitation, hallucinations, hyperreflexia, hyperpyrexia, convulsions and either hypertension or hypotension. Orthostatic hypotension is common. Hepatotoxicity may occur and is not related to dosage or duration of therapy. When it does occur, it can be serious and should be considered when selecting anesthestic agents.

Perhaps of greatest interest to the anesthesiologist is the potential for *severe adverse interactions* between MAOIs and other drugs and foods. Patients taking MAOIs must avoid ingestion of foods containing tyramine, such as red wine, aged cheese, chocolate, citrus fruits, beer and pickled herring. Consumption of these foods may result in delivery of large amounts of tyramine (an indirectly acting sympathetic amine) to the adrenergic nerve terminals where it triggers massive release of NE. A hypertensive crisis ensues and episodes of hypertensive intracranial bleeding and death have been reported. Clinical use of the indirectly acting sympathetic amine, ephedrine, should be avoided for the same reason as tyramine. An exaggerated sympathetic response may also be observed in response to directly acting sympathomimetics. When their use is clinically indicated, dosing should be approached with caution. Symptoms of excess sympathetic activity may be treated with alpha-adrenergic blockers, ganglionic blockers or direct-acting vasodilators.

MAOIs are known to intensify CNS depression caused by ethanol, analgesics and general anesthesia. Use of meperidine or perhaps other phenylpiperidine analgesics may precipitate a severe hyperpyrexic reaction resulting in seizure and coma. Release of the catecholamine serotonin may be responsible for this reaction.

Considerable debate has been generated in the anesthesia literature regarding the safety of anesthetizing patients who are taking MAOIs. MAOIs bind irreversibly to monoamine oxidase and reversal of their effect requires generation of new enzyme, a process which may take up to two weeks. Further, cessation of therapy places the patient at risk for severe depression and, potentially, suicide. Recommendations to discontinue MAOI therapy for 2 weeks prior to surgery are based on limited case reports suggesting potent drug interactions (Wong and Ashburn, 1990). A small number of studies found few adverse effects in humans taking MAOIs given analgesics, opioid anesthesia, or regional blocks. Certainly, choice of anesthesia should avoid use of opioids which release catecholamines (meperidine) or histamine (morphine).

DRUGS WHICH DEPLETE STORES OF SYMPATHETIC NEUROTRANSMITTER

Reserpine

Reserpine, an alkaloid derived from the root of *Rauwolfia serpentina*, binds to and destroys storage vesicles in central and peripheral adrenergic neurons. Norepinephrine and serotonin are subsequently destroyed by cytoplasmic monoamine oxidase and the neurons lose their ability to release these neurotransmitters. A combined central and peripheral sympathectomy results. Its peripheral sympatholytic effects are similar to guanethidine, although postural hypotension is not prominent. Recovery of sympathetic function upon cessation of therapy requires re-synthesis of storage vesicles, which may take days to weeks. Undesirable CNS effects include sedation, inability to concentrate, and occasional psychotic depression which may lead to suicide. Reserpine is largely of historical interest as one of the first widely used antihypertensives. It is occasionally used today in low doses in combination with other, newer, antihypertensive drugs.

Metyrosine

Metyrosine inhibits tyrosine hydroxylase, the enzyme which catalyzes the formation of DOPA from tyrosine. Use of metyrosine in disease states such as pheochromocytoma decreases catecholamine biosynthesis by as much as 80%. It is used most often in the treatment of inoperable or malignant pheochromocytomas. Side effects include crystalluria, sedation, extrapyramidal symptoms, diarrhea and anxiety.

DRUGS WHICH INHIBIT PRESYNAPTIC RELEASE OF SYMPATHETIC NEUROTRANSMITTER

Clonidine, Dexmedetomidine, Guanabenz and Guanfacine

Clonidine, dexmedetomidine, guanabenz and guanfacine are all alpha$_2$-adrenoceptor agonists. Briefly, these drugs activate central alpha$_2$-adrenoceptors to reduce central sympathetic outflow. The systemic effect of this is decreased plasma renin activity, decreased plasma EPI and NE levels, and enhanced vagal tone. This accounts for the antihypertensive effect of these drugs. At higher circulating plasma levels, these compounds activate peripheral post-synaptic alpha$_2$-receptors to produce vasoconstriction and an increase in blood pressure. At high doses, clonidine may cause paradoxical hypertension by activation of peripheral alpha$_1$-adrenoceptors.

A *withdrawal syndrome* is known to occur within 18 hours of abrupt cessation of clonidine therapy. Symptoms of this syndrome include hypertension, tachycardia, insomnia, flushing, sweating, headache, apprehension, and tremulousness. It is most likely to occur in patients taking more than 1.2 mg clonidine per day. This syndrome may be observed postoperatively and confused with emergence symptoms.

Dexmedetomidine is a more selective alpha$_2$-antagonist than clonidine. Unlike clonidine, it may be administered intravenously. It has a short plasma half-life (1.5 hours) and onset of activity is rapid (less than 5 minutes). Peak effects occur within 15 minutes.

Both clonidine and dexmedetomidine are under active investigation as *anesthetic adjuncts* due to their prominent sedative effects, ability to decrease MAC in a dose-dependent fashion, reduce perioperative opioid requirements and blunt the sympathetic cardiovascular effects of surgical stimulation (Aantaa and Scheinin, 1993; Butterman and Maze, 1996; DeKock, 1996).

Bretylium

Bretylium, like guanethidine, is taken up by the post-ganglionic adrenergic nerve terminal and concentrated. It initially causes release of NE stores, but later prevents further NE release. As a result, an initial increase in myocardial contractility is followed by blockade of sympathetic cardiovascular reflexes and orthostatic hypotension. Bretylium, unlike guanethidine, does not deplete the nerve terminal of NE stores.

Muscarinic Cholinergic Agonists

Muscarinic cholinergic receptor activation may antagonize adrenergic activity either postsynaptically (at the level of the effector cell) or presynaptically by inhibiting release of NE. Muscarinic cholinergic receptors are found post-synaptically on multiple cell types. Cellular responses to muscarinic receptor activation are often, but not always, antagonistic to adrenergic receptor responses (see Lawson and Meyer, 1997). The particular response of the cell will depend on which biochemical signaling cascade(s) is (are) affected by the muscarinic and adrenergic receptors (Fig 1-5, page 8).

Less well known are the presence and action of presynaptic muscarinic receptors on sympathetic nerve terminals of the myocardium, coronary vessels and peripheral vasculature (Flacke and Flacke, 1986; Fuder, 1985; Vanhoutte and Cohen, 1984). Stimulation of these receptors inhibits release of NE in much the same manner as alpha$_2$-adrenoceptor stimulation (Fig 1–3, page 5). The prejunctional muscarinic receptor may play an important physiological role in tissues such as the heart wherein the sympathetic and parasympathetic (vagal) nerve terminals lie in close proximity. In these tissues, acetylcholine released from parasympathetic terminals may bind to nearby sympathetic terminals and inhibit NE release. The organ response will depend on the rate of NE release prior to muscarinic inhibition. For example, vagal inhibition of left ventricular contractility is accentuated as the level of sympathetic tone is increased. This interaction is termed *accentuated antagonism*. Its physiological role has yet to be clearly defined because it is unusual for high sympathetic and parasympathetic activity to coexist, except during anesthesia. Muscarinic antagonism of NE release may play a role in mediating vasospastic angina, which tends to occur in young people during periods of high parasympathetic tone, such as sleep. Administration of pro-cholinergic drugs (such as acetylcholinesterase inhibitors) may predispose the anesthetized patient to myocardial ischemia or bronchospasm by a similar mechanism.

SUMMARY

1. *Adrenergic antagonists* act by one or more of five mechanisms: 1) peripheral adrenergic receptor antagonism, 2) autonomic ganglion antagonism, 3) formation of false sympathetic neurotransmitters, 4) depletion of stores of sympathetic neurotransmitter and 5) inhibition of presynaptic release of sympathetic neurotransmitter.

2. *Direct receptor antagonists* include beta-blockers, the most commonly encountered adrenergic antagonists,

with important implications for pulmonary, cardiac and metabolic management of the patient. Use of beta-blockers as well as alpha-blockers in a variety of anesthetic situations is discussed.

3. *Trimethapan* is the autonomic ganglion antagonist most likely to be used by the anesthetist since it may be administered intravenously for rapid induction of hypotension.

4. *Drugs acting on neurotransmitters* include methyldopa and monoamine oxidase inhibitors. The controversy regarding anesthetic management of patients taking MAOIs is discussed. Drugs such as reserpine deplete stores of sympathetic neurotransmitters. Reserpine is occasionally encountered by the anesthetist when used in combination with other drugs for management of hypertension. Drugs which inhibit presynaptic release of sympathetic neurotransmitters include bretylium, alpha$_2$-adrenoceptor agonists, and muscarinic agonists.

REFERENCES

Aantaa, R. and Scheinin M. Alpha$_2$-adrenergic agents in anaesthesia. *Acta Anaesthesiol Scand*, 1993; 37:443-448.

Bockman CS, Jeffries WB and Abel PW. Binding and functional characterization of alpha$_2$-adrenergic receptor subtypes on pig vascular endothelium. *J Pharm & Exp Ther*. 1993; 267:1126-1133.

Burnstock G. Integration of factors controlling vascular tone. *Anesthesiology*, 1993; 79:1368-1380.

Butterman, A.E. and Maze M. Alpha$_2$-adrenergic agonists in anesthesiology. *Semin Anesthesia*, 1996; 15:27-40.

Cubeddu LX. New alpha$_1$-adrenergic receptor antagonists for the treatment of hypertension: role of vascular alpha-receptors in the control of peripheral resistance. *Am Heart J*, 1988; 116:133-162.

Deacon SP, Karunanuyake A and Barnett D. Acebutolol, atenolol and propranolol and metabolic responses to acute hypoglycemia in man. *Br Med J*, 1977; 2:1255-1257.

DeKock, M. Alpha$_2$-adrenoceptor agonists: clonidine, dexmedetomidine, mivazerol. *Current Opinion Anesthesiol*, 1996; 9:295-299.

Dorn GW 2nd, Oswald KJ, McCluskey TS et al. Alpha$_{2A}$-adrenergic receptor stimulated calcium release is transduced by Gi-associated G(beta-gamma)-mediated activation of phospholipase C. *Biochemistry* 1997; 36:6415-6423.

Eisenbach JB and Castro MI. Maternally administered esmolol produces fetal β-adrenergic blockade and hypoxemia in sheep. *Anesthesiology*, 1989; 71:718-722.

Faber JE. *In situ* analysis of alpha-adrenoceptors on arteriolar and venular smooth muscle in rat skeletal microcirculation. *Circ Res*, 1988; 62:37-50.

Flacke WE and Flacke JW. Cholinergic and anticholinergic agents. In: Smith NT, Corbascio AN (Eds). *Drug Interaction in Anesthesia*. Lea & Febiger, Philadelphia, 1986, p160.

Frishman WH and Weksler BB. Effects of beta-adrenoceptor blocking agents on platelet function. In: Frishman WH (Ed). *Clinical*

Pharmacology of the Beta-adrenoceptor Blocking Drugs, 2nd ed. Appleton-Century-Crofts, Norwalk, Conn, 1984, pp 273-298.

Fuder H. Selected aspects of presynaptic modulation of noradrenaline release from the heart. *J Cardiovasc Pharmacol* 1985; 7(suppl 5):S2-S7.

Goetzman BW, Sunshine P, Johnson JD et al. Neonatal hypoxic and pumonary vasospasm: response to tolazoline. *J Pediatr,* 1976; 89:617-621.

Goldberg LI. Pharmacological basis for the use of dopamine and related drugs in the treatment of congestive heart failure. *J Cardiovasc Pharm,* 1989; 14(Suppl 8):S21-S28.

Grandy DK and Civelli O. G protein-coupled receptors: the new dopamine receptor subtypes. *Current Opinions Neurobiol,* 1992; 2:275-281.

Helfman SM, Gold MI, DeLisser EA and Herrington CA. Which drug prevents tachycardia and hypertension associated with tracheal intubation: lidocaine, fentanyl, or esmolol? *Anesth Analg,* 1991; 72:482.

Hoffman BB and Lefkowitz RJ. Adrenergic receptor antagonists. In: Gilman AG, Rall TW, Nies AS, Taylor P (Eds) *The Pharmacological Basis of Therapeutics,* McGraw-Hill, Inc. New York, 1990, pp 221-243.

Hohlfeld J, Liebau S and Forstermann U. Pertussis toxin inhibits contractions but not endothelium-dependent relaxations of rabbit pulmonary artery in response to acetylcholine and other agonists. *J. Pharm Exp Ther.* 1990; 252:260-264.

Jackman WM, Clark M, Friday KJ et al. Ventricular tachyarrhythmias in the long QT syndromes. *Med Clin North Am,* 1984; 68:1079-1109.

Jones CJH and DeFily DV, Patterson JL & Chilian WM. Endothelium-dependent relaxation competes with α_1- and α_2-adrenergic constriction in the canine epicardial coronary microcirculation. *Circulation,* 1993; 87:1264-1274.

Jouppila P, Kirkinew PS, Koivula A and Ylikorkala O. Labetalol does not alter the placental and fetal blood flow or maternatl prostanoids in preeclampsia. *Br J Obstet Gynaecol,* 1986; 93:543-547.

Kuchel OG and Kuchel GA. Peripheral dopamine in pathophysiology of hypertension — interaction with aging and lifestyle. *Hypertension,* 1991; 18:709-721.

Larson CP Jr, Sheur LM and Cohen SE. Maternally administered esmolol decreases fetal as well as maternal heart rate. *J Clin Anesth,* 1990; 2:427-429.

Lawson NW and Meyer DJ Jr. Autonomic Pharmacology. In: Barash PG, Cullen BF & Stoelting RK (Ed). *Clinical Anesthesia,* 3rd ed. Lippincott-Raven, Philadelphia, 1997, pp 243-309.

Mironneau J and Macrez-Lepretre N. Modulation of Ca^{2+} channels by $alpha_{1A}$- and $alpha_{2A}$-adrenoceptors in vascular myocytes: involvement of different transduction pathways. *Cell Signalling,* 1995; 7:471-479.

Murad F. Drugs used for the treatment of angina: organic nitrates, calcium-channel blockers, and β-adrenergic antagonists. In: Gilman AG, Rall TW, Nies AS, Taylor P (Eds) *The Pharmacological Basis of Therapeutics,* McGraw-Hill, Inc. New York, 1990, pp 764-783.

Murdock CJ, Hickey GM, Hockings BE et al. Effect of $alpha_1$-adrenoreceptor blockade on ventricular ectopic beats in acute myocardial infarction. *Int J Cardiol,* 1990; 26:45-58.

Ohgushi M, Yasue H, Kugiyama K et al. Contraction and endothelium dependent relaxation via alpha-adrenoceptors are variable in various pig arteries. *Cardiovasc. Res.,* 1993; 27:779-784.

Osnes JB, Aass H and Skomedal T. Adrenoreceptors in myocardial regulation: concomitant contribution from both α- and β-adrenoreceptor stimulation to the inotropic response. *Basic Res Cardiol,* 1989; 84(Suppl. 1):9-17.

Pickles CJ, Symonds EM and Pipkin FB. The fetal outcome in a randomized double-blind controlled trial of labetalol versus placebo in pregnancy induced hypertension. *Br J Obstet Gynaecol,* 1989; 96:38-43.

Rubin PC. Beta-blockers in pregnancy (editorial). *Br J Obstet Gynaecol,* 1987; 94:292-293.

Schmitz W, Kohl J, Neumann J et al. On the mechanism of positive inotropic effects of alpha-adrenoreceptor agonists. *Basic Res Cardiol,* 1989; 84(Suppl 1):23-34.

Seiler C, Hess OM, Schoenbeck M et al. Long-term follow-up of medical versus surgical therapy for hypertrophic cardiomyopathy: A retrospective study. *J Am Coll Cardiol,* 1991; 17:634-642.

Shanes JG. Beta-blockade — rational or irrational therapy for congestive heart failure? *Circulation,* 1987; 76:971-973.

Sizemore GW and Winternitz WW. Autonomic hyper-reflexia–suppression with alpha-adrenergic blocking agents. *N Engl J Med,* 1970; 282:795.

Stoschitzky, K. and W. Linder. Time to reassess chiral aspects of beta-adrenoceptor antagonists. Clinical evidence for harmful effects of the non-beta-blocking d-enantiomers. *Trends Pharmacol Sci,* 1997; 18:306-7.

Stanaszek WF, Kellerman D, Brogden RN and Romankiewicz JA. Prazosin update. A review of its pharmacological properties an therapeutic use in hypertension and congestive heart failure. *Drugs,* 1983; 25:339-384.

Vanhoutte PM and Cohen RA. Effects of acetylcholine on the coronary artery. *Fed Proc* 1984; 43:2878-2880.

Vanhoutte PM and Miller VM. Alpha$_2$-adrenoceptors and endothelium-derived relaxing factor. *Am. J. Med.,* 1989; 87:1S-5S.

Waagstein F, Bristow MR, et al. Beneficial effects of metoprolol in idiopathic dilated cardiomyopathy. *Lancet,* 1993; 342:1441-1446.

Waldo AL, Camm AJ, de Ruyter H, et al. Effect of d-sotalol on mortality in patients with left ventricular dysfunction after recent and remote myocardial infarction. The SWORD Investigators. Survival With Oral d-Sotalol. *Lancet,* 1996; 348:7-12.

Wong KC and Ashburn MA. Monoamine oxidase inhibitors and anesthesia. Literature Scan: *Anesthesiology Current Insights.* World Medical Communication, Cedar Knoll, NJ, 1990.

Yusuf S, Wittes J and Friedman L. Overview of results of randomized clinical trials in heart disease: 1. Treatments following myocardial infarction. *JAMA* 1988; 260:2088-2093.

CHAPTER 5

Calcium Channel Antagonists and other Agents Decreasing Calcium Influx

Lionel H. Opie and Gaisford G. Harrison

CALCIUM CHANNEL ANTAGONISTS IN ANESTHETIC PRACTICE

Calcium channel antagonists (CCAs, also called calcium channel blockers or CCBs) have direct relevance to three aspects of clinical anesthetic practice.

i.   Their wide use in the treatment of hypertension, angina pectoris and supraventricular tachyarrhythmias, predicates that many patients presenting for anesthesia will be on chronic medication with these agents. Inherent in their mechanism of action is the possibility of adverse interactions with anesthetic agents and adjuvants.

ii.   Peri-anesthetic, CCAs have a place in the management of supraventricular arrhythmias and acute hypertension.

iii. The properties of CCAs give them a potential role in protection of the heart from postischemic reperfusion injury.

MECHANISMS OF ACTION AND PHARMACODYNAMICS OF CCAS

Mechanism of Action

Calcium ions play a decisive role in the electrical activity of the heart and in the excitation-contraction coupling (ECC) of cardiac, vascular smooth and skeletal muscle (see Fig. 1-13) (Foëx, 1993; Butterworth, 1994). The sarcolemma (SL) is relatively impermeable to calcium ions which are actively

pumped out of the myocyte ensuring a low resting cytosolic calcium ion concentration (10^{-7}M) in the face of a 10^4
fold extracellular concentration gradient. Cytosolic entry of
calcium ions through voltage-operated calcium channels
(Fig 1-14, page 20) is the crucial event triggering calcium-
induced-calcium-release from the sarcoplasmic reticulum
(SR) ryanodine receptor channel and thereafter the contractile
process — the actin-myosin interaction — in cardiac muscle.
Beta-adrenoceptor stimulation by increasing cyclic AMP formation provides a second mechanism for increasing myoplasmic calcium ion concentration, so enhancing the force of
contraction in the myocardium (Fig 1-5, page 8). The efficiency of the contractile process is further enhanced in this
case by the increased rate of myofibrillar relaxation secondary to an enhanced reuptake of calcium into the sarcoplasmic
reticulum (SR) under the influence of cyclic AMP.

In addition to its direct involvement in the contractile
process, the increase in myoplasmic calcium ion concentration, through its activation of many of the enzymes
involved in glycolysis and mitochondrial production of
ATP, plays a further supportive role by the provision of the
substrates required to fuel the contraction process.

CCAs directly inhibit calcium entry into effector cells
by binding with specific sites in the calcium channel proteins — specifically the voltage-dependent "slow current"
L-channels. In practice, this group of drugs has no effect on
other types of calcium channels such as the T, N nor P
types (Terrar, 1993), even though a selective T–channel
blocker has become experimentally available (Ertel et al,
1997).

Pharmacological Actions of CCAs

CCAs are structurally classified into three major categories
— the dihydropyridines (DHPs), the benzothiazepines and
the phenylalkylamines — each of which binds to a specific
calcium channel site (Fig 1-14). The prototype — or first
generation — compounds of these categories are respectively nifedipine (class Ia or DHP binding site), diltiazem
(class Ib or D binding site) and verapamil (class Ic or V
binding site) (Spedding and Paoletti 1992). Second generation agents are the long-acting DHPs, of which the forerunner was amlodipine. From the functional point of view (Fig
5-1), the two major groups are the DHPs (dihydropyridines,
nifedipine-like agents which include amlodipine and felodipine) and the non-DHPs (verapamil and diltiazem).

Despite their structural diversity and binding differences, CCAs display a common core of pharmacological
actions which differ between agents only in the varying
intensity with which each is expressed. These effects are: (i)
a negative inotropic effect on cardiac contractility (non
DHPs > DHPs); (ii) negative chronotropic and dromotropic
effects on the SA node and AV nodal conducting tissue
(non DHPs >> DHPs); and (iii) vasodilation — this effect
being more marked on arterioles than on veins, and
includes the coronary vasculature (DHPs > non DHPs).

Thus, of these effects, the first two are the predominant
properties of the non-DHPs verapamil and diltiazem,

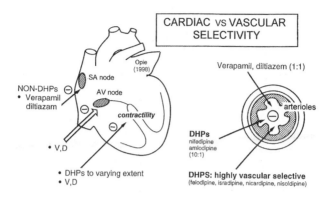

Fig 5-1. Non-DHP vs DHP calcium antagonists. The non-DHPs (dihydropyridines) such as verapamil and diltiazem, act both on the heart and on the arterioles at approximately equal concentrations. Such non-DHPs have negative chronotropic, dromotropic and inotropic effects, thus resembling beta-blockers. The DHPs are more vascular selective, some of them being highly so. (Fig. copyright © LH Opie, 1998).

whereas in the case of the DHP such as nifedipine and amlodipine, vasodilation is the most prominent (Fig 5-1).

Essential to the rational therapeutic use of CCAs is a knowledge of the ratio that the vasodilatory potency of individual agents bears to the negative inotropic effect of the same agent on the myocardium (vasodilation to negative inotropic ratio). In the case of the human myocardium, Godfraind et al (1992) found that these ratios for the prototype CCAs were — nifedipine 10:1, diltiazem 1:1, and verapamil 1:1. Even greater vascular selectivity (up to 1000:1) is displayed by more recently introduced nifedipine-like compounds. In clinical use, verapamil is the most negatively inotropic agent, closely followed by diltiazem.

In terms of clinical application, these observations provide the basis for considering a clinical division of the CCAs into two groups, the dihydropyridines (DHPs), nifedipine and its analogues, and the non-DHPs, verapamil, diltiazem, and their derivatives (Fig 5-1). The properties of the former render them more appropriate for the therapy of hypertension and hypertensive heart disease and the latter to that of ischemic heart disease and supraventricular tachyarrhythmias.

Though highly active on vascular smooth muscle, CCAs have little or no effect on other smooth muscle such as that of the bronchi or gut (exception: verapamil often causes constipation). This difference probably reflects variations between tissues in either the structure or function of their calcium channels.

Also crucial to the therapeutic applicability of CCAs is the fact that skeletal muscle does not react to conventional CCAs. As a result skeletal muscle weakness is not an undesired side-effect of their administration. This difference in response between skeletal muscle and the myocardium probably results from differences in their mechanism of excitation-contraction coupling. In the myocardium, the precontractile rise in myoplasmic calcium ion concentration comes both from the transsarcolemmal calcium influx through the calcium channels and the calcium-induced calcium release from the sarcoplasmic reticulum (SR) that it triggers (Fig 5-2). By contrast, in skeletal muscle, depolarization-activated calcium release from the SR is the principal source of the myoplasmic calcium rise. The calcium channel involved in the latter process is called the *ryanodine receptor*. It is unaffected by the CCAs which act only on the sarcolemmal channels (Terrar, 1993). Also, there appear to be some differences between the sarcolemmal calcium channels in the heart and skeletal muscle, both in their structure and their distribution. In the case of myocardial cells, these channels are found all over the surface of the sarcolemma but are confined to T-tubular clefts in the case of skeletal muscle. There are also important differences between the release mechanism of calcium in the myocardium and in vascular smooth muscle (Fig 5-2).

Calcium Channel Antagonists vs Beta-blockers

The fact that myocardial beta-adrenoceptor stimulation helps to enhance myocardial contractility by increasing the opening probability of the calcium channel (Fig 1-5) means that there could be a close overlap between the cardiac

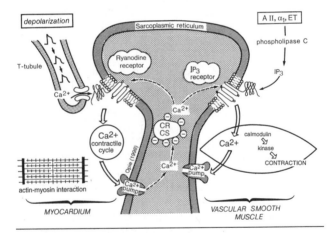

Fig 5-2. Contrasts between myocardium and vascular smooth muscle in calcium release mechanisms. *In the myocardium (left side of figure), the small amount of calcium that has entered the cell through the calcium channel during voltage depolarization, releases much more calcium from the sarcoplasmic reticulum via the calcium release channel. This process is called calcium-induced calcium release, and the release channel forms part of the ryanodine receptor in the membrane of the SR. The subsequent rise of calcium in the cytosol triggers cardiac contraction. Relaxation occurs when the cytosolic calcium level falls as calcium is taken up again (re-uptake) by the energy-requiring calcium pump of the sarcoplasmic reticulum. Next, within the SR, this calcium interacts with the storage proteins, calsequestrin (CS) and calrectulin (CR), thence to be released again. In contrast, in vascular smooth muscle, the contractile cycle responds to stimulation of vasoconstrictor receptors (AII = angiotensin II; α_1 = alpha$_1$-adrenergic activity; ET = endothelin). Activation of phospholipase C leads to release of inositol trisphosphate (IP$_3$), which acts on its receptor to release calcium from the sarcoplasmic reticulum. Whether the IP$_3$ path for calcium release operates in the normal myocardium is controversial (Fig. copyright © LH Opie, 1998).*

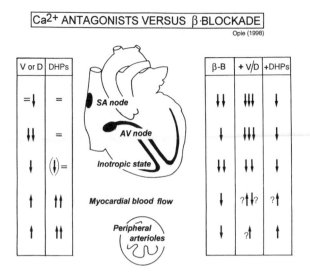

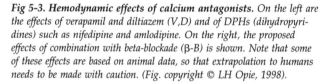

Fig 5-3. Hemodynamic effects of calcium antagonists. On the left are the effects of verapamil and diltiazem (V,D) and of DPHs (dihydropyridines) such as nifedipine and amlodipine. On the right, the proposed effects of combination with beta-blockade (β-B) is shown. Note that some of these effects are based on animal data, so that extrapolation to humans needs to be made with caution. (Fig. copyright © LH Opie, 1998).

effects of CCAs and those of beta-adrenoceptor antagonists. Beta-receptor antagonism increases the number of dephosphorylated calcium channels, and hence decreases the probability of calcium channel opening. By contrast, CCAs increase the number of blocked channels. Taken together, the combined effects of both types of drugs would lessen the number of open calcium channels (Reuter, 1984) and lead to certain possible interactions (Fig 5-3).

During clinical anesthesia, such combination should be strenuously avoided for, together with the negative ino-, dromo- and chronotropic effects of the modern volatile agents and the possibility of hypoxia or ischemia secondary to hypotension, it would constitute a serious danger to the patient.

In vascular and bronchial smooth muscle, however, there is a critical difference between the actions of CCAs and beta-adrenoceptor blockade. Here beta-blockade decreases cyclic AMP inhibition of myosin light chain kinase (MLCK), the enzyme crucial to smooth muscle contraction but without a major function in cardiac contraction. Consequently beta-blockade promotes contraction of smooth muscle, in contrast to the relaxation induced by CCAs — an action which can initiate life-threatening bronchospasm in the asthmatic patient.

A further important difference between the actions of CCAs and beta-adrenoceptor blockers is the metabolic neutrality of the former. They do not impair glucose metabolism, nor alter the blood lipid profile. By contrast, beta-blockers — as also diuretics — when chronically given may increase the insulin resistance noted in some hypertensive patients and change the lipid profile unfavorably (Pollare et al, 1989).

Side Effects and Contra-indications

The so-called "side-effects" of these agents are largely exaggerated expressions of their main pharmacological actions, including interaction with other cardioactive drugs. Reflex tachycardia, facial flushing and headache are found especially with the DHPs, and excessive bradycardia, AV block and impaired myocardial function especially with the non-DHPs. Peripheral edema, often found with the DHPs, is thought to be the result of more powerful arteriolar than venular dilation. Cardiac diseases with "fixed cardiac output" states such as aortic stenosis or hypertrophic obstructive cardiomyopathy constitute strong contra-indications to the use of CCAs, especially the DHPs because their powerful peripheral vasodilation increases the outflow gradient. Left ventricular dysfunction is a standard contra-indication, with however some exceptions (See section on Congestive Heart Failure). For the non DHPs, markedly impaired impulse formation or conduction depression are contraindications. Nifedipine and other DHPs are specifically contra-indicated in the setting of unstable angina or acute myocardial infarction, unless accompanied by beta-blocker therapy (Opie and Messerli 1995). An increase in surgical bleeding (Wagenknecht et al, 1995) has been found with the non-standard DHP agent nimodipine that is paradoxically licensed for use in subarachnoid hemorrhage. In addition, observational studies in the elderly suggest increased perioperative bleeding possibly through an interaction with ketorolac (Zuccala et al, 1997).

Long-term Safety

Recent concerns raised in relation to the long term safety of CCAs, have included increased mortality, cancer and bleeding. For an in depth discounting of the supposed dangers, see the report of the WHO-ISH committee (1997) and the review by Opie (1996). In reality, most of these adverse effects have been derived from observational studies which may be subject to serious bias by selection, and largely related to the effects of short acting nifedipine often inappropriately used. Examples are severe hypertension when excess doses may drop the BP too suddenly (Grossman et al, 1996), or in the very old when this powerful agent was given even though the initial BP was virtually normal (Pahor, 1995). The basis for the meta-analysis showing an increased mortality with high-dose short-acting nifedipine was the incorrect use in unstable angina without a beta-blocker (Furberg, 1995; 1996). When correctly used with due care for their known pharmacological properties, calcium antagonists remain relatively safe drugs.

CCAs AND PRE-ANESTHETIC ASSESSMENT

CCAs are likely to be part of the medical management of many patients suffering from chronic cardiovascular disease who present for anesthesia for surgery, whether cardiac or non-cardiac. Current philosophy in anesthetic practice is that such treatment, when optimum, should not be inter-fered with — or interfered with as little as possible — by the procedures of anesthesia and surgery. To this end, the anesthesiologist must be conversant with the treatment regime involved, possible interactions with anesthetic agents and adjuvants, as well as the means to control these. Such disease states and the use of CCAs in their treatment will now be reviewed.

Angina and Ischemic Heart Disease

As a group, CCAs diminish myocardial oxygen demand by decreasing afterload, and by coronary vasodilation which both relieves exercise-induced coronary vasoconstriction and promotes collateral blood flow to the ischemic zone. In the case of the non-DHPs, verapamil and diltiazem, their negative inotropic action and reduction in heart rate also contribute to their antianginal effect.

In the treatment of *Prinzmetal's vasospastic angina* (a relatively rare condition) the potency of all CCAs as dilators of coronary vasculature is of proven benefit, but in *unstable angina* with threat of myocardial infarction or in early phase myocardial infarction the DHP CCAs should not be given without beta-blockade (HINT Study, 1986; Opie and Messerli 1995). In unstable angina, intravenous diltiazem is bettter than an intravenous nitrate (Gobel et al, 1995).

CCAs are not introduced in the early stages of *acute myocardial infarction,* yet both verapamil and diltiazem have shown promising results in the postinfarct management of patients who did not have prior heart failure (Fischer Hansen, 1994). Beta-blockers are preferred for post-infarct protection.

In *postinfarction LV ischemic dysfunction*, the DHP nisol-dipine has been shown to improve exercise time and indices of diastolic dysfunction (DEFIANT study, 1992).

In *silent ischemia* in association with overt angina, com-bination therapy by nifedipine with beta-adrenergic block-ade (atenolol) has improved hard end-points such as cardiac death, myocardial infarction and unstable angina (Dargie et al, 1993).

Hypertension and Hypertensive Heart Disease

Until recently, there are no real outcome studies with CCAs showing reduction in hard end-points such as stroke. None-theless, the CCAs, and predominantly the long-acting DHPs, have featured prominently in the therapy of hyper-tension and hypertensive heart disease. Specifically decreas-ing systemic vascular resistance (SVR), they act rapidly and do not cause marked secondary sympathetic stimulation during long-term administration (in contrast to the short-term effects following abrupt vasodilation) (Foex, 1987).

Two important outcome studies with the DHPs in hypertension in the elderly have argued for safety and effi-cacy (STONE, 1996; Syst-Eur 1997). The better designed double-blinded study, Syst-Eur, randomized 4695 patients with systolic hypertension to twice daily DHP nitrendipine or placebo. Over a median follow-up period of two years, the primary end-point, stroke, was reduced by 42%, while cardiac events fell by 26%. Cancer and bleeding rates were unchanged though with small numbers, so real differences could still exist. On the basis of this study, the new American recommendation is that either diuretics (preferred) or long-acting DHPs may be used in isolated systolic hypertension (JNC VI, 1997).

CCAs may be safely used in combination therapy with diuretics, nitrates and ACE inhibitors provided that excess hypotension is avoided. Several combination tablets of CCAs and ACE inhibitors are now available for use in hypertension, eg verapamil-trandolapril, amlodipine-benazepril, felodipine-enalapril. With beta-blockers, the DHPs combine better because of their lesser effect on the SA and AV nodes, and lesser negative inotropic effect (Fig 5-3). Combination therapy may allow the use of lower doses of the individual drugs thereby improving therapeutic efficiency with a lessened incidence of side-effects.

Congestive Cardiac Failure

The use of CCAs in congestive heart failure is questionable. Though the non-DHPs, verapamil and diltiazem, are contraindicated by their negative inotropic effect, a case can be made for the long acting DHPs which reduce systemic vascular resistance and so the afterload. Such changes could facilitate myocardial ejection and improve subendocardial perfusion. For this purpose only, the best tested CCAs are the second generation DHP agent such as amlodipine and felodipine (see Chapter 8). Thus amlodipine, when added to standard triple therapy for severe heart failure, did not decrease mortality in the PRAISE study (PRAISE, 1996). Felodipine has also not increased mortality in the VeHeft-III trial (Cohn et al, 1997). Nisoldipine has been safely used in the DEFIANT studies in selected patients with post-infarct left ventricular dysfunction without clinical heart failure (DEFIANT, 1992 & 1997). The new non-DHP agent, mibefradil, was withdrawn when the results of the large MACH-trial in heart failure were analyzed (MACH-1, 1997).

Supraventricular Tachyarrhythmias

Of the CCAs, the non-DHPs, verapamil and diltiazem, alone depress AV nodal conduction and are, consequently, powerful inhibitors of re-entrant supraventricular tachycardia (SVT). With an onset which displays "frequency dependence" (Opie et al, 1995), ventricular response rates in atrial fibrillation and flutter are also rapidly controlled. When verapamil is administered intravenously to control supraventricular tachyarrhythmias, clinical management is facilitated by the fact that the AV nodal depression induced long outlasts the adverse hemodynamic effects of the drug (Singh et al, 1980).

By contrast, however, these drugs have no effect on recurrent sustained ventricular tachycardia (VT) and because of the myocardial depression they induce, their use may be lethal. Before treatment is commenced therefore, it is crucial that the ECG of SVT (narrow complex QRS) be carefully distinguished from that of VT (wide complex QRS) for which condition, it must be re-emphasised, verapamil and diltiazem are contraindicated.

In the Wolff-Parkinson-White syndrome, these drugs do not affect the refractoriness of accessory conduction pathways (bypass tract). Nonetheless, one limb of the re-entry circuit goes through the slow fibers of the AV node, so that verapamil and diltiazem usually work when given acutely. However, when chronically used in this syndrome, their administration can predispose to the development of anterograde conduction along the bypass tract with risk of VT or fibrillation, so that their use becomes contraindicated.

CCAs: DOSAGE SCHEDULES AND PHARMACOKINETICS

The kinetics and dosage schedules of first, second and third generation CCAs are recorded in Tables 5-1 and 5-2. Table 5-3 records those for urgent IV peri-anesthetic use. For the latter, the four drugs used — verapamil, diltiazem, nifedipine (no intravenous formulation) and nicardipine — all have elimination half-lives of the order of 6 hours.

PERI-ANESTHETIC USE OF CCAs

Two complications which may occur during clinical anesthesia and immediately thereafter — supraventricular tachyarrhythmias and acute severe hypertension — may be effectively treated with CCAs (Fig 5-4). The former may be

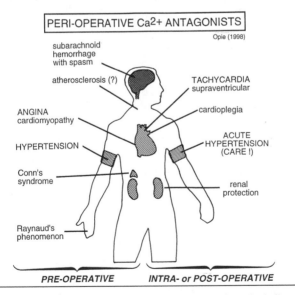

Fig 5-4. *Perioperative use of calcium antagonists:* the major indications are angina pectoris and hypertension. **Intra- or post-operative** use includes supraventricular tachycardia and acute hypertension. Note that abrupt blood pressure (BP) reduction by nifedipine capsules needs care and caution, so that controlled BP reduction by intravenous nicardipine is preferred. (Fig. copyright © LH Opie, 1998).

Calcium Channel Antagonists

Table 5-1. First generation calcium channel antagonists for oral use (including long acting preparations)

Agent	Dose	Pharmacokinetics and metabolism	Side-effects and contra-indications	Interactions & Precautions
Nifedipine • capsules (Adalat, Procardia)	5–10 mg initial; then 10–20 mg 3 x daily titrated; in Prinzmetal's angina up to 30 mg 4 x daily	Poor sublingual but good gastric absorption; bite and swallow best for quick effect, <10min. High first pass metabolism; inactive metabolites. t½ 3 h. Poor trough-peak ratio	Rapid vasodilation elicits reflex tachycardia, flushing, hypotension. Headache and ankle edema. C/I: severe aortic stenosis, obstructive cardiomyopathy, LV failure, unstable angina, AMI.	Fentanyl: added LV depression to beta-blockade. Cimetidine, liver disease, grape fruit juice increase blood levels. Reduce dose in elderly.
• tablets	10–40 mg twice daily	Slow absorption prolongs t½–11 h	Reflex tachycardia & flushing less marked. Headache, ankle edema C/I as above	As above
• prolonged release (Procardia XL, Adalat CC or LA)	30–90 mg once daily	Stable 24h blood levels. Slow onset, about 6h	Few acute vasodilatory S/E Headache, ankle edema. Same C/I.	As above
Verapamil • tablets	240–480 mg daily in 2 or 3 doses (titrated)	Peak plasma levels within 1–2 h. Low bioavailability (10–20%), high first pass metabolism to active norverapamil. Excretion: 75% renal, 25% GI. t½ 3–7h	Constipation. Depression of SA, AV nodes and myocardium. C/I sick sinus syndrome, digitalis toxicity, excess β-blockade, LV failure. Care in obstructive cardiomyopathy. Liver or renal disease increases blood levels.	Cardiodepression: inhalation anesthetics, β-blockers, disopyramide, quinidine, flecainide. Increased levels of digoxin, quinidine, theophylline, carbamazepine, cyclosporine. Sensitizes to neuromuscular blockers.
• Slow release (SR) forms (Verelan, Isoptin SR, Calan SR)	same, single dose, sometimes 2 doses. (SR)	Peak effect 1–2 h (Isoptin SR, Calan SR) or 7–9 h (Verelan). t½ 5–12 h and 12 h (Verelan longest)	As above	As above; long action requires extra care with beta-blockade or nodal disease
• Timed release (Covera-HS)	Same, single bed-time dose	Dual delivery system, first with delayed onset 4–5 h to blunt morning rise in BP & heart rate; second extended release	As for verapamil	As above
Diltiazem • tablets (Cardizem, Tildiem, Tiazem)	240–360 mg daily in 3 or 4 doses	Onset time: 15–30 min. Peak time: 1–2h, t½ 5h. Bioavailability — 45% (first pass hepatic effect) Active metabolite accumulates. 65% GI loss.	Similar to verapamil but no constipation. S/E: transient liver damage, erythema multiforme, exfoliative dermatitis. C/I: heart failure	Similar to verapamil, little/no effect on digoxin levels. Cimetidine increases diltiazem levels. Increased propranolol levels (binding site displacement)
• slow release (Cardizem SR, CD; Dilacor XR)	As above in 1 or 2 (SR) doses	Slower onset, longer t½, 24 h BP reduction, otherwise similar	As above	As above; longer action requires extra care with beta-blockade or nodal disease

C/I = contraindication; GI = gastrointestinal

Table 5-2. Second generation long acting calcium channel antagonists for oral use

Agent	Dose	Pharmacokinetics and metabolism	Side-effects and contra-indications	Interactions & Precautions
Amlodipine (DHP) (Norvasc, Istin)	5–10 mg once daily	t max, 6–12h. Extensive but slow hepatic metabolism, 90% inactive metabolites. 60% renal. t½ 35–50h. Steady state in 7–8 days	Edema, dizziness, flushing, palpitation. C/I: severe aortic stenosis, obstructive cardiomyopathy, unstable angina, AMI*. Care in CHF class II or III; may benefit nonischemic cardiomyopathy.	Prolonged t½ up to 56h in liver failure. Reduce dose, also in elderly and in heart failure. Grape fruit juice: caution but interaction not established.
Felodipine ER (DHP) (Plendil)	5–10 mg once daily	t max, 3–5h*. Complete hepatic metabolism (P-450) to inactive metabolites 75% renal loss, t½ = 22–27h	Edema, headache, flushing. C/I as above except no evidence for benefit in CHF (mortality neutral).	Reduce dose with cimetidine, age, liver disease. Anticonvulsants enhance hepatic metabolism. Grape fruit juice markedly inhibits metabolism.
Isradipine (DHP) (DynaCirc CR)	5–20 mg once daily	t max, 2h. Complete hepatic metabolism to inactive metabolites, 75% renal, 25% GI loss. t½ 8.4h. Food delays absorption	Headache, edema, dizziness, fatigue. C/I: severe aortic stenosis, obstructive cardiomyopathy, LV failure, unstable angina AMI*.	Fentanyl: co-dosage of calcium and beta-blocker, risk of hypotension. As for nifedipine. Propranolol bioavailability increased. Avoid grape fruit juice.
Nisoldipine (DHP) (Sular, Syscor)	10–60 mg once daily	t max, 6–12h. Hepatic metabolism by cytochrome P 450. Urinary excretion. Very high plasma protein binding. Trough-peak ratio of 70–100%	Edema, headache, dizziness. C/I: severe aortic stenosis, obstructive cardiomyopathy, LV failure, unstable angina AMI*. May use in post-MI LV dysfunction if no clinical CHF	Reduce dose in elderly or in liver disease or with cimetidine. High fat meal increases absorption; grapefruit juice markedly interferes with liver breakdown.

* Saltiel, Drugs 1988; 36: 387–428; AMI = acute phase myocardial infarction; CHF = congestive heart failure

successfully controlled with intravenous verapamil or diltiazem, the latter with nifedipine or preferably with intravenous nicardipine.

Supraventricular Tachyarrhythmias

Verapamil and diltiazem are still regarded by many as the
drugs of choice for the control of SVT, although their place
is now challenged by the much shorter acting adenosine.
Verapamil and diltiazem continue to be used for the reduction of the ventricular response rate in atrial fibrillation
and/or flutter. However, an exception must be made when
these arrhythmias complicate the use of *hypothermic anesthetic techniques*. Because of the myocardial depression
inherent with hypothermia, a life-threatening depression of
cardiac output may follow administration of CCAs in this
situation. Further, as previously noted, before treatment is
embarked upon there must be certainty of the diagnosis of
SVT in contra-distinction to VT, and, of course, such treatment must be ECG monitored.

For the acute therapy of SVT or atrial flutter/fibrilla-
tion, *verapamil* given as an IV bolus of 5–10 mg (0.1–0.15
mg/kg) over a minute has an onset of action within 1 to 2
minutes, provided that there is no major myocardial
depression. This may be accompanied by a short-lived
hypotensive effect which dissipates within 20 minutes, with
the depression of AV nodal conduction persisting. If necessary this bolus dose may be repeated after 10 minutes.
Thereafter, if required, treatment may be continued by a
continuous infusion of 5µg/kg/min for 30–60 minutes. For
intravenous diltiazem dosage, see Table 5-3.

Alternative strategies. The recently introduced very
short-acting beta-blocker, *esmolol* (elimination half-life 9
minutes), though it also carries the risk of myocardial
depression, has the virtue of allowing a faster retreat from
any unfavorable reaction.

In the important differentiation between SVT and VT,
IV *adenosine* (ultra short-acting, half-life 10 seconds) provides both a therapeutic and diagnostic test. Adenosine
stops SVT but leaves VT unchanged, any complicating
myocardial depression being obviated by its ultra short
half-life. When the ECG diagnosis is equivocal, or the
hemodynamic state in doubt, adenosine is preferred to
CCAs.

Acute Severe Hypertension

During *coronary artery bypass grafting*, acute hypertension with tachycardia may accompany sternotomy especially when high-dose opioid anesthetic techniques are used
(van Wezel, 1989). Likewise, during emergence from
anesthesia, though elevations in blood pressure are not
uncommon and are seldom of clinical consequence, rarely,
in 3–9% of patients substantial hypertension of the order of
>180/110 mmHg is observed. Its occurrence is often asso-
ciated with previous or poorly controlled hypertensive disease (60% of patients) or widespread atherosclerotic
vascular pathology and often follows surgery such as

Drug	Indication	Dose	Pharmacological effects	Precautions
Verapamil (Isoptin)	1. Paroxysmal supraventricular tachycardia* 2. Reduction of ventricular response rate in atrial fibrillation or flutter*	IV 5–10 mg, may repeat after 10 min. IV infusion 1 mg/min to total of 10 mg. IV infusion (myocardial depression) 0.0001 to 0.005 mg/kg/min.	Bolus drops BP within 1–2 min, peak effect 5–12 min. Effect on AV node 10 min to 6 h. If risk of hypotension pretreat with calcium gluconate (90 mg).	C/I ventricular tachycardia, WPW, sick sinus syndrome, AV block, LV depression or prior therapy with IV beta-blocker or IV digoxin or digoxin toxicity. Care in obstructive cardiomyopathy.
Diltiazem (Cardizem injectable, Cardizem Lyo-ject Syringe)	As above	IV 0.25 mg/kg (~20 mg) over 2 min; then after 15 min 0.35 mg/kg (~25 mg) over 2 min then infuse at 5–15 mg/h; constant infusions at 3, 5, 7, 11 mg/h give steady state levels similar to oral doses of 120, 180, 240, 360 mg daily	SVT usually reverts within 3 min. In atrial flutter or fibrillation, heart rate reduction within 2–7 min, lasts for hours after end of infusion. Hypotension may last for hours.	As above.
Nicardipine (Cardene IV)	Perioperative hypertension Licensed in USA for short term treatment of hypertension	Solution of 0.1 mg/ml (not in sodium bicarbonate or Ringer's); individualize dose; for gradual BP fall, 5–15 mg/h; for more rapid BP fall, higher doses. Must monitor BP carefully.	High first pass metabolism inactivates drug possibly in proportion to liver blood flow. BP starts to fall within 10 min. After infusion, BP effect halves after about 30 min with persisting effect up to 50 h.	C/I in severe aortic stenosis, obstructive cardiomyopathy. Caution in LV disease, may be less depressant than nifedipine. Excess hypotension if beta-blockade plus anesthesia.
Nifedipine (Procardia, Adalat capsules)	Perioperative hypertension (off label use)	5–10 mg capsules, pierced and swallowed or contents washed down nasogastric tube. Poor absorption if given sublingually†	BP starts to fall within 10 min; risk of excess hypotension.	As above. Avoid in congestive heart failure. Prefer intravenous agents.
Nimodipine (Nimotop)	To reduce ischemic defects due to subarachnoid hemorrhage due to ruptured congenital aneurysms; possibly cerebral anti-ischemic protection	30 mg capsule, pierced and swallowed or contents washed down nasogastric tube. In UK: IV infusion 1 mg/h increased after 2h to 2 mg/h; less if hypotension	BP fall within minutes (time not clearly defined).	As for nifedipine capsules. Caution with cerebral edema. Avoid in peri-operative period (bleeding)

* WPW = Wolff-Parkinson-White syndrome; SVT= supraventricular tachycardia; † van Harten et al, 1987. Lancet 2: 1363; IV = intravenous

coronary artery bypass grafting or carotid endarterectomy (Bertrand, 1989). Such hypertension may lead to acute LV failure, myocardial ischemia or infarction, cardiac arrhythmias or intracerebral hemorrhage, depending on the patients underlying medical status. Commonly associated factors include pain, hypoxia, hypercapnea, fluid overload and emergence delirium. While such acute hypertension demands aggressive evaluation and rapid treatment, the therapeutic approach should be tempered by the realisation that in the peri-operative period more clinical disasters follow profound hypotension than severe hypertension. It is recommended that treatment of the hypertension per se be commenced if the systolic pressure exceeds 180 mmHg and/or the diastolic 110 mmHg, or if the post-operative blood pressure exceeds the preoperative by more than 20%, or if signs of cardiac or neurological compromise develop.

Nifedipine is often effective (Sodoyama et al, 1983), although there is no proper outcome study with this agent. Capsules (5–10 mg) with ends perforated may be swallowed when the patient is fully conscious, or the contents may be sucked into a syringe and administered down a nasogastric tube when one is in situ. Contrary to common belief, sublingual administration of nifedipine leads to poor absorption and low blood levels (van Harten et al, 1987). Recent serious doubts about safety (Grossman et al, 1997) should be seen in perspective. These authors collected 16 cases of serious side-effects, and the only two who died were given nifedipine for unstable angina (contraindicated) rather than for severe hypertension, while the third who developed sinus arrest had pulmonary hypertension with an initial blood pressure of only 110/70 mmHg. Yet when carefully given to monitored patients with severe hypertension, Jennings et al (1986) found nifedipine to be safe and effective. Nifedipine capsules, being powerfully hypotensive, should be given only with great caution in the elderly (Pahor et al., 1995). It should be considered that a 5 mg dose (half the contents of a 10 mg capsule) is often as effectively hypotensive as 10 mg (Maharaj and van der Byl, 1992), the latter dose or higher being used in all of the cases with reported adverse side-effects (Grossman et al, 1996).

Nicardipine, being less cardiodepressant than nifedipine and available as an intravenous formulation (continuous infusion, 3µg/kg/min), offers a more elegant manner of BP control (van Wezel, 1989). A negative inotropic effect has been noted in about 10% of patients (David et al, 1991).

When the hypertension is accompanied by tachycardia, short-acting beta-blockade with *esmolol* is indicated (see Chapter 7).

Other drugs commonly used for this condition are *labetalol* (5 mg increments intravenously until control is achieved, followed by infusion of 2.5–7.5 mg per hour) or *hydralazine* (10–20 mg infused slowly). *Sodium nitroprusside* requires great care because the blood pressure may drop abruptly and coronary steal phenomenon may occur after coronary artery bypass grafting.

INTERACTIONS OF CCAs AND ANESTHETICS

Cardiovascular Interactions

While their detailed cardiovascular pharmacodynamic pro-files are varied (Forrest, 1989; Jones, 1990; Hartman et al, 1992), all the modern volatile anesthetic agents — halothane, ethrane, isoflurane, sevoflurane and desflurane — display a central core of actions exactly similar to those of CCAs (Terrar, 1993 and see Chapter 2) namely (i) nega-tive inotropic effect on myocardial contractility; (ii) varying depressive chrono- and dromotropic effects on sinoatrial activity and AV nodal conduction; and (iii) reduction of systemic vascular resistance secondary to vasodilation. Further, these actions are secondary to the effects these agents have on calcium fluxes across cellular and organelle membranes (Franks and Lieb, 1994; Wide et al, 1993; Lee et al, 1994). It is not surprising, therefore, that serious interac-tions (Fig 5-5) may become manifest when patients on chronic medication with CCAs, especially when combined with beta-adrenoceptor blockade, are submitted to anesthe-sia with any of these agents (Merin et al, 1987). Likewise, similar interactions may be expected when for any reason CCAs are administered acutely during the course of general anesthesia with any of these volatile agents. Such interac-tions manifest as exaggerated, life-threatening and often dif-ficult to control depression of cardiovascular function — the precise functional depression depending in large mea-sure on the 'vasodilation to negative inotropic ratio' which characterizes the particular CCA involved. Any or all of the modalities of inotropy, SA nodal pacing, AV nodal conduc-tion (to the extent of complete heart block or asystole) and SVR can be affected.

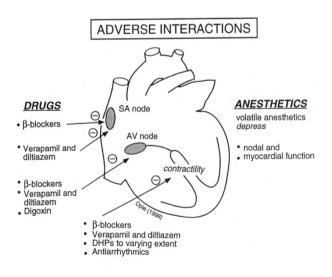

Fig 5-5. Adverse interactions. *Possible adverse interactions between volatile anesthetics and drugs acting on the SA (sino-atrial) and AV (atrioventricular) nodes or on contractility. DHPs = dihydropyridines. (Fig. copyright © LH Opie, 1998).*

Whether such interactions are additive or synergistic, no generalisations can be made. From the point of view of clinical management, the answer varies with the agents involved and the observed parameters on which the judgement is based. While most interactions appear to be additive, ethrane has been noted to be associated with the more severe interactions — inter-reactions that could then be regarded as synergistic (Atlee et al, 1988; Lynch, 1988; Kapur et al, 1984).

In contrast to the volatile anesthetics, no specific interactions are documented between the CCAs and the most commonly used intravenous anesthetic agents thiopentone, etomidate, propofol or high-dose opioid anesthesia (Bronheim and Thys, 1993).

Potassium Homeostasis

Also of relevance to these cardiovascular interactions, especially those concerned with chrono- and dromotropy, is the manner in which CCAs influence the response to potassium homeostasis. CCAs have been shown to increase the sensitivity of the myocardium to hyperkalemia — a condition characterized by intraventricular conduction defects even to the extent of causing complete heart block (Nugent et al, 1984). Moreover, in CCA-treated animals, smaller doses of potassium were shown to produce hyperkalemic effects than was the case with controls and such effects were only partially corrected by intravenous calcium. This must be borne in mind during clinical anesthesia when patients on CCA medication require massive transfusion of stored blood e.g. during cardiac or major vascular surgery or surgery for multiple trauma.

Non-cardiovascular Interactions

Enhancement of neuromuscular blockade. As the CCAs (especially verapamil) may reduce calcium and/or sodium conductance at presynaptic sites as well as modifying the intracellular presynaptic calcium ion pool, the possibility arises that they may enhance or prolong the actions of neuromuscular blocking drugs (Durant et al, 1984). Clinically relevant enhancement of neuromuscular blockade (NMB) by both nondepolarizing and depolarizing NMB agents has been documented by many observers (Foex, 1987). These observations carry the implication that peri-anesthetic *"train of 4" monitoring* of NMB is important in patients receiving CCAs and postoperative observation of such patients should be particularly vigilant to avoid the risk of unrecognized neuromuscular blockade.

Interactive reduction of MAC. Verapamil has been shown to reduce by 25% the Mean Anesthetic Concentration (MAC) of halothane — an action attributed to its actions on Na^+ as well as Ca^{2+} channels (Maze et al, 1983). The relevance of this observation to the even greater reduction of MAC associated with the CCA like actions of adenosine is speculative (Kress and Tass, 1993).

MANAGEMENT OF ADVERSE INTERACTIONS

The key to the successful management of the above adverse drug interactions is early detection through adequate and appropriate monitoring of the components of cardiovascular function, followed by a timeous and appropriate response. For such response the following strategies have been advocated (Fig 5-6).

(a) Intravenous atropine may be sufficient to counter bradycardia or mild degrees of heart block.

(b) An intravenous bolus of calcium chloride may help but often as a temporary measure only. In the case of verapamil, whereas the drop in blood pressure may be reversed, its AV nodal effects are not (Lehot et al, 1987). Similarly, the circulatory depression caused by nifedipine and beta-adrenoceptor blockade is only partially reversed by calcium administration (De Wolf et al, 1984), so that further measures may be needed.

(c) Catecholamine infusion can be of use but may fail in the face of severe CCA overdosage when the calcium channels are heavily blocked. Logically, a calcium infusion could be added, yet this combination with catecholamines may promote ventricular arrhythmias and possibly an excessive increase in afterload from the adrenergic vasoconstrictive effect.

(d) Phenylepherine, a pure alpha$_1$-adrenergic agonist, has been successfully used in patients receiving combina-

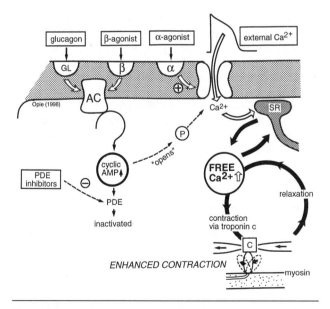

Fig 5-6. Measures to increase cytosolic calcium. For overdose of calcium channel antagonists or adverse interactions between these drugs and β-blockers, several different measures can be used to induce a rise of cytosolic Ca^{2+} concentration and hence to increase contractility. PDE = phosphodiesterase; SR = sarcoplasmic reticulum; GL = glucagon receptor; α = alpha-adrenoreceptor; β = beta-adrenoreceptor. (Fig. copyright © LH Opie, 1998).

tion therapy with CCAs and beta-blockade (Massagee et al, 1987).

(e)   Glucagon, a hormone which links to adenylate cyclase and to cyclic AMP by a receptor which is independent of the beta-adrenoceptor, is a practical alternative or addition to the above. It antagonizes the myocardial depression caused by verapamil, diltiazem and nifedipine (Zaritsky et al, 1988).

(f)   Amrinone and milrinone, powerful phosphodiesterase inhibitors, also increase cytosolic cyclic AMP levels independently of the beta-adrenoceptor and have been shown to reverse the effects of verapamil whether alone or in combination with beta-blockade (Makela and Kapur, 1987).

CCAs AND ORGAN PROTECTION

Myocardial Protection

Protection of the ischemic myocardium during cardiopulmonary bypass is achieved by the use of a variety of cardioplegic solutions, local myocardial cooling and whole body hypothermia. As reperfusion injury is thought to be initiated by increased calcium flux into the ischemic myocardium with consequent cell damage, the use of CCAs could be expected to be beneficial (Fleckenstein-Grun, 1994). Verapamil and diltiazem protect myocardial ATP stores during cardiac arrest and lead to more normal myocardial function thereafter (Yamamoto et al, 1983; Balderman et al, 1984). In a prospective randomised study on patients undergoing coronary bypass grafting, nifedipine infusions (not commercially available) given for 24h from the onset of extracorporeal circulation had beneficial effects, the incidence of myocardial infarction fell, and perioperative necrosis was reduced (Seitelberger et al 1991). Furthermore, CCAs have been shown to reduce experimental reperfusion stunning (du Toit and Opie, 1992). However, fear of the negative inotropic effects of these agents in the postcardioplegic period has prevented their widespread clinical use.

Cerebral Protection?

This use of CCAs may be considered only in highly selected cases of brain ischemia. Drugs with a degree of selectivity for cerebral vasodilation, such as *nimodipine*, experimentally inhibit vasospasm induced by spasmogenic agents such as serotonin, catecholamines, histamine, thromboxane or whole blood. Clinical studies in selected patients with subarachnoid hemorrhage show that the addition of nimodipine to other measures — low molecular weight dextran and supportive care — speeds up neurological recovery and decreases mortality without adverse effects on the cardiovascular system (Gelmers, 1988). In contrast, when nimodipine was given with the aim of preventing neurological side-effects after cardiopulmonary bypass, then there was an increased mortality, explained by excess bleeding (Wagenknecht et al, 1995), so that in the view of the present authors, nimodipine is clearly contraindicated during cardiothoracic surgery.

After cardiac arrest, because of a vasoconstrictive increase in cerebral vascular resistance and glial cell swelling, neurological recovery may be hindered by cerebral hypoperfusion once normal circulation has been restored (Rolfsen and Davis, 1989). Administered after circulation has been re-established following cardiac arrest, both nicardipine (Iwatsuki et al, 1987) and nimodipine (Forsman et al, 1989) have been shown to improve neurological outcome. When considering long-term 1 year prognosis, nimodipine gave no advantage over placebo despite an early decrease in the incidence of recurrent ventricular fibrillation (Roine et al, 1990).

MAGNESIUM: A CCA-LIKE AGENT

The cardiovascular pharmacological actions of magnesium and adenosine mirror those of the CCAs. However, in contrast to the classical CCAs, their 'calcium antagonism' is the indirect secondary response to other primary mechanisms. Accordingly discussion of the general pharmacology of magnesium sulfate is appended here. For convenience that of adenosine is included with that of other agents acting on smooth muscle (Ch.6). The specific antiarrythmic use of both these agents is covered in Ch.7.

Long regarded as of little importance in clinical anesthesia (other than for its conventional use in eclampsia) magnesium, in its role as the "physiological CCA" (Iseri and French, 1984) has been shown, of recent years, to have actions which add greatly to the armamentarium of cardiovascular drugs of the anesthesiologist and intensivist (James, 1992). Magnesium's actions relevant to anesthetic practice stem from its effects on cytosolic calcium concentration by competing with calcium ions for their entry through calcium channels, and in the regulation of transmembrane pumps which extrude calcium from the cytosol by competing with calcium for various protein kinase binding sites. The result, when there is hypermagnesemia, is a basic core of cardiovascular pharmacological actions which mirror those of the conventional CCAs while at the same time enjoying the advantage of easy clinical controllability because of its moderately large volume of distribution, rapid renal-elimination and consequently short half-life.

Mechanisms of Action and Pharmacodynamics

(a) *Peripheral vasodilation.* Peripheral vasodilation is the most prominent of magnesium's cardiovascular actions and it may account for the mild tachycardia often found. The vasodilation stems both from its direct CCA-like effect on the peripheral vasculature (Altura, 1987), and from an indirect action, depression of calcium-mediated autonomic transmitter release. At higher dosage levels the latter effect can produce ganglionic blockade (Mordes and Whacker, 1978).

(b) *Negative inotropic effect.* Negative inotropic effects do not appear to be a troublesome accompaniment of magnesium therapy when used alone (James, 1992). Sustained severe myocardial depression, however, has been documented following the combined use of diltiazem and magnesium (Wallis et al, 1986).

(c) *Antiarrhythmic effects.* These result from several mechanisms (also see Ch.7). First, there is inhibition of the release of catecholamines from the adrenergic nerve terminals so that catecholamine-induced arrhythmias are counteracted (Mayer et al, 1989). A similar mechanism may explain why magnesium is effective in a variety of other arrhythmias (Iseri, 1986) including those induced by bupivacaine overdose (Solomon et al, 1990). Secondly, magnesium appears to be specifically effective in torsades de pointes, a particularly dangerous arrhythmia fortunately seldom met in anesthetic practice (Tzivoni et al, 1988). Torsades is predisposed to by chronic depletion of magnesium and/or potassium, and also by the use of certain agents that prolong the action potential duration such as sotalol or quinidine. While, intravenous infusion of magnesium will terminate the arrhythmia, optimal clinical practice predicates that torsades de pointes should be prevented by pre-anesthetic correction of magnesium and/or potassium depletion (Gambling et al, 1988).

(d) *Nervous system effects.* Effects on the neuromuscular junction are a manifestation of magnesium's depressive effect on calcium-mediated transmitter release. Here, induced hypermagnesemia (at plasma levels of greater than 2.5 mmol/l) produces dose-dependent presynaptic inhibition of acetylcholine release with consequent depression of neuromuscular transmission (Krendal, 1990). At 5 mmol/l the degree of neuromuscular block is substantial, greatly enhancing the action of muscle relaxant drugs as well as other conditions which depress neuromuscular transmission such as myasthenia gravis or Lambert-Eaton syndrome (Ghonheim and Long, 1970; Sinatra et al, 1985; Skaradoff et al, 1982). While the actions of both non-depolarizing and depolarizing relaxants are affected, Baraka and Yazigi (1987) found no prolongation of the action of a single dose of succinyl choline in magnesium-treated pre-eclamptic mothers.

Pharmacokinetics and Dosage of Magnesium

The above pharmacological effects require a circulating blood level of magnesium ion of 2 to 4 mmol/l (physiological levels 0.7 to 1.0 mmol/l). This is achieved through the intravenous administration of a solution of magnesium sulfate by continuous infusion while monitoring appropriate cardiovascular parameters e.g. BP, ECG, central venous pressure (James, 1992). In the presence of normal renal function, the following dosage schedule is required: loading dose magnesium sulfate 40–60 mg/kg; continuous maintenance infusion 15–30 mg/kg/hour. This rate of infusion may be adjusted to levels appropriate to the clinical requirements.

Peri-anesthetic use of Magnesium

Pheochromocytoma. Induced hypermagnesemia finds a particular application in the anesthetic management of patients undergoing resection of pheochromocytomas (James, 1992). Inclusion of continuous infusion of magnesium sulfate in the anesthetic technique effectively controls the acute hypertensive (and possibly arrhythmic) response of these patients to maneuvers that stimulate and/or enhance catecholamine release. Such events include induction of anesthesia, endotracheal intubation and the surges of catecholamine release which accompany surgical handling of the tumor. When the latter is excessive, supplementation with an additional short-acting vasodilator such as sodium nitroprusside may be required. Following resection of the tumor, magnesium sulfate infusion is discontinued. At this time, especially in patients who have been on heavy dosage of adrenergic blocking agents preoperatively, some adrenergic inotropic support may be required. To avoid possible problems with reversal of neuromuscular blockade when infusion of magnesium has been prolonged and dosage high, it is recommended that the shorter acting relaxant, vecuronium be used.

Cardiac and vascular surgery. In terms of arrhythmia prevention, the need for correction of hypomagnesemia preoperatively, already noted, is of particular importance in the anesthetic management of cardiopulmonary bypass surgery. Again the value of magnesium as an antiarrhythmic in the anesthetic management of this branch of surgery is well documented (Iseri, 1990; England et al, 1992). In addition to catecholamine-induced arrhythmias, intractable ventricular tachycardia and torsades de pointes, magnesium is of value also in controlling the arrhythmias associated with digitalis and hypokalemia. Magnesium has also been used as a component of cardioplegic solutions for the protection it affords the ischemic myocardium and its counteraction of Ca^{2+}-induced reperfusion injury (Hearse et al, 1981; Yano et al, 1985). The vasodilatory and antiarrhythmic effects of magnesium also find application during the aortic cross clamping phase of resection of abdominal aortic aneurysm — an additional advantage being protection of the spinal cord from ischemic neuronal damage at this time (Amory et al, 1990).

Gestational proteinuric hypertension/Caesarean section. For decades before this condition acquired its present name of gestational proteinuric hypertension (GPH), magnesium has been — and is still being — used successfully in the treatment and prevention of eclampsia. Its therapeutic success, for reasons not long clearly understood, is now thought to depend almost entirely on its vasodilatory properties. Peripherally this lowers the vascular resistance and so reverses the hypertensive manifestations of the condition while centrally its powerful cerebral vasodilatory action reverses the cerebral vasospasm now considered the probable cause of the convulsions characteristic of this condition (Van den Plas et al, 1990; Trommer et al, 1988; Sadeh, 1989).

When patients treated by continuous magnesium infusion present for anesthesia for Caesarean section two disadvantages are: first, the synergism of magnesium and neuromuscular blocking agents — both depolarizing and non-depolarizing; and second, the sensitivity of such patients because of magnesium-induced vasodilation to blood and fluid loss with consequent, possibly excessive, hypotension (Liao, 1990).

Use in critical care medicine. While it is self-evident that magnesium should enjoy the same attention as the other physiological ions in management of the electrolyte homeostasis of patients requiring intensive care, in certain conditions the pharmacological properties of hypermagnesemia may have application. In *acute myocardial infarction,* a beneficial effect on the incidence and severity of early postinfarction arrhythmias has been attributed to magnesium by some workers (Rasmussen, 1989; Bertschat, 1989), while another reports a reduction in mortality (Schechter, 1990). However, enthusiasm for the apparent myocardial protective effects of magnesium in the early post infarction phase have now been dampened by the negative outcome of a recent large and authoritative clinical trial (ISIS-4 study, 1994). Nonetheless, a careful review of the experimental data strongly suggests that magnesium should be given at the time of reperfusion and not thereafter, as was the case in ISIS-4. There will therefore be another trial (MAGIC, MAGnesium In Coronary thrombosis) in which the emphasis will be on the early administration of magnesium (Antman, 1995). In *tetanus,* less well known and still insufficiently evaluated, is the use of magnesium in the treatment of that most serious complication of tetanus — autonomic dysfunction (Lipman et al, 1987).

Interaction between magnesium and anesthetic agents. Interaction of magnesium administration with anesthetic agents appears to be confined to a non-specific summation of their respective effects on systemic vascular resistance and so the level of hypotension.

SUMMARY

1.   *Mechanisms of action of CCAs.* These agents directly impede transsarcolemmal calcium entry into myocardial and vascular smooth muscle cells by inhibition of "slow current" L-calcium channels. This causes: (i) a negative inotropic effect on myocardial contraction; (ii) negative chronotropic and dromotropic effects on the SA node and AV nodal conduction, and (iii) vasodilation. The latter is more prominent on arteriolar (including coronary circulation) than venous vasculature. Recently T-channel blockade has been identified as a mechanism of sinus node slowing and vasodilation.

2. *DHPs vs non-DHPs.* While CCAs include agents derived from three chemical structures, for practical clinical purposes they can be classified into two groups with chiefly cardiac and vascular actions. Vasodilation is the predominant action of the dihydropyridine (DHP) group represented by nifedipine and its derivatives such as amlodipine. Nodal and myocardial effects are most prominent with the 'non-DHP' drugs verapamil and diltiazem. Sometimes the CCAs are divided into the first generation agents, verapamil, nifedipine and diltiazem and their recent long-acting forms. The second generation agents are the recently developed DHPs that are either long-acting (amlodipine) or more vascular selective (felodipine, nisoldipine) and/or in long acting formulations (isradipine).

3. *Clinical properties.* Regarding the non-DHPs major indications are angina, ischemic heart disease, supraventricular tachycardia (SVT), and hypertensive heart disease. Diltiazem is reasonably well tested in unstable angina, and verapamil less so. Verapamil has better evidence for post-infarction cardioprotection, with some evidence for the use of diltiazem after non-Q-wave infarcts. DHPs have as major indications hypertension and effort angina. They are not well tested in unstable angina, nor post-infarct. Short acting nifedipine capsules are contraindicated in unstable angina or early infarction.

4. *Combination therapy.* Both DHPs and non-DHPs may be combined with beta- blockers or with ACE inhibitors or nitrates. Because of their negative inotropic and added nodal inhibitory effects, caution must be exercised when non-DHPs are combined with beta-adrenergic blockade.

5. *Cautions and contraindications.* Non-DHPs are contraindicated by any condition associated with depressed LV function or nodal or AV conduction defects, such as sick sinus syndrome or heart block of varying severity. Contraindications to the DHPs include any condition associated with fixed cardiac output state such as LV outflow obstruction (aortic stenosis, hypertrophic obstructive cardiomyopathy). Depressed LV function is a relative contraindication, with the safest drugs being amlodipine and felodipine. Unstable angina or early myocardial infarction are specific contraindications to nifedipine capsules unless beta-blockade is also given. DHPs as a group are not well tested in unstable angina nor in myocardial infarction. Nimodipine is now contraindicated in the peri-operative period because of an observed increased incidence of surgical bleeding (Wagenknecht et al 1995). In addition, caution is required in the elderly because there may be increased perioperative bleeding with CCAs as a group, possibly through an interaction with ketorolac.

6. *Volatile anesthetic agents*: halothane, en-, iso-, des-, and sevoflurane share many properties with the CCAs. When anesthetized with any of these agents, patients

134 Calcium Channel Antagonists

on chronic medication with the latter may suffer additive or synergistic depression of cardiovascular function. This caveat applies particularly to those on combined CCA/beta-adrenoceptor blocker therapy.

7. *Peri-anesthetic use.* CCAs (verapamil or diltiazem) are directly indicated for the therapy of: (i) paroxysmal supraventricular tachycardia (PSVT) and (ii) reduction of ventricular rate in atrial fibrillation or flutter. Contraindications include WPW. For acute hypertension — use intravenous nicardipine but not nifedipine for careful control of the rate of BP drop. For the above indications, treatment with adenosine (PSVT) or the short acting beta-blocker, esmolol, may be preferred.

8. *Excess effects of CCAs.* Countermeasures to CCA overdosage or exaggerated interaction with volatile anesthetics should aim to increase cytoplasmic calcium levels. The following intravenous agents can be can be used: (i) atropine; (ii) calcium chloride; (iii) catecholamine infusion; (iv) phenylephrine; (v) glucagon; (vi) phosphodiesterase inhibition by amrinone or milrinone. In life-threatening situations a combination of agents with actions mediated by different cellular mechanisms is logical.

9. *Magnesium* may be regarded as a physiological CCA when infused to plasma levels of 2–4 mmol/l. The principal pharmacological effects are: peripheral and cerebral vasodilation, and inhibition of calcium-mediated transmitter release in the autonomic nervous system (including the adrenal medulla), and at the neuromuscular junction. Consequent on the latter is an antiarrhythmic effect on the heart and depression of neuromuscular transmission. These properties find their most useful application to anesthetic practice during resection of pheochromocytoma, cardiopulmonary bypass surgery, and in the obstetric/anesthetic management of gestational proteinuric hypertension. The most important adverse reaction is its inhibitory effect on neuromuscular transmission with enhancement of the action of neuromuscular blocking agents. This must be anticipated and controlled.

REFERENCES

Altura BM. Magnesium-calcium interaction in contractility of vascular smooth muscle: magnesium versus organic calcium channel blockers on myocardial tone and agonist-induced responsiveness of blood vessels. *Canad J Physiol Pharmacol* 1987; 65: 729–745.

Amory DW, Jasaitis D, Wright C. Use of magnesium to protect against spinal cord ischemia. *Anesthesiology* 1990; 73: A732.

Antman EM. Magnesium in Acute MI Timing is critical. *Circulation* 1995; 92: 2367–2372.

Atlee JL, Hartman SR, Brownlee, SW, Kreigh C. Conscious state comparisons of the effects of the inhalational anaesthetics and diltiazem, nifedipine or verapamil on specialised atrioventricular conductive times in spontaneously beating dog hearts. *Anesthesiology* 1988; 68: 519–528.

Balderman SC, Chan AK, Gage AA. Verapamil cardioplegia: improved myocardial preservation during global ischemia. *J Thorac Cardiovasc Surg* 1984; 88: 57–66.

Baracka A, Yazigi A. Neuromuscular interaction of magnesium with succinyl choline — vercuronium sequence in eclamptic parturients. *Anesthesiology* 1987; 67: 806–808.

Bertrand ML. Post-operative circulatory complications, In: Nunn JF, Utting JE, Brown BR (eds), *General Anaesthesia*, 5th edition, Butterworth, London, 1989, 1160–1166.

Bertschat F, Ising H, Gunther T, et al. Antiarrhythmic effects of magnesium infusions in patients with acute myocardial infarction. *Magnesium Bulletin* 1989; 11: 155–158.

Bronheim D, Thys DM. *Cardiovascular Drugs in Principles and Practice of Anesthesiology,* Vol 2. Rogers MC, Tinker JH, Corvino BC, Long-Necker DE (eds). Mosby Year Book Inc, Chicago, 1993, 1541–1574.

Butterworth JF, Zaloga GP. Calcium and magnesium as vasoactive drugs. In: Skarvan K (ed). *Balliere's Clinical Anaesthesiology,* Balliere Tindall 1994; 8: 109–136.

Cohn JN, Ziesche S, Smith R, et al. Effect of the calcium antagonist felodipine as supplementary vasodilator therapy in patients with chronic heart failure with enalapril (V-HeFT III Study). *Circulation* 1997; 96: 856–863.

David D, Du Bois C, Loria Y. Comparison of nicardipine and sodium nitroprusside in treatment of paroxysmal hypertension following aorto-coronary bypass surgery. *J Cardiothorac Vasc Anesth* 1991; 5: 357–361.

DEFIANT Research Group (Doppler Flow and Echocardiography in Functional cardiac Insufficiency: Assessment of Nisoldipine Treatment). Improved diastolic function with the calcium antagonist nisoldipine (coat-core) in patients postmyocardial infarction: results of the DEFIANT study. *Eur Heart J* 1992; 13: 1496–1505.

DEFIANT-II Study. Doppler flow and echocardiography in functional cardiac insufficiency: Assessment of nisoldipine therapy. Results of the DEFIANT-II study. *Eur Heart J* 1997; 18: 31–40.

De Wolf A, Marquez J, Nemoto E, et al. Cardiovascular effects of isoflurane, enflurane and halothane anesthesia with calcium and beta-blockade in the monkey. *Anesthesiology,* 1984; 61: A13

Durant NN, Nguyen K, Katz RL. Potentiation of neuromuscular blockade by verapamil. *Anesthesiology* 1984; 60: 298–303.

Du Toit EJ, Opie LH. Modulation of severity of reperfusion stunning in isolated rat hearts by agents altering calcium flux at onset of perfusion. *Circ Res* 1992; 70: 960–967.

England MR, Gordon G, Salem M, Chernow B. Magnesium administration and dysrhythmias after cardiac surgery: a placebo-controlled double-blind randomised trial. *JAMA* 1992; 268: 2395–2402.

Ertel S, Ertel EA and Clozel J-P. T-type CA^{2+} channels and pharmacological blockade: potential pathophysiological relevance. *Cardiovasc Drugs Ther* 1997; 11: 723–739.

Fischer Hansen J. Postinfarct prophylaxis by calcium antagonists. In: Opie LH (ed). *Myocardial Protection by Calcium Antagonists.* Authors' Publishing House/Wiley-Liss, New York, 1994, 98–111.

Fleckenstein-Grun G. Intracellular calcium overload — A cytotoxic principle: cellular protection by calcium antagonists. In: Opie LH (ed), *Myocardial Protection by Calcium Antagonists. Wiley Liss/Authors' Publishing House, New York 1994, 29–45.*

Foëx P. Channel blockers. In: Feldman SA, Scurr CF, Paton W (eds). *Drugs in Anesthesia: Mechanisms of action.* Edward-Arnold Publishers, London, 1987, 353–380.

Forrest JB. Comparative pharmacology of inhalational anesthetics. In: Nunn JF, Utting JE, Brown BR (eds), *General Anesthesia,* 5th ed. Butterworths, London, 1989, 60–72.

Forsman M, Aarseth HP, Skulbert A, et al. Effects of nimodipine on cerebral blood flow and cerebrospinal fluid pressure after cardiac arrest. Correlation with neurological outcome. *Anesth Analg* 1989; 68: 436–443.

Franks NP Lieb WR. Molecular and cellular mechanisms of general anesthesia. *Nature* 1994; 36: 607–614.

Furberg CD and Psaty BM. Corrections to the nifedipine meta-analysis. (Letter). *Circulation* 1996; 93: 1475–1476.

Furberg CD, Psaty BM and Meyer JV. Nifedipine dose-related increase in mortality in patients with coronary heart disease. *Circulation* 1995; 92: 1326–1331.

Gambling DR, Birmingham CL, Jenkins LC. Magnesium and the anesthetist. *Canad J Anesth* 1988; 35: 644–654.

Gelmers HJ, Gorter K, DeWeerdt CJ et al. A controlled trial of nimodipine in acute ischaemic stroke. *N Engl J Med* 1988; 318: 203–207.

Ghonheim MM, Long JP. The interaction between magnesium and other neuromuscular blocking agents. *Anesthesiology* 1970; 32: 23–27.

Göbel EJ, Hautvast RW, and Gilst WH, et al. Randomised, double-blind trial of intravenous diltiazem versus glyceryl trinitrate for unstable angina pectoris. *Lancet* 1995; 346: 1653–1657.

Godfraind T, Salomone S, Dessy C, et al. Selectivity scale of calcium antagonists in human cardiovascular system based on in vitro studies. *J Cardiovasc Pharmacol* 1992; 20 (Suppl 5): S34–S41.

Grossman E, Messerli FH, Grodzicki T, Kowey P. Should a moratorium be placed on sublingual nifedipine capsules given for hypertensive emergencies and pseudoemergencies. *JAMA* 1996; 276:1328–1331.

Hartman JC. Pagel PS, Proctor LT, et al. Influences of desflurane, isoflurane and halothane on regional tissue perfusion in dogs. *Canad J Anaesth* 1992; 39: 877–887.

Hearse DJ, Braimbridge MV, Jynge P. *Protection of the Ischaemic Myocardium: Cardioplegia.* Raven Press, New York, 1981.

HINT Research Group (Holland Interuniversity Nifedipine/Metoprolol Trial). Early treatment of unstable angina in the coronary care unit: a randomised double-blind placebo-controlled comparison of recurrent ischaemia in patients treated with nifedipine or metoprolol or both. *Br Heart J* 1986; 56: 400–413.

Iseri LT. Role of magnesium in cardiac tachyarrhythmias. *J Cardiol* 1990; 65: 47K–50K.

Iseri LT. Magnesium and cardiac arrhythmias. *Magnesium* 1986; 5:111–126.

Iseri LT, French JH. Magnesium: nature's physiologic calcium blocker. *Am Heart J* 1984; 108: 188–193.

ISIS-4 Collaborative Group. A randomised factorial trial assessing early oral captopril, oral mononitrate, and intravenous magnesium sulphate in 58050 patients with suspected acute myocardial infaction. *Lancet* 1995; 345: 669–685.

Iwatsuki N, Ono K, Koga Y, Amaha K. Prevention of postischemic hypoperfusion after canine cardiac arrest by nicardipine. *Crit Care Med* 1987; 15: 313–317.

James MFM. Clinical use of magnesium infusion in anesthesia. *Anesth Analg* 1992; 74: 129–136.

Jennings A, Jee LD, Smith JA, et al. Acute effect of nifedipine on blood pressure and left ventricular ejection fraction in severely hypertensive outpatients. Predictive effects of acute therapy and prolonged efficacy. *Am Heart J* 1986; 111: 557–563

JNC VI. Joint National Committee on Prevention, Detection, Evaluation and Treatment of High Blood Pressure. The Sixth Report of the Joint National Committee on Prevention, Detection, Evaluation and Treatment of High Blood Pressure. *Arch Intern Med* 1997; 157: 2413–2446.

Jones RM. Desflurane and sevoflurane: Inhalational anesthetics for this decade. *Br J Anaesth* 1990; 65: 527–536.

Kapur PA, Bloor BC, Flacke WE, Orwin SK. Comparison of cardiovascular responses to verapamil during influrane, isoflurane and halothane anesthesia in the dog. *Anesthesiology* 1984; 61: 156–160.

Krendal DA. Hypermagnesemia and neuromuscular transmission seminars in neurology. *Semin Neurol* 1990; 10: 42–45.

Kress HG, Tass PWL. The effects of second messenger calcium in neurones and non-muscular cells. *Br J Anaesth* 1993; 71: 47–58.

Lee DL, Zhang J, Blanck JJ. Effects of halothane on voltage-dependent calcium channels in isolated Langendorff perfused rat hearts. *Anesthesiology* 1994; 81: 1212.

Lehot JJ, Leone BJ, Foëx P. Calcium reverses global and regional myocardial dysfunction caused by the combination of verapamil and halothane. *Acta Anaesth Scand* 1987; 31: 441–447.

Liao JC, Lijima T, Palahniuk RJ. Effect of magnesium sulphate on hemodynamics and reflex sympathetic vasoconstriction. *Anesthesiology* 1990; 73: 942A.

Lipman J, James MFM, Erskine J, et al. Autonomic dysfunction in severe tetanus: magnesium sulphate as an adjunct to deep sedation. *Crit Care Med* 1987; 15: 987–988.

Lynch C. Combined depressant effects of diltiazem and volatile anesthetics on contractility in isolated ventricular myocardium. *Anesth Analg* 1988; 67: 1036–1046.

MACH-I and Levine TB. For the MACH-I Investigators. The design of the Mortality Assessment in Congestive Heart Failure Trial. *Clin Cardioil* 1997; 20: 320–326.

Maharaj B and van der Byl K. A comparison of the acute hypotensive effects of two different doses of nifedipine. *Am Heart J* 1992; 124: 720–725.

Makela VHM, Kapur PA. Amrinone and verapamil-propranolol induced cardiac depression during isoflurane anesthesia in dogs. *Anesthesiology* 1987; 66: 792–797.

Massagee JT, McIntyre RW, Kates RA, et al. Effects of preoperative calcium entry blocker therapy on alpha-adrenergic responsiveness in patients undergoing coronary revascularization. *Anesthesiology* 1987; 67: 485–491.

Mayer DB, Miletich DJ, Feld JM, Albrecht RF. The effects of magnesium salts on the duration of epinephrine-induced ventricular tachyarrhythmias in anesthetized rats. *Anesthiology* 1989; 71: 23–28.

Maze M, Mason DM, Kates RE. Verapamil decreases MAC for halothane in dogs. *Anesthesiology* 1983; 59: 327–329.

Merin RG, Chelly JE, Hysing ES, et al. Cardiovascular effects and interaction between calcium blocking drugs and anesthetics in chronically instrumented dogs. IV. Chronically administered oral verapamil and halothane, influrane and isoflurane. *Anesthesiology* 1987; 66: 140–146.

Mordes JP, Wacker WEC. Excess magnesium. *Pharmacol Rev* 1978; 29: 273–300.

Nugent M, Tinker JH, Moyer TP. Verapamil worsens the rate of development and hemodynamic effects of acute hyperkalemia in halothane anesthetized dogs: effect of calcium therapy. *Anesthesiology* 1984; 60: 435–439.

Opie LH, Frishman WH, Thadani U. Calcium channel antagonists. In: Opie LH (ed), *Drugs for the Heart,* 4th edition. WB Saunders Company, Philadelphia, 1995, 50–82.

Opie LH, Messerli FH. Nifedipine and mortality. Grave defects in the dossier. *Circulation* 1995; 92: 1068–1073.

Opie LH. Calcium channel blockers for hypertension – dissecting the evidence for adverse effects. *Am J Hypertens* 1997; 10:565–577.

Pahor M, Guralnik JM, Corti M, et al. Long term survival and use of antihypertensive medications in older persons. *J Am Geriat Soc* 1995; 43: 1191–1197.

Pollare T, Lithell H, Selinus I, Berne C. Sensitivity to insulin during treatment atenolol and metropolol: a randomised, double-bind study of the effects on carbohydrate and lipoprotein metabolism in hypertensive patients. *Brit. med. J* 1989; 298:1152–1157.

PRAISE Study. Packer M, O'Connor C, et al. for the Prospective Randomized Amlodipine Survival Evaluation Study Group. Effect of amlodipine on morbidity and mortality in severe chronic heart failure. *N Engl J Med* 1996; 335: 1107–1114.

Rasmussen HS. Clinical intervention studies on magnesium in myocardial infarction. *Magnesium* 1989; 8: 316–325.

Reuter H. Ion channels in cardiac cell membranes. *Ann Rev Physiol* 1984; 45: 473–484.

Roine RO, Kaste M, Kinnunen A, et al. Nimodipine after resuscitation from out-of-hospital ventricular fibrillation. *JAMA* 1990; 264: 3171–3177.

Rolfsen ML, Davis WR. Cerebral function and preservation during cardiac arrest. *Crit Care Med* 1989; 17: 238–292.

Sadeh M. Action of magnesium in the treatment of preeclampsia-eclampsia. *Stroke* 1989; 20: 1273–1275.

Schechter M. Beneficial effect of magnesium in acute myocardial infarction. *Magnesium Bulletin* 1990;12: 1–5.

Seitelberger R, Zwolfer W, Huber S et al. Nifedipine reduces the incidence of myocardial infarction and transient ischemia in patients undergoing coronary bypass grafting. *Circulation* 1991; 83: 460–468.

Sinatra RS, Phillip BK, Naulty JS, Ostheimer GW. Prolonged neuromuscular blockade of vecuranium in a patient treated with magnesium sulphate. *Anesth Analg* 1985; 64: 1220–1222.

Singh BH, Collet JT, Chew CYC. New perspectives in the pharmacological therapy of cardiac arrhythmias. *Prog Cardiovasc Dis* 1980; 22: 243–301.

Skaradoff MN, Roaf ER, Datta S. Hypermagnesemia and anesthetic management. *Canad J Anaesth* 1982; 29: 35–41.

Sodoyama O, Ikeda K, Matsuda I, et al. Nifedipine for control of postoperative hypertension. *Anesthesiology* 1983; 59: A18.

Solomon D, Bunegin I, Albin M. The effect of magnesium sulphate administration on cerebral and cardiac toxicity of bupivacaine in dogs. *Anesthesiology* 1990; 73: 341–346.

Spedding M, Paoletti R. Classification of calcium channel antagonists: progress report. *Cardiovasc Drugs Ther* 1992; 6: 35–39.

STONE Study. Gong L, Zhang W, et al. Shanghai Trial of Nifedipine in the Elderly. *J Hypertens* 1996; 14: 1237–1245.

Syst-Eur Trial, Staessen JA, Fagard R, et al. Randomised double-blind comparison of placebo and active treatment for older patients with isolated systolic hypertension (Syst-Eur Trial). *Lancet* 1997; 350: 754–764.

Terrar DA. Structure and function of calcium channels and the actions of anesthetics. *Br J Anaesth* 1993; 71: 39–46.

Trommer BL, Homer D, Mikhael MA. Cerebral vasospasm and eclampsia. *Stroke* 1988; 19: 326–329.

Tzivoni D, Banai S, Schuger C, et al. Treatment of torsade de pointes with magnesium sulphate. *Circulation* 1988; 77: 392–397.

Van den Plas L, Dive A, Dooms G, Mahieu P. Magnetic resonance evaluation of severe neurological disorders in eclampsia. *Neuroradiology* 1990; 32: 47–49.

Van Harten J, Burggraaf K, Danhof M, et al. Negligible sublingual absorption of nifedipine. *Lancet* 1987; 2: 1363–1365.

Van Wezel HB, Kookem JT, Visser GA, et al. The efficacy of nicardipine and sodium nitroprusside in preventing post-sternotomy hypertension. *J Cardiol Anesth* 1989; 3: 707.

Wagenknecht LE, Furberg CD, Hammon JW, et al. Surgical bleeding: Unexpected effect of a calcium antagonist. *Brit. Med. J.* 1995: 310: 776–777.

Wallis DE, Gierke LW, Scanlon PJ, et al. Sustained postischemic cardiodepression following magnesium-diltiazem cardioplegia. *Proc Soc Exp Biol Med* 1986; 182: 375–385.

WHO-ISH Committee. Ad Hoc Subcommittee of the Liaison Committee of the World Health Organisation and the International Society of Hypertension. Effects of calcium antagonists on the risks of coronary heart disease, cancer and bleeding. *J Hypertens* 1997; 15: 105–115.

Wide DW, Davidson BA, Smith MD, Knight PR. Effects of isoflurane and enflurane on intracellular calcium mobilization in isolated cardiac myocytes of the rat. *Anesthesiology* 1993; 79; 73–82.

Yamamoto F, Manning AS, Braimbridge MV, Hearse DJ. Cardioplegia and slow calcium-channel blockers. *J Thorac Cardiovasc Surg* 1983; 86: 252–261.

Yano Y, Milam DF, Alexander JC. Terminal magnesium cardioplegia: protective effect in isolated rat heart model using calcium accentuated ischemic damage. *J Surg Res* 1985; 39: 529–534.

Zaritsky AL, Horowitz M, Chernow B. Glucagon antagonism of calcium channel blocker-induced myocardial dysfunction. *Crit Care Med* 1988; 16: 246–251.

Zuccala G, Pahor M, Landi F, et al. Use of calcium antagonists and need for perioperative transfusion in older patients with hip fracture; observational study. *BMJ* 1997; 314: 643–644.

CHAPTER 6

Vascular Smooth Muscle and Vasodilators

Bruce Leone

Vasodilators are used widely in the management of patients with arterial hypertension, congestive heart failure and angina. They are also used extensively in the management of hypertensive crises, especially during the perioperative period, and they play a major role in the control of acute myocardial ischemia. The major classes of vasodilators include the nitrovasodilators, the ACE inhibitors and the angiotensin receptor antagonists. Calcium channel antagonists are discussed in chapter 5.

NITRIC OXIDE DONORS

In 1980 Furchgott and Zawadski demonstrated that the vasorelaxant action of acetylcholine in isolated aortic rings was mediated by a diffusible factor released from the endothelium (Furchgott and Zawadski, 1980). In 1987 Palmer and colleagues, using a chemiluminescence assay, showed that nitric oxide was at least one of the relaxing factors (Palmer et al, 1987). The *nitrovasodilators* are a group of pharmacological agents producing their pharmacological effects by releasing nitric oxide. This group includes nitroglycerin, sodium nitroprusside, isosorbide mono- and dinitrate, SIN-1, amyl nitrite and K^+ channel opening agents such as nicorandil.

Mechanism of action of nitric oxide

Nitric oxide is synthesized from the guanidino-nitrogen of the L-arginine (Fig 6-1). This transformation is controlled by an enzyme, nitric oxide synthase, which can be stimulated by a number of physical and chemical signals and is inhibited by arginine analog (most commonly L-NAME and L-NMMA). After release from the endothelial membrane, nitric oxide diffuses across the extracellular space into the smooth muscle cell and utilizes the soluble guanylate cyclase, leading to an increase in the intracellular concentration of cyclic GMP which activates a protein kinase resulting in smooth muscle relaxation (Fig 6-1). Cyclic GMP also stimulates calcium efflux and calcium uptake by intracellu-

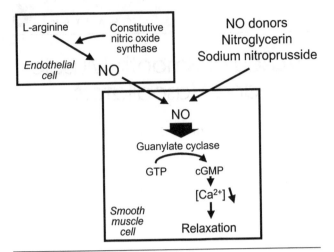

Fig 6-1. The central role of nitric oxide (NO) in the control of vasorelaxation.

lar stores. It may also inhibit calcium influx by decreasing the production of diacyl glycerol (DAG) and inositol 1,4,5 triphosphate (IP$_3$) resulting in a decrease in protein kinase C activity.

Release of NO. The most important physiological stimulus for the release of nitric oxide is the increase of shear stress that can be produced by elevated flow velocity or viscosity of the blood (Pohl et al, 1986). However, nitric oxide is continuously released by the endothelium to regulate the level of vascular tone. Some authors have demonstrated that a vasoconstrictor influence is required for basal NO release (Adeagbo et al, 1994). NO can also be released from non-adrenergic non-cholinergic nerves that innervate certain blood vessels (Toda and Okamura 1991).

Inhaled NO. Inhalation of NO provides selective vasodilation of the pulmonary circulation since NO absorbed into blood is rapidly inactivated by hemoglobin. However, high doses of NO administered to anesthetized rabbits induce acute effects on blood pressure and bleeding times.

Perioperative use of NO. Inhaled NO in patients undergoing surgery is successfully used in several instances:

1. Adult valvular patients with high pulmonary resistance and right ventricular failure, during weaning off assisted ventilation (Girard et al, 1992; Fullerton et al, 1997).

2. Right ventricular failure after cardiac transplantation (Girard et al, 1993).

3. Pulmonary transplantation: NO may be of use in helping to avoid the use of extra-corporeal bypass.

4. Surgery for congenital heart defects with pulmonary hypertension (Journois et al, 1993; Matsui et al, 1997).

5. Persistent pulmonary hypertension of the newborn (Roberts et al, 1992; Roberts et al, 1997).

6. Acute Respiratory Distress Syndrome (Rossaint et al, 1993; Manketlow et al, 1997; Zapol, 1996).

Sodium Nitroprusside

Pharmacodynamics and mechanisms of action

Sodium nitroprusside's action is due to the release of nitric oxide (Fig 6-1). Despite the fact that sodium nitroprusside has been widely used for many years, the precise mechanism by which it releases nitric oxide has only recently been elucidated. Nitroprusside releases nitric oxide in the presence of light. When exposed to reducing agents, large quantities of nitric oxide are released. Red cell membranes and smooth muscle cell membranes have these reducing capacities (Bates et al, 1981). It is noteworthy that tolerance does not develop with nitroprusside.

Pharmacological action

Hemodynamic effects. Nitroprusside is a rapidly acting intravenous antihypertensive agent. The hypotensive effects are due to vasodilatation, and its effect on the arteriolar vascular bed is at least as potent as that in the venous system. The hemodynamic consequences of nitroprusside administration are a decrease in both preload and afterload and a reduction in blood pressure. Nitroprusside reduces ventricular filling pressures by directly increasing venous compliance, resulting in a redistribution of blood volume from central to peripheral veins: peripheral vascular resistance is decreased and aortic compliance is increased as a consequence of arteriolar dilation. Nitroprusside also dilates pulmonary arterioles and reduces right ventricular afterload. These hemodynamic effects are titratable and can be interrupted abruptly by stopping the infusion. A reflex tachycardia and a transient rise in cardiac output may accompany the vasodilatory effects of intravenously administered nitroprusside.

The combined decrease in preload and afterload improves myocardial energetics by reducing wall tension. Moreover, nitroprusside has a direct coronary vasodilator effect. However, in patients with coronary disease, the arteriolar vasodilatation may result in coronary steal by diverting coronary blood flow from muscle supplied by partially occluded vessels to non ischemic territories (Oates et al, 1995).

Toxicity. A special problem with nitroprusside is the formation of toxic metabolites: thiocyanate and cyanide ions. The metabolism of nitroprusside includes the release of cyanides from the molecule, its transformation to thiocyanate by liver rhodanese and elimination by the kidney. This conversion is enhanced if exogenous sulfur, usually thiosulfate, is supplied thereby reducing blood cyanide levels. Thiocyanate toxicity is indicated by unexplained abdominal pain, mental status changes, or convulsions. Cyanide toxicity may appear as an increasing drug requirement, acidosis, and increasing venous PO_2 and oxygen content denoting an increasing inability of the cells to use oxygen. The mean elimination half-life of thiocyanate is 3 days in patients with normal renal function. The use of nitroprusside is contraindicated in patients with hepatic or renal failure (Tinker and Michenfelder, 1976).

Nitroglycerin

Pharmacodynamics and mechanisms of action

The first therapeutic use of glyceryl trinitrate was proposed by Murrel in 1879 "as a remedy for angina pectoris". Since this first description, organic nitrates have remained the main treatment of angina pectoris.

Mechanism of action. Nitroglycerin is one of the few therapeutic agents which undergoes biotransformation to its active form at the site of action. Current hypotheses as to the mechanism of action of organic nitrates are that these compounds undergo biotransformation in vascular smooth muscle cells to an activator of guanylate cyclase, resulting in increased accumulation of cyclic GMP and relaxation. Several nitrogen-oxide-containing products are presumably formed from organic nitrates: nitric oxide, inorganic nitrite (NO_2^-) and intermediates like S-nitrosothiols, thionitrates and sulfinyl nitrites. Multiple biotransformation systems for organic nitrates contribute to NO formation (Fig 6-1).

Tolerance to nitroglycerin. The efficiency of nitroglycerin is decreased after 18 to 24 hours. This is in part due to a decrease in the formation of nitric oxide from nitroglycerin. The administration of thiols does enhance vasodilation produced by nitroglycerin both in vivo and in vitro, but this is not specific for tolerance. Thiol-donating compounds enhance the effect of nitroglycerin even in the non-tolerant state (Münzel et al, 1989).

Pharmacological action of nitroglycerin

Hemodynamic effects. The nitroglycerin relaxes both arterial and venous smooth muscle cells. Low concentrations of nitroglycerin predominantly dilate veins. Nitroglycerin may increase the venous pooling resulting in a decrease in left ventricular end-diastolic pressure and volume: the decrease in systemic vascular resistance is mild at these low doses. Higher doses of organic nitrates cause further venous pooling and decrease arteriolar resistance, predominantly decreasing systolic blood pressure and cardiac output. An activation of compensatory sympathetic reflexes results in tachycardia and peripheral arteriolar vasoconstriction.

Effects on coronary blood flow. Several studies demonstrate that nitrates are potent dilators of both normal and atherosclerotic coronary arteries, thereby increasing coronary blood flow. Brown and colleagues demonstrated that approximately 75% of stenoses dilated in response to nitroglycerin and suggested that this resulted from dilation of the normal portion of the artery in eccentric stenoses (Brown et al, 1994). Collateral flow to ischemic regions is increased and a redistribution of blood flow to subendocardial tissue occurs. Finally, despite a potent vasodilatory effect on large coronary arteries, the net increase in coronary blood flow is submaximal and brief (Fam et al, 1968).

This suggests that nitroglycerin has only a minor effect on the smaller coronary arteries. Other studies demonstrated that the lack of effect on small coronary arteries was due to an incapacity to convert nitroglycerin to its more vasoactive metabolites (Sellke et al, 1991; Kurz et al, 1991). These studies support an important role for intracellular thiols as a co-factor in an enzymatic process of conversion of nitroglycerin to active metabolites. Nitroglycerin preferentially dilates large coronary arteries and has a poor effect on coronary resistance. These effects may explain the absence of steal phenomenon, an effect that is usually observed with agents (such as dipyridamole) which act on small coronary arteries.

Effects on myocardial oxygen requirements. The hemodynamic effects of nitroglycerin on the systemic circulation explain the reduction in myocardial oxygen demand. The major determinants of myocardial oxygen consumption include left ventricular wall tension, heart rate and contractility. Nitroglycerin affects mainly ventricular wall tension by increasing venous capacitance, which in turn decreases venous return to the heart and thereby decreases left ventricular wall tension and myocardial oxygen consumption. An additional benefit of reducing preload is the increased left ventricular perfusion favouring the subendocardium. Organic nitrates do not directly affect the inotropic state. However, an improvement in the lusitropic state of the heart may be seen, with more rapid early diastolic filling.

Dosage and pharmacokinetics

Nitroglycerin remains the treatment of choice for episodes of angina pectoris and is effective for short term angina prophylaxis. The nitrates in common use include nitroglycerin, isosorbide dinitrate (ISDN) and isosorbide 5-mononitrate (ISMN).

When administered sublingually an effective concentration of nitroglycerin rapidly appears in the circulation because sublingual administration avoids first pass metabolism. The metabolism of nitroglycerin is mainly via the hepatic enzyme glutathione organic nitrate reductase. The clinical effects dissipate in 30 to 60 minutes.

Nitroglycerin is available as an oral sustained release tablet (Table 10-7). This formulation is widely used clinically. Transdermal nitroglycerin patches are also available for the prophylactic treatment of patients with angina pectoris. Applicable each day, patches must be left in place 24 hours. However, the efficacy of the nitroglycerin patches may be improved by limiting transdermal dosing to 12 hours per day, thus avoiding the development of tolerance.

Oral ISDN is the most frequently prescribed nitrate. However, the problem of tolerance still remains with this type of formulation if frequent daily doses are prescribed. With eccentric dosing, the medication is given in a fashion that provides a period of washout and tolerance is largely prevented.

ISMN is the metabolite of ISDN. It has an excellent bio-availability after oral administration and does not undergo a first pass hepatic metabolism. This property offers the advantage of more predictable clinical effects. Immediate and sustained release ISMN are available but for both formulations, tolerance has been clearly documented. The most recent preparation of ISMN is a controlled release preparation that has been shown to provide high plasma levels of ISMN during the first 12 hours following administration, but with low plasma levels during the following 12-hour period. This preparation was designed to provide a period of low nitrate exposure to prevent the development of tolerance.

The effects of intravenous nitroglycerin have been well described for many years (Sorkin et al, 1984). When nitroglycerin is administered by a continuous intravenous infusion, the hemodynamic effects appear in 90 seconds and are dose dependent. Only 1% of the nitroglycerin infused is detected in the plasma compartment because of a high volume of distribution. The hemodynamic effects disappear in a few minutes following the discontinuation of an intravenous infusion.

Perianesthetic use of nitrates

During the perioperative period, several indications for the use of nitrates have been proposed:

1. *Treatment of myocardial ischemia peri- and post-operatively:*

   a) Myocardial ischemia associated with ventricular arrhythmia especially when anesthesia is increased by halogenated anesthetics.

   b) Myocardial ischemia with an increase in pulmonary wedge pressure persisting with an increased inspired fraction of halogenated anesthetics.

   c) Coronary artery spasm

   d) Myocardial ischemia occurring without any change in blood pressure and heart rate during deep anesthesia levels (Slogoff and Keats, 1985).

2. *Intraoperative prevention of myocardial ischemia:*

   The intravenous administration of nitroglycerin has been proposed to provide prophylaxis against myocardial ischemic episodes during vascular surgery (Coriat et al, 1984).

3. *Improvement of left ventricular function in patients with coronary disease postoperatively:*

   The administration of a continuous intravenous infusion of nitroglycerin prevents decreases in ejection fraction in coronary patients during recovery from anesthesia (Coriat et al, 1986).

4. *Control of aortic pressure and pulmonary wedge pressure during aortic cross-clamping:*

   The venodilation induced by nitroglycerin is beneficial during aortic cross-clamping. It prevents the increase in pulmonary wedge pressure after clamping during abdominal aortic aneurysm repair (Attia et al, 1976). The short half-life of nitroglycerin allows rapid dissipation of hemodynamic effects and mitigates against a fall in systemic pressure after unclamping.

5.   *Treatment of hypertensive episodes intraoperatively:*

The use of nitroglycerin has been proposed to treat acute increase in blood pressure intra- and postoperatively in different situations:

a)   During coronary artery surgery (Kaplan and Jones, 1979).

b)   During non-cardiac surgery in severely hypertensive patients.

c)   During eclampsia, nitroglycerin is effective in preventing the hypertensive response to endotracheal intubation (Hood et al, 1985).

However, since the hypotensive properties of nitroglycerin are mainly due to a decrease in venous return, its use must be cautious in potentially hypovolemic patients and in patients with hypertrophic cardiopathy. Nitroglycerin can be administered intravenously either as a continuous infusion (0.5-3.0 mg/kg/min) or bolus (0.5 mg).

6.   *Treatment of postoperative cardiogenic pulmonary edema:*

Intravenous nitroglycerin is indicated for the treatment of cardiogenic pulmonary edema, especially in patients with coronary heart disease, because of its beneficial effects on left ventricular preload and myocardial energetic balance.

RENIN-ANGIOTENSIN SYSTEM

Physiology

The renin-angiotensin system (RAS) plays a central role in the maintenance of blood pressure and regulation of volume, particularly during anesthesia.

The RAS is defined as a biochemical cascade (Fig 6-2). A highly specific proteolytic enzyme, renin, cleaves an ineffective peptide precursor, angiotensinogen, to generate a decapeptide, angiotensin I (AI). AI is converted to an octapeptide, angiotensin II (AII), by a non specific carboxypeptidase, the angiotensin-converting enzyme (ACE). AII is the effective final product of enzymatic reactions.

In addition to its role in the RAS, the ACE (also named kininase II) inactivates the vasodilatory and natriuretic bradykinin. Thus ACE increases blood pressure in producing the vasoconstrictor and salt retaining AII and by degrading a vasodepressor and salt-excreting molecule: bradykinin.

Angiotensin II is a powerful vasoconstrictor acting on both arteries and veins. The angiotensin II-induced vasoconstriction is the result of direct activation of the angioten-

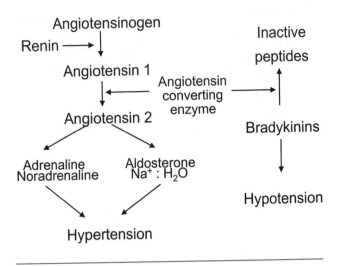

Fig 6-2. Role of the renin-angiotensin-aldosterone system in the control of blood pressure.

sin II AT_1 receptor and potentiation of the effects of the sympathetic nervous system.

Angiotensin II interacts with at least two known angiotensin membrane receptors, type 1 and type 2 (AT_1 and AT_2) (Timmermans et al, 1993). The physiological effects of AII, such as vasoconstriction, aldosterone stimulation and salt and water homeostasis seem to be mediated via stimulation of the G-protein-coupled AT_1 receptor, which then activates phospholipase C to generate diacylglycerol (DAG) and inositol triphosphate (IP_3). IP_3 releases calcium from intracellular stores which results in smooth muscle cell contraction (Fig 4-3, page 94). Calcium and DAG activate enzymes including protein kinase C and calcium calmodulin kinases that catalyse phosphorylation. The role of AT_2 receptors is less clear. They may be involved in proliferation and differentiation of smooth muscle cells.

Angiotensin facilitates norepinephrine (NE) release from sympathetic nerves, as well as the release of both NE and epinephrine into the bloodstream, by both a direct effect to release neuro-effector stores and an indirect effect by adrenergic ganglion stimulation (Fig 1-4, page 6). By activation of central receptors, AII can increase sympathetic outflow from the brain to both the vasculature and myocardium.

Although plasma renin originates mainly from kidneys, other organs such as brain, heart, adrenals and blood vessels also produce renin. Almost all angiotensin I and II is generated within tissue rather than in plasma (Dzau, 1987). AII is released in the circulation and binds to specific receptors on target organ tissue, acting like a diffuse endocrine system. Thus, a complete renin-angiotensin system can be found locally in vascular smooth muscle. Clearly, angiotensin release by vascular smooth muscle cells may have important influences on autocrine and paracrine functions.

Role of RAS in anesthesia and surgery

Anesthesia and surgery have significant effects on the RAS. The surgery by itself is responsible for stimulation of the

RAS as part of a general increase in different hormones involved in the "stress response" (Traynor and Hall, 1981).

The RAS participates in the regulation of blood pressure during anesthesia using halothane or isoflurane (Kataja et al, 1988). The role of RAS in the regulation of blood pressure is enhanced by sodium or volume depletion, which may occur during the perioperative period (Miller et al, 1978).

Activation of RAS is well known to occur during controlled hypotension (Miller et al, 1977), cardiopulmonary bypass (Taylor et al, 1977), and aortic cross-clamping (Grindlinger et al, 1981).

ACE Inhibitors

Hemodynamic effects

ACE inhibitor (ACEI) effects depend on the underlying pathophysiologic state and degree of RAS activation. ACEIs lower blood pressure mainly by reducing peripheral vascular resistance with no change in cardiac output (Haber, 1976). ACEIs have relaxant effects not only on arterioles but also on large arteries and veins, explaining the decrease in cardiac filling pressures. ACEIs increase the parasympathetic tone, but the sympathetic response to baroreflex stimulation is maintained (Cody et al, 1981).

Dosage and pharmacokinetics

A large number of ACEIs are now available for clinical use. The main differences between these molecules are in potency, the need for a conversion from a prodrug to an active compound, and pharmacokinetics.

Captopril has a short onset of action when given orally (30 minutes) and its effect on blood pressure lasts 3 to 4 hours.

The administration of ACEIs as prodrugs such as enalapril implies that the prodrug must be de-esterified after absorption into the active compounds (Table 10-6). The onset of action of these drugs is typically delayed (1 to 4 hours) and the duration of the blood pressure lowering effect is prolonged (from 12 to more than 24 hours).

Enalaprilat is available for intravenous administration at a dosage of 0.625 to 1.25 mg over 5 minutes and may be repeated every 6 hours.

Therapeutic use of ACE inhibitors

Hypertension. ACEIs lower blood pressure, except in primary hyperaldosteronism, and are first-line drugs in the treatment of essential hypertension. In addition to their effect on blood pressure, this class of antihypertensive drug prevents the effect of angiotensin on migration and proliferation of vascular and cardiac smooth muscle cells (Jackson, 1995).

Left ventricular systolic dysfunction. Large, prospective, randomized, placebo-controlled clinical trials have shown that ACEIs given to patients with systolic dysfunction, prevent and delay the progression of heart failure, decrease the incidence of sudden death and myocardial infarction, decrease hospitalization and improve quality of life (CONSENSUS Trial Study Group, 1987).

Myocardial infarction. Studies have shown that the overall mortality was reduced when ACE inhibitors are given shortly after infarction (Ambrosioni et al, 1996).

Progressive renal impairment. ACEIs have been shown to delay the impairment of renal function in diabetic nephropathy (Lewis et al, 1993).

Adverse effects

Hypotension. This adverse effect occurs in patients with elevated plasma renin activity during the initial dosing of the drug. Thus, in patients with congestive heart failure or salt depletion, treatment must be initiated with small doses of ACE inhibitors.

Cough. This is the most frequent adverse effect of ACE inhibitors. It is observed in 5 to 20% of patients and is not related to the dose. It is probably due to an accumulation of bradykinin in the lungs.

Hyperkalemia. Increased serum potassium may be observed in patients with renal failure, in patients taking potassium sparing diuretics, beta adrenoceptor blockers, or non-steroidal anti-inflammatory drugs (NSAIDs).

Acute renal failure. ACE inhibitors can induce renal insufficiency in patients with bilateral renal stenosis or stenosis of the renal artery of a single remaining kidney. Renal insufficiency has also been observed in patients with normal renal arteries but with other risk factors, such as hypovolemia induced by diuretics and salt depletion, congestive heart disease, age, and treatment with NSAIDs.

Interactions with anesthesia

Concerns regarding potential hemodynamic instability (hypotension and bradycardia) have been reported in patients undergoing general anesthesia in whom ACEIs were given before surgery (Kataja et al, 1989).

In hypertensive patients treated with ACEIs, it has also been suggested that the decrease in blood pressure during induction of anesthesia may be amplified by the diastolic dysfunction observed in these patients (Colson et al, 1992).

Perianesthetic use of ACEIs

Despite the adverse reactions observed during induction of anesthesia in patients treated with ACEIs, the use of these drugs has been proposed in several instances.

Some studies have examined the ability of ACEIs to attenuate the pressor response during tracheal intubation but ACEIs were either ineffective (Murphy et al, 1989) or resulted in hypotension or bradycardia (McCarthy et al, 1990).

The use of ACEIs has been proposed during controlled hypotension. It has been shown that the dose of sodium nitroprusside required to achieve target mean arterial blood pressure was decreased when patients were pretreated pre-operatively with ACEIs (Woodside et al, 1984).

ACEIs have been used to prevent the impairment of renal hemodynamics during cardiopulmonary bypass for coronary bypass (Colson et al, 1990).

Angiotensin II Receptor Antagonists

The development of other drugs acting on the RAS, particularly on the angiotensin receptor, was pursued for several reasons. Firstly, because despite their efficacy in the treatment of hypertension and congestive heart failure, ACEIs are implicated in adverse effects of which cough is the most frequent. This is due to the fact that ACE is not a specific enzyme and has other substrate besides angiotensin I, including bradykinin, substance P, neurokinins, and luteinizing hormone releasing hormone (LHRH).

Angiotensin receptor (AT_1) antagonists, a new class of pharmacologic blockers of the RAS, have been shown to be safe and effective antihypertensive agents.

Pharmacodynamic and mechanism of action

AT_1 receptor antagonists block the pressor and functional responses to angiotensin II both in vitro and in vivo. AT_1 non-peptide receptor antagonists display no intrinsic properties, unlike the peptide *saralasin*, the first AT_1 receptor antagonist. *Losartan* is a potent, orally active, specific and competitive AT_1 receptor antagonist. This agent causes reactive increase in plasma renin, angiotensin I and II with a fall in aldosterone. *Valsartan, candesartan,* and several other AT_1 blockers are now available. All are licensed for hypertension and at present not for heart failure in the US.

Pharmacokinetics and dosage

Losartan is well absorbed when given orally. This drug undergoes a hepatic first pass metabolism by a p450 cytochrome. Losartan is partially metabolized into an active metabolite and inactive metabolites. Losartan is given orally once a day at a dose ranging from 25 to 50 mg (Goa and Wagstaff, 1996).

Therapeutic use

Hypertension. Losartan 50 mg once a day lowers blood pressure in patients with mild to moderate hypertension over 24 hours (Ikeda et al, 1997).
Congestive heart failure. Angiotensin II receptor antagonists may have some advantages over ACEIs. With losartan, first dose hypotension may be avoided. Angiotensin II receptor antagonists will antagonize A II generated via non-ACE pathways, and losartan may avoid renal side effects. However, large scale trials showing a reduction of mortality in heart failure are thus far available only for ACE inhibitors and not for AT_1 blockers.

ADENOSINE

Adenosine is a purine nucleoside recently used in the clinical setting for its anti-arrhythmic and vasodilatory properties.

Chemistry, pharmacodynamics and mechanism of action

Adenosine is formed by the dephosphorylation of adenosine monophosphate (AMP) via the catalytic action of 5'nucleotidase (Fig 6-3). AMP may be produced from the degradation of ATP and ADP intracellularly or may be formed from extracellular sources, such as platelets and endothelium. Adenosine may also be produced by the breakdown of S-adenosyl-homocysteine to adenosine and homocysteine.

The biological actions of adenosine are the result of interactions with receptors on the cell membrane:

a)   adenosine 1 and 2 receptors modulate the activity of the cyclic AMP system, independently of beta-adrenergic activity (Van Calker et al, 1979).

b)   adenosine may activate an acetylcholine-sensitive potassium receptor causing a hyperpolarization of the cell membrane by increasing potassium conductance through its channel in the atrium, sinus node and AV node. This effect is not dependent upon cyclic AMP (Belardinelli et al, 1989).

c)   adenosine blocks the slow inward calcium current during the upstroke of an action potential in the myocyte. This effect is potentiated by a beta-adrenergic stimulation which increases the flow of inward calcium current. This is called the "indirect action" of adenosine (Belardinelli et al, 1988).

Adenosine is transported into the cell by a specific adeno-

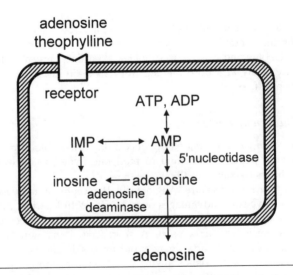

Fig 6-3. Diagrammatic representation of the metabolism of adenosine in cardiac cells.

sine transport system. Adenosine is then either degraded by deamination or phosphorylated to AMP intracellularly.

Physiological action

During ischemia, adenosine is released by the myocardium (Fig 6-4). This is probably the result of the breakdown of ATP to AMP and AMP to adenosine. Since adenosine is a potent coronary vasodilator, it participates in the local regulation of coronary blood flow by dilating the coronary bed perfusing an ischemic territory to improve oxygen delivery to this region. Moreover, it decreases heart rate through its action on the SA node, depresses contractility in the atrium and ventricle, and may decrease the amount of norepinephrine released. As a consequence, myocardial oxygen demand is decreased.

Pharmacological effects of adenosine

In the SA node, adenosine has a negative chronotropic effect and may cause sinus bradycardia and sinus arrest when used at high dose (DiMarco et al, 1983).

The effect of adenosine in the AV node results in a dose-dependent increase in the interval between atrial and bundle of His conduction.

There is little direct effect on ventricular myocytes in the absence of catecholamines. Through its indirect effect, adenosine depresses ventricular contractility when cyclic AMP levels are elevated. This indirect cardiac effect is anti-adrenergic, as it counteracts the positive chronotropy, dromotropy and inotropy induced by circulating catecholamines.

Vascular properties of adenosine

Adenosine induces relaxation of vessels by increasing cyclic AMP formation through the stimulation of A_2 receptors.

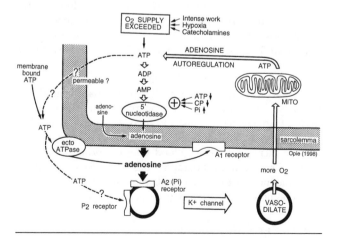

Fig 6-4. Adenosine as vasodilator. *Adenosine formed from ATP in conditions of increased myocardial work of hypoxia is thought to interact with a vascular A_2 receptor (see Table 7-1) to cause vasodilation. ATP may act as an additional dilator. CP = creatine phosphate, Pi = inorganic phosphate. (Fig. copyright © L.H. Opie, 1998)*

Depending on the vessel studied, adenosine causes either an endothelium-dependent or independent dilation.

The vasodilatory properties of adenosine have been shown in several vascular territories. In the coronary circulation, it increases coronary blood flow and has been associated with steal phenomenon.

Bolus injections of adenosine induce negative chronotropic and dromotropic effects on SA and AV nodes but no change in blood pressure; continuous administration exerts different hemodynamic effects. In anesthetized patients, adenosine has been used to induce and maintain hypotension during surgery (Owall et al, 1987). Hypotension induced by adenosine infusion is the result of a decrease in systemic vascular resistance coupled with an increase in cardiac output without tachycardia or pressure rebound at the end of the infusion. Adenosine dilates cerebral vessels inducing an increase in cerebral blood flow. This precludes its use in patients with intracranial hypertension. Adenosine also has vasodilatory effects on the pulmonary vascular bed (Morgan et al, 1991).

Dosage and pharmacokinetics

Adenosine must be administered intravenously in order to elicit a pharmacological response. It is metabolized very quickly in the blood, with a plasma half-life of 1 to 7 seconds. Adenosine is prepared in 2 ml vials containing either 6 or 12 mg of adenosine (see page 181).

Therapeutic use of adenosine

Diagnostic and treatment of supraventricular tachycardia. Adenosine is useful in the emergency management of AV nodal re-entrant supraventricular tachycardia and specific types of ventricular tachycardia (DiMarco et al, 1983; Lerman et al, 1986; Griffith et al, 1988). The dosage that is effective for these indications ranges from 3 to 30 mg in rapid bolus.

Blood pressure control during anesthesia. Induced hypotension or control of hypertensive episodes can be obtained by a continuous intravenous infusion of adenosine at rates ranging from 50 to 350 mg/kg/min (Sollevi et al, 1984; Owall et al, 1987).

Pulmonary hypertension. Adenosine can act as a selective pulmonary vasodilator, especially when infused centrally.

Coronary artery disease. Intracoronary or intravenous injections of adenosine are also used to assess coronary flow reserve. During thallium-201 cardiac imaging, adenosine is used to increase coronary blood flow in normally perfused areas. Stress echocardiography has also been performed using adenosine to induce wall motion abnormalities and thus diagnose myocardial regions at risk for ischemia.

Adenosine antagonists

Methylxanthines, including *theophylline* and *aminophylline*, act as competitive antagonists for the adenosine receptors. Thus aminophylline antagonizes the electrophysiological actions of adenosine in vivo and vitro. The inhibitory effect of xanthine derivatives results from the binding to both adenosine 1 and 2 receptors.

Adenosine transport blockers

Dipyridamole potentiates the electrophysiological effects of adenosine. Dipyridamole can block the cellular uptake of adenosine and thus prolong its effect. Several calcium antagonists, including *verapamil, nitrendipine and nifedipine*, inhibit the transport of adenosine into cells and may thereby potentiate its actions. *Benzodiazepines* may interact with adenosine by inhibiting the adenosine transport system and reducing adenosine deaminase activity. These mechanisms may explain the potentiation of cardiac response to adenosine by benzodiazepines in vivo. *Quinidine* attenuates the electrophysiological effects of adenosine. *Indomethacin* is able to potentiate the actions of adenosine by inhibiting the adenosine transport system.

SUMMARY

1. *Applications of vasodilator drugs.* These drugs have wide application to the management of patients suffering from essential hypertension, ischemic heart disease and angina, as well as congestive cardiac failure (CHF). Relevant to the application of particular vasodilator agents are the differences they display in their effects on venous, as compared to arteriolar, blood vessels or large vessel conductance as compared to smaller resistance vessels.

2. *The major classes of vasodilator agents* include the nitrovasodilators, ACE inhibitors and angiotensin receptor antagonists, adenosine, α-adrenoreceptor blocking drugs and calcium channel antagonists. The latter two major groups are discussed separately in chapters 4 and 5.

3. *Nitrovasodilators.* Their action is mediated through the production of NO at endothelial level. NO itself may be administered by inhalation, its primary application being the release of primary vasoconstriction in various cardiac surgical conditions and ARDS. Other nitrovasodilators such as nitroglycerin, isosorbide dinitrate (ISDN) and isosorbide mononitrate (ISMN) find their application in the treatment of angina and reduction of preload and in higher dose afterload in the treatment of CHF. Nitrate tolerance is a troublesome feature of chronic nitrate medication.

4. *Renin-angiotensin system.* Drugs which decrease the effects of enhanced activity of the renin-angiotensin system, ACE inhibitors and angiotensin receptor antagonists, find application in the treatment of essential hypertension (chapter 8) and CHF (chapter 10). In the treatment of mild to moderate CHF, ACE inhibition, together with diuretics, has surplanted the prime use of digoxin. During the perioperative period ACE

inhibitors can enhance the effects of anesthetic and other drugs which produce hypotension and bradycardia.

5. *Adenosine* acting through dual mechanisms causes vasodilatation and the effects of calcium channel antagonism, but with evanescent pharmacokinetics and a half-life of only 10 seconds. While used primarily for its antiarrhythmic properties in the management of supraventricular tachycardia (SVT), its vasodilator properties, administered by continuous infusion, are of use for the induction of hypotension in hypotensive anesthetic techniques. Given directly into the pulmonary artery, these vasodilatory effects have applications in the control of pulmonary hypertension.

REFERENCES

Adeagbo ASO, Tabrizchi R and Triggle CR. The effects of perfusion rate and NG-nitro-L-arginine methyl ester on cirazoline- and KCl-induced responses in the perfused mesenteric arterial bed of rats. *Br J Pharmacol* 1994; 111:13-20.

Ambrosioni E, Borghi C and Magnani B. The effect of the angiotensin-converting enzyme inhibitor zofenopril on mortality and morbidity after anterior myocardial infarction. *N Engl J Med* 1996; 332:80-85.

Attia RR, Murphy JD, Snider M, et al. Myocardial ischemia due to infrarenal crossclamping during aortic surgery in patients with severe coronary artery disease. *Circulation* 1976; 53:961-965.

Bates JN, Baker MT, Guerra R and Harrison DG. Nitric oxide generation from nitroprusside by vascular tissue: evidence that reduction of the nitroprusside anion and cyanide loss are required. *Biochem Pharmacol* 1991; 42: 5157-5165.

Belardinelli L, Giles W and West A. Ionic mechanisms of adenosine actions in pacemaker cells from rabbit heart. *J Physiol (Lond)* 1988; 405:615-633.

Belardinelli L, Linden J and Berne R. Cardiac effects of adenosine. *Prog Cardiovasc Dis* 1989; 32:73-97.

Brown BG, Bolson EL and Dodge HT. Dynamic mechanisms in human coronary stenosis. *Circulation* 1984; 70:917-922.

Cody RJ, Bravo EL, Fouad FM and Tarazi RC. Cardiovascular reflexes during long term converting enzyme inhibition and sodium depletion. The responses to tilt in hypertensive patients. *Am J Med* 1981; 71:422-426.

Colson P, Ribstein J, Mimran M et al. Effect of angiotensin-converting enzyme inhibition on blood pressure and renal function during open heart surgery. *Anesthesiology* 1990; 72:23-27.

Colson P, Saussine M, Seguin JR, et al. Hemodynamic effects of anesthesia in patients chronically treated with angiotensin-converting enzyme inhibitors. *Anesth Analg* 1992; 74:805-808.

CONSENSUS Trial Study Group. Effects of enalapril on mortality in severe congestive heart failure: results of the Cooperative North Scandinavian Enalapril Survival Study (CONSENSUS). *N Engl J Med* 1987; 316:1429-1435.

Coriat P, Daloz M, Bousseau D, et al. Prevention of intraoperative myocardial ischemia during non-cardiac surgery with intravenous nitroglycerin. *Anesthesiology* 1984; 61:193-196.

Coriat P, Mundler O, Bousseau B, et al. Response of left ventricular ejection fraction to recovery from general anesthesia: measurement by gated radionuclide angiography. *Anesth Analg* 1986; 65:593-600.

Dzau V. Implication of local angiotensin production in cardiovascular physiology and pharmacology. *Am J Cardiol* 1987; 59:59A-65A.

Fam WM and Mc Gregor M. Effects of nitroglycerin and dipyridamole on regional coronary resistance. *Cir Res* 1968; 22:649-659.

Fullerton DA, Jaggers J, Piedalue F, et al. Effective control of refractory pulmonary hypertension after cardiac operations. *J Thorac Cardiovasc Surg* 1997; 113:363-370.

Furchgott RF and Zawadski JV. The obligatory role of endothelial cells in the relaxation of arterial smooth muscle by acetylcholine. *Nature* 1980; 288:373-376.

Girard C, Lehot JJ, Pannetier JC, et al. Inhaled nitric oxide after mitral replacement in patients with chronic pulmonary hypertension. *Anesthesiology* 1992; 77:880-883.

Girard C, Durand PG, Vedrinne C, et al. Inhaled nitric oxide for right ventricular failure after heart transplantation. *J Cardiothorac Anesth* 1993; 7:481-485.

Goa KL and Wagstaff AJ. Losartan potassium: a review of its pharmacology, clinical efficacy and tolerability in the management of hypertension. *Drugs* 1996; 51:820-845.

Griffith MJ, Ward DE, Linker NJ and Camm AJ. Adenosine in the diagnosis of broad complex tachycardia. *Lancet* 1988; 1:672-675.

Grindlinger GA, Vegas AM, Williams GH, et al. Independence of renin production and hypertension in abdominal aortic aneurysmectomy. *Am J Surg* 1981; 141: 472-477.

Haber E. The role of renin in normal and pathological cardiovascular homeostasis. *Circulation* 1976; 54:849-861.

Hood DD, Dewan DM, James FM, et al. The use of nitroglycerine in preventing the hypertensive response to tracheal intubation in severe pre-eclampsia. *Anesthesiology* 1985; 63:329-332.

Ikeda LS, Harm SC, Arcuri KE, et al. Comparative antihypertensive effects of losartan 50 mg and losartan 50 mg titrated to 100 mg in patients with essential hypertension. *Blood Press* 1997; 6:35-43.

Jackson EF, Garrison JC. Renin and angiotensin. In: Goodman & Gilman's: *The Pharmacological Basis of Therapeutics*. Ninth Edition, McGraw-Hill, New York, 1995; pp 733-758.

Journois D, Pouard P, Mauriat P, et al. Inhaled nitric oxide as a therapy of pulmonary hypertension following surgery for congenital heart defects. *J Thorac Cardiovasc Surg* 1993; 107:1129-1135.

Kaplan J and Jones EL. Vasodilator therapy during coronary artery surgery. *J Thorac Cardiovasc Surg* 1979; 77:301-309.

Kataja JHK, Kaukinen S, Viinamaki OVK, et al. Hemodynamic and hormonal changes in patients pretreated with captopril for surgery of the abdominal aorta. *J Cardiothorac Vasc Anesth* 1989; 3:425-432.

Kataja J, Viinamaki O, Punnonen R and Kaukinen S. Renin-angiotensin-aldosterone system and plasma vasopressin in surgical patients anesthetized with halothane or isoflurane. *Eur J Anaesth* 1988; 5:121-129.

Kurz MA, Lamping KG, Bates JN, et al. Mechanisms responsible for the heterogeneous coronary microvascular response to nitroglycerin. *Circ Res* 1991; 68:847-855.

Lerman BB, Elardinelli L, West GA, et al. Adenosine sensitive ventricular tachycardia: evidence suggesting cyclic AMP-triggered activity. *Circulation* 1986; 74:270-280.

Lewis EJ, Hunsicker LG, Bain RP and Rohde RD. The effect of angiotensin converting enzyme inhibition on diabetic nephropathy. *N Eng J Med* 1993; 329:1456-1462.

Manktelow C, Bigatello LM, Hess D and Hurford WE. Physiologic determinants of the response to inhaled nitric oxide in patients with acute respiratory distress syndrome. *Anesthesiology* 1997; 87:297-307.

Matsui J, Yahagi N, Kumon K, et al. Effects of inhaled nitric oxide on postoperative pulmonary circulation in patients with congenital heart disease. *Artif Organs* 1997; 21:17-20.

McCarthy GJ, Hainsworth M, Lindsay K, et al. Pressor responses to tracheal intubation after sublingual captopril. A pilot study. *Anesthesia,* 1990; 45:243-245.

Miller ED, Ackerly JA and Peach MJ. Blood pressure support during general anesthesia in a renin-dependent state in the rat. *Anesthesiology* 1978; 48:404-408.

Miller ED, Ackerly AJ, Vaughan RED, et al. The renin-angiotensin system during controlled hypotension with sodium nitroprusside. *Anesthesiology* 1977; 47:257-262.

Morgan JM, McCormack DG, Griffith MJ, et al. Adenosine as a vasodilator in primary pulmonary hypertension. *Circulation* 1991; 19:60-67.

Münzel T, Holtz J, Mülsch A, et al. Nitrate tolerance in epicardial arteries or in the venous system is not reversed by N-acetylcysteine in vivo, but tolerance-independent interactions exists. *Circulation* 1989; 79:188-197.

Murphy JD, Vaughan RS and Rosen M. The effects of enalaprilat on the cardiovascular responses to postural changes and tracheal intubation. *Anaesthesia* 1989; 44:816-821.

Oates JA. Antihypertensive agents and the drug therapy of hypertension. In: Goodman & Gilman's: *The Pharmacological Basis of Therapeutics.* Ninth Edition, McGraw-Hill, New York, 1995; pp 780-808.

Owall A, Gordo E, Lagerkranser M, et al. Clinical experience with adenosine for controlled hypotension during cerebral aneurysm surgery. *Anesth Analg* 1987; 66:229-234.

Palmer RMJ, Ferrige AG and Moncada S. Nitric oxide accounts for the biological activity of endothelium-derived relaxing factor. *Nature* 1987; 327:524-526.

Pohl U, Holtz J, Busse R and Bassenge E. Crucial role of endothelium in the vasodilator response to increased flow in vivo. *Hypertension* 1986; 8:37-44.

Roberts JD, Polaner DM, Lang P and Zapol WM. Inhaled nitric oxide in persistent pulmonary hypertension of the newborn. *Lancet* 1992; 340:818-819.

Roberts JD Jr, Fineman JR, Morin FC 3rd et al. Inhaled nitric oxide and persistent pulmonary hypertension of the newborn. The Inhaled Nitric Oxide Study Group. *N Engl J Med* 1997; 336:605-610.

Rossaint R, Falke KJ, Lopez F, et al. Inhaled nitric oxide in adult respiratory distress syndrome. *N Engl J Med* 1993; 328:399-405.

Sellke FW, Tomanek RJ and Harrison DG. L-Cysteine selectively potentiates nitroglycerin-induced dilation of small coronary microvessels. *J Pharmacol Exp Ther* 1991; 258:365-369.

Slogoff S and Keats AS. Does perioperative myocardial ischemia lead to postoperative myocardial infarction? *Anesthesiology* 1985; 62:107-114.

Sollevi A, Lagerkranser M, Irestedt L, et al. Controlled hypotension with adenosine in cerebral aneurysm surgery. *Anesthesiology* 1984; 61:400-405.

Sorkin EM, Brogden RN and Romankiewicz JA. Intravenous glyceryl trinitrate (Nitroglycerin). A review of its pharmacological properties and therapeutic efficacy. *Drugs* 1984; 27:45-80.

Taylor KM, Morton IJ, Brown JJ, et al. Hypertension and the renin-angiotensin system following open heart surgery. *J Thorac Cardiovasc Surgery* 1977; 74:840-845.

Tinker JH and Michenfelder JD. Sodium nitroprusside: pharmacology, toxicology and therapeutics. *Anesthesiology* 1976; 45:340-354.

Toda N and Okamura T. Role of nitric oxide in neurally induced cerebroarterial relaxation. *J Pharmacol Exp Ther* 1991; 258:1027-1032.

Timmermans PB, Wong PC, Chiu AT, et al. Angiotensin II receptors and angiotensin II receptor antagonists. *Pharmacol Rev* 1993; 45:205-251.

Traynor C and Hall GM. Endocrine and metabolic changes during surgery: anaesthetic complications. *Br J Anaesth* 1981; 53:153-160.

Van Calker D, Muller M, and Hamprecht B. Adenosine regulates via two different types of receptors. The accumulation of cyclic AMP in cultured brain cells. *J Neurochem* 1979; 33:995-1005.

Woodside J, Garner L, Bedford EF, et al. Captopril reduces the dose requirements for sodium nitroprusside induced hypotension. *Anesthesiology* 1984; 60:413-417.

Zapol WM. Inhaled nitric oxide. *Acta Anaesthesiol Scand* 1996; Suppl 109:81-83.

CHAPTER 7

Arrhythmias and their Management in the Peri-Operative Period

John L. Atlee and Gaisford G. Harrison

PART I: ARRHYTHMIAS AND ION CHANNELS: MECHANISMS OF ARRHYTHMOGENESIS

The function of the heart is to generate sufficient cardiac output to meet the changing needs of the body. To do this effectively, atrial and ventricular contraction must be initiated and properly synchronized to each other by the specialized cardiac conducting system, which continually generates and propagates impulses required for contraction in cardiac muscle. The timing and speed of impulse generation and propagation are regulated by the autonomic nervous system. If this normally orderly process is disrupted or occurs at an inappropriate rate, an arrhythmia is present. While anesthetic drugs can appreciably alter normal cardiac electrophysiological behavior, intrinsic stability of the system is normally preserved. With heart disease or physiological imbalance, however, anesthetic agents may be pro- or antiarrhythmic.

CARDIAC ELECTROPHYSIOLOGY

Abnormal electrophysiological phenomena result from the effects of disease, drugs or other imbalances that alter the ionic and electrical properties of normal myocardial fibers. However, before we can consider these abnormal phenomena we must first examine the basis for normal cardiac electrophysiology.

Ion currents, channels and gating

Unlike nerve, where action potentials (APs) resemble a sudden spike, most cardiac APs can be divided into five distinct phases (Fig 7-1): *phase 0* — rapid depolarization; *phase 1* — initial rapid repolarization; *phase 2* — plateau;

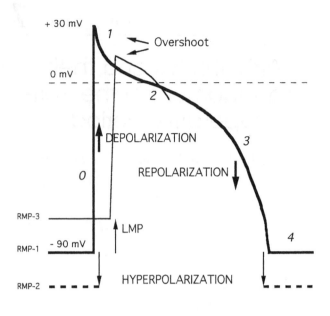

Fig 7-1. Phases of the cardiac action potential (AP). *Schematic of cardiac AP from a quiescent Purkinje fiber showing the five AP phases and terminology used to describe the transmembrane potential (TMP) changes. With depolarization, the TMP is more positive; and with repolarization, more negative. With hyperpolarization, the resting membrane potential (RMP) is more negative than normal. If the RMP is reduced by the effects of disease, loss of membrane potential (LMP) has occurred. Overshoot describes that portion of the AP during phase 0 or 1 when the TMP is positive to O mV.*

(From JL Atlee's 'Arrhythmias and Pacemakers', WB Saunders Company, Philadelphia, 1996, with permission)

phase 3 — final rapid repolarization; *phase 4* — electrical diastole or resting potential in quiescent fibers. Automatic fibers of the sinoatrial (SA) or atrioventricular (AV) nodes lack a plateau phase, and also a stable diastolic membrane potential. Instead, they spontaneously depolarize to threshold potential for generation of an AP (Fig 7-2).

Ion channels are large glycoproteins that span the cell membrane bilayer (GAMBIT members, 1994). With an appropriate stimulus, they form pores that permit ions to cross the cell membrane rapidly, thereby creating ion currents. Some channels open only after a delay following the stimulus, and others rectify (notably, K^+ channels). By *rectification* is meant that ions are conducted more effectively in one direction across the membrane than the other. Stimuli for channel opening include membrane voltage changes, chemical mediators and mechanical deformation. Chemical mediators may act directly or through receptors and second messengers (Bosnjak, 1997).

The process whereby an ion channel protein changes its conformation in response to an external stimulus is termed gating (GAMBIT members, 1994). Channel gating is not necessarily synonymous with channel opening. Channel gating kinetics can be very rapid, with major changes in channel function occurring in less than a millisecond, or quite slow (seconds). Once open, channel proteins may stay

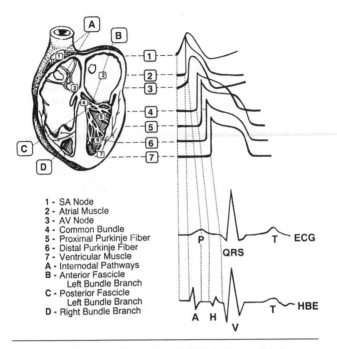

1 - SA Node
2 - Atrial Muscle
3 - AV Node
4 - Common Bundle
5 - Proximal Purkinje Fiber
6 - Distal Purkinje Fiber
7 - Ventricular Muscle
A - Internodal Pathways
B - Anterior Fascicle
    Left Bundle Branch
C - Posterior Fascicle
    Left Bundle Branch
D - Right Bundle Branch

Fig 7-2. Pacemaker and conduction system. Depiction of the heart showing the approximate location of the primary pacemaker (SA node), atrial preferential (internodal) conducting pathways, AV node, bundle branches, left anterior and posterior fascicular branches, and the terminal Purkinje network. Representative AP from each of these locations are shown to the right. Note that the duration of AP from the fascicular branches (proximal Purkinje fibers) is longer than those of fibers from the terminal Purkinje network (distal Purkinje fibers). In turn, the timing of AP from the above locations is shown in relation to events of the surface electrocardiogram (ECG) and His bundle electrograms (HBE).

(From JL Atlee's 'Arrhythmias and Pacemakers', WB Saunders Company, Philadelphia, 1996, with permission)

open until closed by another signal, or they may close even in the face of a maintained stimulus (i.e. inactivate). Inactivated channels usually do not reopen until they have recovered from inactivation, a time- and/or often voltage-dependent process.

Ion channels can be voltage- or ligand-gated. A number of channel types have been purified, cloned, and sequenced from heart and other excitable cells (Pong, 1992; Caterall et al, 1994; Bosnjak and Lynch, 1998). They share considerable homology, especially in the intramembranous segments. Therefore, it is not surprising that some channel-active drugs interact with more than one channel type in the heart (Na^+, K^+, Ca^{2+}), or the same channel type in other tissues. Given the recent progress in determining ion channel structure and function at the molecular level, it is becoming possible to determine key structural differences and drug-binding sites, and to tailor drugs that are channel- and tissue-specific.

Resting potential (Phase 4)

Resting membrane potential (RMP) varies considerably among cardiac cell types along with conduction velocity and other AP characteristics (Sperelakis, 1979). Cells such as atrial or ventricular muscle and Purkinje fibers have a more negative RMP (80-90 mV). Because their AP upstrokes (phase 0) are dependent mainly on fast-inward (Na^+) current, they are termed *fast response fibers*. SA or AV node fibers have less a negative RMP (50-70 mV). Because their AP upstrokes are more dependent on slow-inward (Ca^{2+}) current, they are termed *slow response fibers*.

Potassium is the major ion determining RMP, because during phase 4 the cell membrane is quite permeable to K^+ but relatively impermeable to other ions (GAMBIT members, 1994; Atlee 1996; Bosnjak and Lynch, 1998). While providing very stable electrical behavior, the K^+ gradient is maintained at considerable energy expense (5-10% of myocardial O_2 utilization) by the membrane-bound Na^+-K^+ ATPase (sodium pump) fueled by hydrolysis of ATP (Fig 7-3). This pump generates net outward positive current (i.e. is electrogenic), since it transports three Na^+ out of the cell for two K^+ into the cell against their respective electrochemical gradients, which helps to make the RMP more negative. Also, depending on the membrane potential at a given moment and the Na^+ and Ca^{2+} concentrations inside and outside the cell, a Na^+/Ca^{2+} exchanger that does not require ATP, can run in either direction to transport Na^+ or Ca^{2+} into or out of the cell (Fig 7-3). During the RMP phase, the Na^+/Ca^{2+} exchanger eliminates one Ca^{2+} for three entering Na^+ thereby generating net inward (depolarizing) current. Finally, in parallel with the Na^+/Ca^{2+} exchanger, an ATP-dependent Ca^{2+} transport system also exists in the cell membrane (Fig 1-13, page 18), which, however, is responsible for elimination of only a fraction of Ca^{2+} from the cell.

Action potential (Phases 0-3)

AP upstroke — rapid depolarization (phase 0). The ionic basis for phase 0 depends on the fiber type. In fast response tissue (atrial or ventricular muscle, Purkinje fibers) with more negative RMP, rapid AP upstroke velocities and distinct overshoots, phase 0 is due to the rapid influx of Na^+. In slow response fibers (SA and AV nodes) with less negative maximum diastolic potential, reduced upstroke velocities and little or no overshoot, phase 0 is largely dependent on the predominantly Ca^{2+} inward current. To propagate to adjacent fibers, the depolarizing stimulus must be of sufficient strength to depolarize the cell to threshold potential (TP, about -65 mV in normal Purkinje fibers). Smaller depolarizing stimuli do not result in normally propagated AP, but rather produce smaller *electronic potentials* that are incapable of propagation or propagate slowly. These are similar to those that result from stimulation during the relative refractory period of the AP (Fig 7-3).

AP repolarization and plateau (phases 1-3). A number of currents contribute to the AP during the repolarization and plateau phases (Fig 7-3) (Atlee, 1996; Bosnjak and Lynch, 1998). *Phase 1* – Inactivation of inward Na^+ and Ca^{2+} currents (I_{Na-Ca}) combines with the transient outward K current (I_{to}) to produce a net efflux of positive charges.

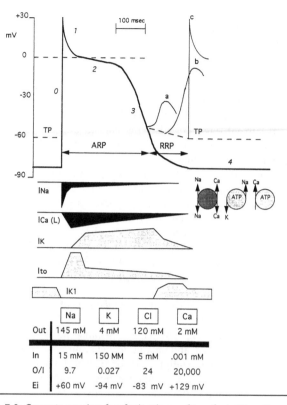

Fig 7-3: Currents causing depolarization and repolarization. *Representation of the five AP phases of a quiescent Purkinje fiber, along with the major ionic currents (I_{Na}, $I_{Ca(L)}$, I_K, I_{to}, I_{K1}) responsible for AP depolarization and repolarization. Inward currents are shown in black and outward ones in gray, with the relative timing and magnitude of each shown only as rough approximations. The five AP phases are the result of selective membrane permeability to individual ions, changes in intracellular ion concentrations during inscription of the AP, and active or passive ion-exchange mechanisms that restore intracellular concentrations of ions during phase 4. Individual ion concentrations outside (Out) and inside (In) the cell during phase 4 are shown below, along with their respective outside/inside ratios (O/I) during phase 4 and ionic equilibrium potentials (Ei). Finally, during the relative refractory period (RRP), only small electronic potentials ("a" and "b") that cannot be propogated occur. At the end of the RRP, a normal AP ("c") capable of propagation occurs. Note that the TP is more positive during the RRP.*
(From JL Atlee's 'Arrhythmias and Pacemakers', WB Saunders Company, Philadelphia, 1996, with permission).

Also there may be briefly reversed flux through the Na^+-Ca^{2+} exchanger (I_{Na-Ca}) and inactivation of T-type (transient) Ca^{2+} inward current. T-type calcium channels, conducting the T-type inward calcium current, are activated first during the depolarization process at about -55 mV, whereas the L-channels are activated soon thereafter at about -30 mV. Whereas T-channels are transient in their opening, L-channels are more long-lasting. However, T-channels are not found in normal ventricular tissue. *Phase 2* – During the plateau, membrane conductance for all ions is reduced. A number of currents contribute to hold plateau potential around 0 mV. Particularly in proximal Purkinje fibers, with prominent AP plateaus, a small Na^+ "window current" (not shown in Figure 7-3) contributes to the AP plateau. This may be due to different populations of Na^+ channels with different inactivation kinetics, or different modes of operation of the same channel (Zipes, 1997). A slowly decaying L-type (long lasting) Ca^{2+} inward current also contributes. While inward rectifier (I_{K1}) K^+ channels are blocked during the plateau, the voltage dependent K^+ current (I_K) becomes active to provide progressively more outward current (Fig 7-3). Also, the current dependent on the Na^+/Ca exchanger, I_{Na-Ca}, may help to maintain plateau potential by providing net inward current (3 Na^+ in for 1 Ca^{2+} out). *Phase 3* — the delayed (I_K) and inward rectifier K^+ currents (I_{K1}) are responsible for final rapid repolarization. Increasing activation of (I_K), persistence of any remaining I_{to}, along with time- and voltage-dependent inactivation of L-type I_{Ca}, all contribute to early phase 3 repolarization. As the membrane potential becomes negative to -30 to -40 mV, I_{K1} conducts an increasing outward current (especially with high $[K+]_o$) to accelerate repolarization toward the end of phase 3.

Refractoriness. During the AP plateau, fibers cannot be reexcited regardless of stimulus strength. They are absolutely refractory (Fig 7-3). This is because most Na^+ channels are inactivated and unable to generate enough current for phase 0. Repolarization must occur before the Na^+ channels can reopen. In fast response fibers, restoration of the normal membrane potential is usually sufficient for full recovery, fibers are relatively refractory, and only small non-propagated or slowly propagating APs are elicited with stimulation. In slow response fibers or depressed fast response fibers (i.e. fast response fibers with reduced RMP due to disease or imbalance), the relative refractory period may extend several hundred milliseconds beyond full recovery of excitability.

IMPULSE GENERATION

Automaticity

Automatic (pacemaker) fibers have an unstable membrane potential during phase 4. After reaching a maximum diastolic potential (MDP) following phase 3, they begin to depolarize toward threshold potential (TP) to form the pacemaker potential (phase 4 depolarization). Pacemaker rate is affected by changes in the rate of phase 4 depolarization, MDP and TP (Fig 7-4). Automaticity results from a net reduction in outward current movement during phase 4. The mechanism varies among cell types, depending most on MDP (Baumgarten and Fozzard, 1992; Fozzard and Arnsdorf, 1992; Anumonwo and Jalife, 1995; Atlee 1996; DiFrancesco et al, 1995; Bosnjak and Lynch, 1998). Critical to the pacemaker potential are the absence or presence of distinct ionic conductances. In contrast to atrial and ventricular muscle, pacemaker fibers have virtually no resting I_{K1} conductance to fix RMP near the K^+ equilibrium potential, so that diastolic membrane potential is more unstable. Quite modest inward currents can then depolarize these

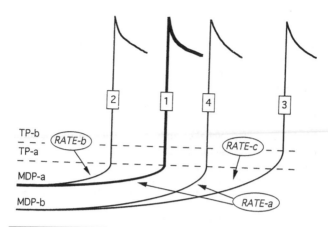

Fig 7-4. Automatic Purkinje fiber. Schematic of mechanisms whereby the rate of pacemaker discharge in an automatic Purkinje fiber may be altered, TP, threshold potential; MDP, maximum diastolic potential; Rate, rate of diastolic (phase 4) depolarization. 1, Normal automaticity (MDP-a; TP-a; Rate-a). 2, The rate of automaticity is increased (Rate-b) following catecholamines. Since MDP and TP are unchanged, TP is reached sooner. 3, The rate of automaticity has been decreased (Rate-c) by exposure to acetylcholine. Also, MDP is hyperpolarized (MDP-b), and TP reduced (TP-b). Automaticity is slowed since it takes longer to achieve TP. 4, With simultaneous cholinergic and sympathetic stimulation, MDP remains hyperpolarized (MDP-b), but TP and the rate of phase 4 depolarization are restored to normal. Automaticity is faster than in 3, but slower than in 1 because MDP-b is further from TP-a than MDP-a.

(From JL Atlee's 'Arrhythmias and Pacemakers', WB Saunders Company, Philadelphia, 1996, with permission)

fibers. Activation of a K^+ hyperpolarizing current (e.g. by acetylcholine or adenosine) will oppose such depolarization.

Pacemaker currents

There are no less than 3, and possibly 4, pacemaker currents, providing a factor of safety (Fig 1-6, page 9). 1) I_K due to deactivation of the delayed rectifier current; 2) I_{Na-Ca} the background inward current from the Na^+/Ca^{2+} exchanger over the range of potentials for phase 4 depolarization; 3) I_f, an inward pacemaker current carried by a relatively nonspecific cationic channel (Na^+influx/K^+ efflux); and 4) T- and L-components of I_{Ca} are activated to cause inward currents at -55 and -30mV respectively.

Automaticity of secondary pacemakers

Secondary pacemakers include subsidiary atrial, AV junctional (nodal), and Purkinje fibers. Purkinje fibers have the highest MDP (-85 to -90 mV), and nodal fibers the lowest (-60 to -70 mV). Subsidiary atrial pacemaker fibers have MDP intermediate between those of nodal and Purkinje fibers. In those subsidiary pacemaker fibers, with greater (i.e. more negative) MDP values, I_f is more active. I_K and the exchanger (Na^+-Ca^{2+}) background currents play a similar role in initiating phase 4 depolarization as in SA node cells, and the calcium currents $I_{Ca(T)}$ and $I_{Ca(L)}$ contribute when activated at membrane potentials of above -55 and

-30 mV during depolarization, respectively. However, given the higher MDP of secondary pacemaker fibers compared to SA node, quantitative differences are expected in the relative amounts of the various currents activated. For example, I_f contributes most to the Purkinje fiber pacemaker potential.

Control of pacemaker activity

Modulation of pacemaker activity is achieved by the autonomic nervous system, along with the intracellular chemical environment (Ca^{2+}, H^+, ATP) and intercellular mechanisms (Irisawa and Brown, 1993; Anumonwo and Jalife 1995) (Fig 7-4). Acetylcholine (ACh) slows SA node discharge rate by:

1) membrane hyperpolarization due to stimulation of ACh-activated K^+ current — $I_{K(ACh)}$.

2) shift of l_f activation to more negative voltages (antagonized by atropine).

3) inhibition of I_{Ca}.

β-adrenergic stimulation increases SA node discharge rate by (i) stimulation by the second messenger cyclic AMP that phosphorylates L-type Ca^{2+} channels, thereby increasing membrane permeability to Ca^{2+} (Fig 1-5, page 8); and by (ii) increasing I_f by shifting the site of pacemaker activation to cells with a more negative voltage range.

Individual pacemaker fibers of the SA node have slightly different natural frequencies, but coordinate their activity to produce a single impulse propagated to the rest of the heart. Such pacemaker synchronization probably involves phase-dependent electrotonic interactions mediated through gap junctions which permit adjacent SA pacemaker fibers to behave as coupled oscillators. Gap junctions are specialized membrane protein structures that form low-resistance pathways for exchange of ions and small molecules between adjacent cardiac cells.

IMPULSE PROPAGATION

Conduction

Current source and sink

Membrane factors determining the propagation of conduction include active and passive membrane properties (Fozzard and Arnsdorf, 1992; Atlee, 1996; Bosnjak and Lynch, 1998). The membrane generator (current source) is mostly fast-inward current (I_{Na}) during phase 0. The amount of sodium ions entering depends on the number of open Na^+ channels and the Na^+ electrochemical gradient. I_{Na} provides the positive charges needed to discharge the membrane and neutralize excessive negative charges maintaining RMP. By virtue of its capacitance, passive cell membrane can contain electrical charges and so act as a current sink.

Safety factor of conduction

The rate of rise of AP phase 0, speed of AP propagation, and AP overshoot, amplitude and duration all provide a measure of the ability of the current source to saturate the sink. Conduction is more likely to be successful in fast response fibers with high RMP, AP upstroke velocities and overshoots. These fibers are said to have a high safety factor of conduction. In contrast, conduction is much slower in fibers with lower RMP, slower AP upstroke velocities and overshoots. These fibers have a low safety factor of conduction.

Cable analysis of cardiac conduction

A biologic cable consists of the low-resistance intracellular core surrounded by the relatively high-resistance cell membrane, in turn bathed by low-resistance extracellular fluid. When cell membrane resistance is high, less depolarizing current leaks out so that depolarization occurs more rapidly and further along the fiber. Hence, large Purkinje fibers with low longitudinal resistances conduct far better than smaller muscle fibers. However, there are limitations to cable analysis. Varying structural complexities of cardiac fibers, especially the presence of low resistance gap junctions (Pressler et al, 1995), and varying fiber orientation and geometry (Keener and Panfilox, 1995), play an important role in determining the speed of conduction. For example, cable analysis does not predict the directional dependence of conduction velocity (Spach, 1995).

CELLULAR MECHANISMS FOR ARRHYTHMIAS

An arrhythmia is any cardiac rhythm or conduction disturbance other than normal sinus rhythm at a physiologic rate with 1:1 AV conduction. As such, arrhythmias with adverse outcomes that require significant treatment and/or cardiopulmonary resuscitation can be expected in about 1.6 percent of patients having general anesthesia (Forrest et al, 1990; Forrest et al, 1992; Atlee, 1996) — and so, can have an important impact on anesthetic and surgical outcomes. The most important causes for arrhythmias in perioperative settings include coronary artery, hypertensive and valvular heart disease, physiologic ion imbalance and adverse drug effects (Atlee, 1996). Fundamental to successful arrhythmia management is that treatment of heart disease be optimal, and that identifiable contributing factors be removed or corrected. More specific treatment with drugs or devices has of itself recognized potential to cause complications, but is nonetheless often required. Such treatment is more likely to be successful if targeted at the electrophysiologic mechanisms underlying the arrhythmias (GAMBIT members, 1994).

Loss of membrane potential and the depressed fast response

Many abnormal electrophysiologic phenomena that cause arrhythmias are associated with partial depolarization of fast response fibers, termed *loss of membrane potential* (LMP). Fast response fibers with LMP are termed depressed fast response fibers. Cellular depolarization responsible for LMP can have a variety of causes, including hypoxia, ischemia, myocardial injury, and hyperkalemia. LMP alters the depolarization and repolarization phases of fast response APs so that the AP contours of depressed fast responses more closely resemble those of physiologic slow response fibers as found in the SA or AV nodes (Fig 7-2). Reduced AP upstroke velocity following LMP is explained by incomplete recovery from inactivation of Na^+ channels. Membrane depolarization to -65 mV may inactivate half of the Na^+ channels, and that to -50 mV all the Na^+ channels (Fozzard and Arnsdorf, 1992; Zipes, 1997). At membrane potentials positive to -55 mV, $I_{Ca\ (L,T)}$ will be activated to generate the AP upstroke. Where there are depressed fast responses, AP changes are likely to be heterogeneous due to varying degrees of Na^+ channel inactivation among fibers. This may lead to small, modest or complete conduction impairment in different areas of the heart. Also, refractoriness may outlast full restoration of RMP in depressed fast response fibers, similar to that in slow response fibers. These changes are conducive to reentry of excitation (below). Finally, LMP may contribute to abnormal automaticity and triggered activity (below).

Altered normal and abnormal automaticity

Altered normal automaticity is not the same as abnormal automaticity. Altered normal automaticity occurs in fibers that are normally automatic at their usual high level of MDP, e.g. SA and AV nodes and Purkinje fibers (GAMBIT members, 1994). Enhancement occurs over a range of membrane potentials of from -90 to -65 mV. With altered normal automaticity, the mechanisms for automaticity are believed to remain nearly the same, although the kinetics and magnitude of ionic currents responsible for automaticity have changed (Zipes, 1997). Thus, the rate of pacemaker discharge may increase or decrease, but is still within the expected range.

Abnormal automaticity can only occur when fibers are depolarized from their normal MDP or RMP (i.e. *depolarization-induced automaticity*), e.g. abnormal automaticity might occur in a Purkinje fiber that was depolarized by hypoxia/ischaemia. In contrast to altered normal automaticity, the ionic mechanism for abnormal automaticity is substantially different from that for normal automaticity in the same fiber type, or it occurs in fibers that do not normally exhibit automaticity. Additionally, abnormal automaticity usually occurs at a lower level of membrane potential (≤ 60 mV) than altered normal automaticity in the same fiber type, although there may be no sharp distinction between membrane potential required for the two types of automaticity in partially depolarized Purkinje fibers. Deactivation of the delayed rectifier (I_K) is believed to be the major factor that initiates pacemaker activity at membrane potentials appropriate for abnormal automaticity (GAMBIT members, 1994). That the slow-inward calcium current (I_{Ca}) is also involved, is suggested by experiments in which verapamil, but not lidocaine, suppressed automaticity in partially depolarized

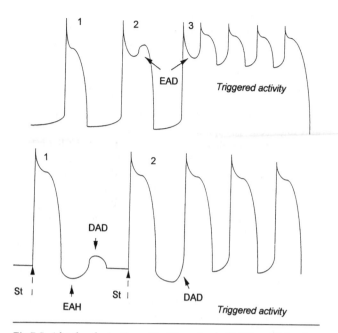

Fig 7-5. Afterdepolarizations. Depiction of early (EAD) and delayed afterpolarizations (DAD) with triggered activity. Top — AP of an automatic Purkinje fiber. The second AP is associated with a subthreshold (EAD) arrow, and the third with a threshold EAD that initiates a series of triggered AP's, terminated by a return to normal membrane potential. Bottom — The first and second AP are stimulated (St). The first is followed by an early hyperpolarization (EAH), that often precedes DAD, and a subthreshold DAD. The second AP initiates a threshold DAD that triggers a series of spontaneous AP. See text for further discussion.

(From JL Atlee's 'Arrhythmias and Pacemakers', WB Saunders Company, Philadelphia, 1996, with permission)

Purkinje fibers (Elharrar, 1980). Abnormal automaticity may cause ventricular and junctional arrhythmias during the early stages (<48 hrs) of myocardial infarction (Janse, 1989; Wit and Janse, 1993).

Afterdepolarizations and triggered activity

The term triggered activity describes cardiac impulse initiation that is dependent on afterdepolarizations (Fozzard and Arnsdorf, 1992; Wit and Rosen, 1992; Zipes, 1997; GAMBIT members, 1994). Afterdepolarizations are oscillations in membrane potential that occur after the AP upstroke (Fig 7-5). Those occurring before full AP repolarization are early afterdepolarizations (EAD), and those afterwards delayed afterdepolarizations (DAD). EADs occur during the plateau or repolarization phases of AP initiated from a high RMP (> -75 mV). Under certain conditions, they may trigger a second AP, which may self-perpetuate as triggered sustained rhythmic activity (Fig 7-5). Triggered activity may continue for a variable number of beats, but terminates when repolarization of the initiating AP restores the normal high level of RMP. EADs are likely to result from abnormalities involving membrane currents responsible for the AP plateau and repolarization, and are believed to be the mechanism for *torsades de pointes* in association with QT interval prolongation (below). K^+ channel activators (pinacidil), Mg^{2+}, α-adrenergic blockade, antiarrhythmics that shorten AP duration (lidocaine), tetrodotoxin and calcium channel antagonists may all oppose EADs and triggered activity, depending on the circumstances which produced them. DADs and triggered rhythmic activity (Fig 7-5) usually occur in circumstances where there is intracellular Ca^{2+} overload. This may occur with adrenergic stimulation and high $[Ca^{2+}]_o$, digoxin excess with Na^+ pump inhibition, or after thrombolytic reperfusion in acute myocardial infarction. DADs are believed to result from transient inward current caused by oscillatory Ca^{2+} induced Ca^{2+} release from the overloaded sarcoplasmic reticulum. The current, carried mainly by Na^+, may result from activation of a non-selective cation channel or be due to electrogenic Na^+-Ca^{2+} exchange. DADs and triggered activity can be inhibited by agents which:

i)   reduce I_{Ca}, such as calcium antagonists and β-blockers; or

ii)   inhibit Ca^{2+} release from the sarcoplasmic reticulum, such as certain experimental agents; or

iii)   reduce I_{Na}, such as lidocaine and thereby reduce intracellular Ca^{2+}.

Re-entry of excitation

The propagating impulse normally dies out after sequential activation of the heart when it encounters refractory tissue or the inexcitable annulus fibrosus. However, sometimes it may persist to reexcite myocardium that is no longer refractory, termed reentry of excitation, reciprocation or circus movement. Essential requirements for reentry are unidirectional conduction block and slowed conduction. Slowed conduction in an alternate pathway facilitates reentry by allowing tissue proximal to the site of unidirectional conduction block time to recover from refractoriness (Fozzard and Arnsdorf, 1992; Janse, 1992; Zipes 1997; Wit and Janse, 1993; GAMBIT members, 1994; Atlee, 1996).

Unidirectional conduction block. Unidirectional conduction block may be caused by regional differences in recovery of excitability, occur at connecting sites between adjacent fibers, or result from geometric factors (Janse, 1992).

Recovery of excitability. Usually, as impulses propagate through tissue with nonuniform refractoriness, propagation fails in tissue with the longest refractory periods. These tissues can be reexcited if the impulse conducts through surrounding tissue with shorter refractoriness and returns to the previously refractory site of former block before arrival of the next impulse from above (Fig 7-6). In the normal heart, there is substantial diastolic time during which excitability is normal, so that uneven refractoriness is usually present only during propagation of rapid or premature beats. Ischemia facilitates reentry by increasing disparity of AP duration and refractoriness in ventricular and Purkinje fibers.

Cellular connections. Sites where the cross-sectional area of interconnected cells suddenly increases may predispose

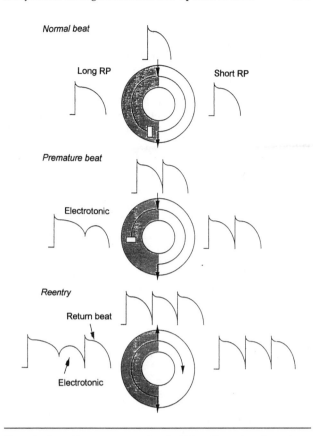

Fig 7-6. Nonuniform recovery of excitability. *Shown is a tissue ring with a zone of fibers (gray) with longer refractory periods (RP). Top — With normal beats, propagation fails in the zone with long RP. Middle — A premature beat produces an electronic potential which blocks proximally. Bottom — The same premature beat returns through the zone with long RP to excite no-longer refractory fibers and initiate re-entry.*

(From JL Atlee's 'Arrhythmias and Pacemakers', WB Saunders Company, Philadelphia, 1996, with permission)

to unidirectional block. One such site is the Purkinje fiber-ventricular muscle junction. Anterograde activation of ventricular muscle occurs only at specific junctional sites, whereas retrograde Purkinje fiber activation can occur at sites where anterograde conduction is not possible (Janse, 1992).

Geometric factors. Unidirectional block of conduction can result from geometric factors:

1) Branching sites or junctions of separate fiber bundles form areas with a low safety factor of conduction.

2) Conduction in the longitudinal direction is several times faster than that in the transverse direction in normal fibers.

3) In fibers with reduced excitability or tissue with uneven conduction and refractoriness (tissue anisotropy), transverse conduction may be faster.

4) There is no consistent relationship between fiber orientation and conduction velocity in the ischemic heart.

Slowed conduction. The SA and especially the AV nodes are potential sites for reentrant tachycardia. Reentry may also occur during slow propagation of rapid or premature beats in anisotropic tissues (Fig 7-6). Variable depression of fast response fibers can lead to slowed conduction in some areas and block in others. The likelihood of reentrant beats or tachycardia is greater in depressed fast response fibers compared to SA or AV nodal tissue because refractoriness is more uneven.

Types of reentry. The simplest form of reentry requires an *anatomically defined circuit.* In such a circuit, duration of refractoriness and conduction velocity determine whether or not reentry can occur. Anatomical reentry requires that a premature beat penetrate the circuit during its excitable gap

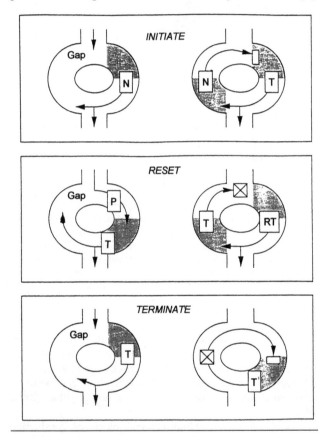

Fig 7-7. Concept of excitable gap. Impulses from outside a re-entry cir-cuit can penetrate it to initiate, reset or terminate re-entry tachycardia. Top — An impulse enters the circuit within the gap of nonrefractory tis-sue between receding (stippled) and advancing wavefronts of a normal beat (N). It continues to circulate as tachycardia (T), since the normal beat is blocked by receding refractoriness of tachycardia. Middle — A pre-mature beat (P) penetrates the gap during tachycardia, entering the ante-rograde and retrograde pathways. It collides with and extinguishes the advancing tachycardia wavefront, but continues in the anterograde path-way resetting the phase of tachycardia (RT). Bottom — The impulse en-ters the circuit just behind the advancing tachycardia wavefront, blocks in the zone of refractoriness, but collides with and extinguishes the advan-cing tachycardia wavefront, thereby terminating tachycardia.

(From JL Atlee's 'Arrhythmias and Pacemakers', WB Saunders Com-pany, Philadelphia, 1996, with permission)

(Fig 7-7). The premature beat could arise from a stimulated or triggered AP, or propagating AP from a protected automatic focus. Tissue anisotropy or zones of depressed conduction reduce the size of an anatomic obstacle required to sustain reentry. *Leading circle reentry* does not require an anatomic obstacle. The premature impulse initiating tachycardia and the tachycardia wavefront propagate circumferentially in perimeter tissue with shorter refractoriness while blocking in central tissue with longer refractoriness. Other types of reentry include *anisotropic reentry* and *reflection*. The former is believed responsible for reentry with chronic transmural myocardial infarction, and relies on differences in fiber geometry and directional conduction velocities in surviving epicardial fibers. The latter describes reentry in adjacent linear fibers, one with a zone of depressed conduction (Janse, 1992; GAMBIT members, 1994). With reflection, propagation occurs in one direction in the normal fiber, with conduction block in the depressed zone of the other. The impulse returns through the no-longer refractory depressed zone to reexcite proximal tissue of both fibers. Finally, *ordered* and *random reentry* are distinguished (Hoffman and Rosen, 1981). Ordered reentry occurs over a relatively fixed pathway, causing a regular rhythm (e.g. atrial flutter). With random reentry, the reentry pathways are continuously changing their size and shape with time, so that the rhythm is irregular (e.g. atrial fibrillation).

Sites for reentry. Clinical studies suggest that only 5 to 10 percent of paroxysmal (reentry) supraventricular tachycardia (PSVT) is due to *SA node reentry*, with the remainder about equally divided between *AV node* and *AV node with accessory pathway* reentry (Zipes, 1997). The cause for AV node reentry could be functional longitudinal dissociation of the AV node into fast (beta) and slow (alpha) pathways, the result of electrophysiologic and not anatomic differences. Alternatively, the human heart has atrial inputs from the crista terminalis and interatrial septum that could serve as the alpha and beta pathways. Yet another possibility is that functional longitudinal dissociation is due to tissue anisotropy within the AV node. Fast conducting bundles of atrial muscle fibers form accessory pathways (AV connections) in patients with the Wolff-Parkinson-White syndrome (WPW). WPW results from ventricular preexcitation (delta wave) with symptomatic tachyarrhythmias. Accessory pathways participate with the atrium, AV node, His-Purkinje system and ventricular myocardium in a type of reentry known as AV reciprocation. Accessory pathways may be concealed (do not cause preexcitation) in some patients, yet still be capable of retrograde impulse transmission to sustain orthodromic AV reciprocating tachycardia (anterograde conduction via AV node; retrograde conduction via accessory pathway).

Atrial reentry may be ordered (atrial flutter, PSVT) or random (atrial fibrillation). It is widely believed that atrial flutter is due to circus movement around the caval orifices, but PSVT due to atrial reentry is relatively rare (<5 per cent of PSVT) (Zipes, 1997). Tachycardia due to macro- or micro-reentry may originate within the *His-Purkinje system*. The former is due to differences in refractoriness between the right and left bundle branches, or bundle branches and ventricular myocardium. The latter is due to the combination of slow conduction and short refractory periods at the Purkinje fiber-ventricular muscle fiber junction. Shortened refractoriness, slowed conduction and increased dispersion of refractory periods are all conducive to the genesis of reentry tachycardia in ischemic ventricular myocardium. With infarcted myocardium, reentry depends more on anatomically defined circuits comprised of surviving normal fibers interspersed with fibrous tissue.

Proarrhythmia and torsades de pointes

Paradoxically class IA, IC and III antiarrhythmic drugs (see below) manifest a property that is self-defeating viz. a proarrhythmic potential — an ability to worsen or exaggerate existing arrhythmia. This proarrhythmia may be associated with drug-induced prolongation of the APD and/or the QT interval — the acquired long QT syndrome (Marcus and Opie, 1995; Atlee, 1996). Class III agents reduce the outward K^+ currents (predominantly the rapidly repolarizing component of I_K, I_{Kr}) that mediate repolarisation. This change results in a prolongation and possible heterogeneity of repolarisation and consequently refractoriness, which in turn provides the milieu for macroreentry. The proarrhythmic effect of class IA and IC agents (particularly the latter) stems from their powerful inhibition of the Na^+ current especially in conduction tissues. Thereafter increasing heterogeneity together with unidirectional block sets the stage for reentry circuits, EADs and the induction of mono- or polymorphic wide complex VT.

Torsades de pointes is a particularly dangerous type of polymorphic VT associated with the acquired long QT syndrome especially in the presence of other causative factors (Table 7-1). Though the background electrophysiological and triggering factors for torsades de pointes are now gen-

Table 7-1. Causes for acquired QT-interval prolongation and torsades de pointes

Antiarrhythmic Drugs	Non-Sedative Antihistaminics
Class IA, IC and III antiarrhythmic agents	Terfenadine, astemizole, cisapride
Psychoactive Agents, CNS Causes	**Miscellaneous Drugs**
Phenothiazines, antihistamines, Tricyclic antidepressants, Haloperidol, Lithium toxicity Subarachnoid hemorrhage, Stroke	Chloral hydrate, Probucol Alpha-adrenergic blockers Doxorubicin, Volatile anesthetics
	Metabolic Causes
	K^+, Mg^{2+} and Ca^{2+} deficient states, Malnutrition, liquid protein diets, Hypothyroidism, hypothermia
Antibiotics	**Cardiac Conditions**
Ampicillin, erythromycin Trimethoprim-sulfamethoxazole	Mitral valve prolapse Cardiomyopathies, myocarditis

erally agreed upon, the mechanisms for the maintenance of the distinctive undulating "twisting of the points" of this type of VT remain speculative (Lazzara, 1997). Treatment includes identification and elimination of causative factors and the administration of magnesium sulphate and class IB antiarhythmics. Electrical defibrillation may be necessary.

In the *congenital long QT syndrome* — the result of defects in the genes expressing the sarcolemmal channels transmitting slow and rapid components of the repolarizing K^+ currents, I_{Ks} and I_{Kr} (Wang et al, 1996; Curran et al, 1995) as well as the Na^+ delayed inactivation channels — there are episodes of torsades de pointes. In this case adrenergic stimulation may act by shortening the APD and enhancing the transition from EADs to torsades de pointes. Accordingly, therapy for this condition should include β-adrenergic blockade.

PART II — SPECIFIC MANAGEMENT: ANTIARRHYTHMIC DRUGS

The most widely accepted classification for antiarrhythmic drugs is that of Vaughan Williams with certain modifications and elaborations (Vaughan Williams, 1984; Task Force of Working Group on Arrhythmias of the European Society of Cardiologists, 1991). In this classification, antiarrhythmic drugs are divided into four groups, based on their electrophysiological properties and the ion channel effects underlying these (Fig 7-8, Table 7-2). In studying this table, particular note should be taken of those drugs which prolong the QT interval (Class IA, IC, III).

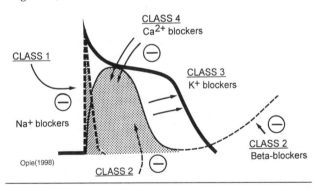

Fig 7-8. The classical four types of antiarrhythmic agents. Class I agents decrease phase zero of the rapid depolarization of the action potential (rapid sodium channel). Class II agents, beta-blocking drugs, have complex actions including inhibition of spontaneous depolarization (phase 4) and indirect closure of calcium channels, which are less likely to be in the "open" state when not phosphorylated by cyclic AMP. Class III agents block the outward potassium channels to prolong the action potential duration and hence refractoriness. Class IV agents, verapamil and diltiazem, and the indirect calcium antagonist adenosine, all inhibit the inward calcium channel which is most prominent in nodal tissue, particularly the AV node. Most antiarrhythmic drugs have more than one action. (Fig. copyright © L H Opie, 1998) (Modified from Fig 20-10, L H Opie, The Heart, Physiology from Cell to Circulation, Lippincott-Raven, Philadelphia, 1998)

Table 7-2. Classification of antiarrhythmic drugs

Class	Drug	Ion Channel Effect	ECG Effect	Repolar- ization Time
IA	Procainamide Disopyramide Quinidine	Na^+ channel block Delayed rectifier block RTC: 300-1500 msec	↑ QTc ↑ QRS	Prolongs
IB	Lidocaine Phenytoin Tocainamide Mexilitine	Na^+ channel block RTC: < 300 msec.	↓ QTc	Shortens
IC	Flecainamide Propafenone Moricizine*	Marked Na^+ channel block RTC: > 1500 msec.	↑ PR ↑↑ QRS	Unchanged
II	Esmolol Propranolol Metoprolol Acebutolol	β Adrenoceptor block. Phase IV inhibited. Indirect Ca^{++} channel block	↓↓ SA rate ↑ PR	Unchanged
III	Bretylium Sotalol* Amiodarone* Ibutilide	K^+ repolarizing current block	↑ QTc	Prolongs markedly
IV	Verapamil Diltiazem	Ca^{++} channel (L) block	↓ SA rate ↑ PR	Unchanged
Similar to class IV	Adenosine MgSO$_4$	K^+ channel (K_{ADO}) opener Hyperpolarization CCA-like	↑ PR ↑ PR (high dose)	Unchanged

* = Multiclass Effects
RTC = Recovery Time Constant
↑ = Increases
↓ = Decreases

In considering the pharmacological effects of these drugs, attention will be focused on those agents that are principally of use during the perioperative period (Table 7-3). Ideally, these will be relatively short-acting, lacking of proarrhythmic potential or gross depressive hemodynamic effect, will have no serious interaction with anesthetic agents and will be available in an intravenous formulation. Intravenous administration of antiarrhythmic drugs must be controlled clinically by continuous monitoring of ECG and BP. These drugs and their dosage are listed in Table 7-3. Antiarrhythmic drugs which are utilized for the long-term control of chronic tachyarrhythmias but which are inappropriate for use, de novo, in the perioperative setting (unavailability of an intravenous preparation, lack of data or published trials or trials have not shown significant benefit) are listed in Tables 7-4A and 7-4B. Recommendations for drug dosage and administration are presented in these tables.

Class I antiarrhythmic agents

Class I antiarrhythmic agents act primarily through inducing varying degrees of Na^+ channel blockade, thereby slowing conduction and counteracting reentrant arrhythmias. The group is subdivided into three divisions based on the precise electrophysiological effects of the individual drugs and their consequent effect on repolarization time.

The groups differ in their time constants for recovery from block — a measure of use dependence, i.e. greater Na^+ channel blockade at faster heart rates for drugs with longer time constants. On this basis they may be classed as fast (<300msec, Class IB drugs), intermediate (300-1500msec, Class IA drugs), and slow (>1500msec, Class IC drugs) Na^+ channel blockers.

Class IA agents

Procainamide (Pronestyl). Of Class IA agents only procainamide is suitable for intravenous administration and use in the perioperative period. A structural analogue of procaine, procainamide is generally effective against a wide variety of supraventricular and ventricular arrhythmias (Marcus and Opie, 1995). For the latter, its place as a second choice after lidocaine for recurrent ventricular tachyarrythmias is now challenged by amiodarone. In common with quinidine and disopyramide, procainamide increases the ERP/APD ratio in fast response fibers.

Properties. Procainamide slows conduction in the AV node, accessory pathways and ventricular muscle. It does not affect SA node activity, but may slow automaticity in latent pacemakers, abnormal forms of automaticity or triggered and catecholamine-induced automaticity. Procainamide displays a slight negative inotropic effect which may become particularly apparent after over-rapid administration. Hypotension and bradycardia may both follow from mild ganglionic blockade and impairment of cardiovascular reflexes. Its principal metabolite, N-acetyl procainamide (NAPA), is pharmacologically active, having primarily a Class III antiarrhythmic action. However, NAPA prolongs the QT interval less than quinidine and disopyramide and accordingly is less proarrhythmic.

Pharmacokinetics. Procainamide is well absorbed following oral administration (bioavailability 80-90%) for chronic administration. An intravenous formulation is available for acute and perioperative use. Renal elimination ($t_{\frac{1}{2}} \beta$ 2-5 hrs) accounts for 50-70% of the administered drug, hepatic acetylation to NAPA being responsible for the remainder. The latter reaction is less in genetically slow acetylators. Accordingly, NAPA plasma levels should be monitored in patients maintained on chronic procainamide medication.

Indications. Procainamide may be used for ventricular tachyarrhythmias in the perioperative period or in early phase acute myocardial infarction (AMI) even in the presence of cardiac failure or low output states. As with other Class IA agents it is effective for atrial tachyarrhythmias and may convert atrial fibrillation of recent onset to sinus rhythm. When used for atrial fibrillation or flutter, the ventricular rate may increase as the atrial rate slows unless this is prevented by the prior administration of digoxin, β-blockers or calcium channel antagonists. Rapid ventricular rates in response to preexcitation via accessory conduction pathways may also be controlled by procainamide.

Table 7-3. Drugs for perioperative arrhythmia (see Fig 7-12)

Class	Drug	Elimination Half Life	Dosage & Administration (Intravenous)	Arrhythmia
IA	Procainamide	3 hrs	Bolus. 100 mg over 2 min followed by 25-50 mg/5min up to total dose 1-2g	SVT, WPW, VT
IB	Lidocaine	1-2 hrs	Bolus 1-2 mg/kg. Infusion 10-50µg/kg/min Not > 24-30 hrs	VT
	Phenytoin	16-24 hrs	Central or large free flowing vein 100 mg/5min. Total dose <15mg/kg Only short infusion	VT (Dig.Tox) CLQTS
IC	Flecainide	13-19 hrs	1-2 mg/kg over 10min then 0.15-0.25 mg/kg/h	SVT, WPW
II	Esmolol	9 min	Bolus 0.25-2.0 mg/kg. Infusion 50-200µg/kg/min	Sympathetic Induced Tachy. & SVT
III	Amiodarone*	IV: PL.conc ↓ to 10% peak levels in 30-45 min	15 mg/min × 10min; 1 mg/min × 6 hrs. 0.5 mg/min × 24 hrs (1 000 mg/24 hrs)	Refractory VT & SVT
	Bretylium*	7-9 hrs	5-10 mg/kg. Dilute to 50 ml minimum. Infuse over 10-30 minutes. May repeat after 1-2 hrs, or infusion 1-2µg/min	Refractory VT
	Ibutilide	2-12 hrs	0.015-0.025 mg/kg. Infused over 10 min. Repeat after 10 min, if required	Atrial Fib/flutter
IV	Verapamil	3-7 hrs	5-10 mg. Over 3-5 minutes. May be repeated after 30 min. Infusion 5µg/kg/min	AV Nodal SVT
	Diltiazem	4-7 hrs	0.25 mg/kg over 2 min; then 5-15 mg/hr	AV Nodal SVT

Table 7-3 continued

Class	Drug	Elimination Half Life	Dosage & Administration (Intravenous)	Arrhythmia
CCA like	Adenosine	10 sec	Central or large free flowing vein. Incremental doses at 1-2 minute intervals, 6-12-18 mg, saline chaser	AV Nodal SVT
	MgSO$_4$	4-8 hrs	Loading bolus 40-60 mg/kg. Thereafter Infusion 15-30 mg/kg/hr.	Torsades de pointes
Unclassed	Digoxin	1.5 days	IV 0.9 mg/m^2 or 0.5 mg IV followed by 0.25 mg oral × 2	Atrial Fib/Flutter
Brady-Arrhythmia	Atropine	2½ hrs	0.2-0.5 mg. Repeated to total 2.0 mg	
	Ephedrine	10-15 min	5 mg aliquots → 50 mg	
	Isoproterenol	2 min	0.5 — 10 µg/kg/min	
	Dobutamine	2.4 min	2.5 — 10 µg/kg/min	
	Glucagon	3 min	40 — 120 µg/kg/min	

* = Multiclass effects
VT = Ventricular tachyarrhythmia
Dig Tox = Digoxin Toxicity
AV = Atrioventricular
PL Conc. = Plasma concentration
SVT = Supraventricular Tachyarrhythmia
WPW = Wolff-Parkinson-White Syndrome
CLQTS = Congenital Long QT Syndrome
Fib/Flutter = Fibrillation/Flutter
IV = Intravenous

Table 7-4 A. Class I antiarrhythmic drugs used for chronic arrhythmias

Drug	Dose (Oral)	Dose (IV)	Pharmacokinetics	Side Effects & Interactions	Precautions and Contraindications
CLASS IA					
Quinidine	1.2-1.6g/day divided doses 4-12 hrly	—	t½ 7-9 hrs PL 2.3-5 µg/ml	nausea, diarrhea, vagolytic, hypotension syncope, enzyme inducers	↑digitalis levels monitor QRS, QT, plasma K⁺
Disopyramide	Loading dose 300 mg 100 — 200 6 hrly	2 mg/kg over 5 min. to max 150 mg. Then 400 µg/kg/hr. — 3000 mg (max) in 1st hr & up to 8000 mg/day.	t½ 8 hrs PL 3-6 µg/ml	vagolytic, urinary retention, negative inotropy hypotension, CHF	CHF. Glaucoma, prostatism, SA node dysfunction
CLASS IB					
Tocainide	Loading 400-800 mg then 2-3/day	0.5-0.75 mg/kg/min for 15 minutes	t½ 13.5 hrs PL 4-10 µg/ml	CNS excitatory. Dizziness, tremor, GI reaction blood dyscrasia. Immune based pulm. fibrosis	
Mexilitine	Loading 400 mg then 100-400 gm × 3/day	100-250 mg at 12.5 mg/min then 0.5 mg/kg/hr	t½ 10-17 hrs PL 1-2 µg/ml	Dizziness, tremor, confusion, nausea, liver damage	Cardiogenic shock, heart block, conduction defects
CLASS IC					
Flecainide	100-200 mg × 2/day, hospitalize	1-2 mg/kg over 10 min then 0.15-0.25 mg/kg/hr	t½ 13-19 hrs PL <1.0 µg/ml	Dizziness, visual disturbance, fatigue, tremor, agents inhibiting SA node or conduction	Sick sinus syndrome, structural heart disease, RBBB, LAHB
Propafenone	150-300 mg × 3/day	2 mg/kg then 2mg/min	t½ 2-10 — 32 hrs PL 0.2-3.0 µg/ml	↑ Digoxin levels, CHF, GI effects	Structural heart disease, SA, AV node or bundle branch abnormality, asthma (relative)
Moricizine*	200-300 mg × 3/day	—	t½ 6-13 hrs	Dizziness, vertigo, headache, nausea	Impaired LV function

t½ = plasma ½ life. PL = therapeutic plasma level   *Multiclass effects. *Proarrhythmic potential and risk of Torsade de Pointes (tp)* — All Class IA, IC and III exhibit proarrhythmia characterised by inter class synergism.
Metabolism and excretion: All of the above (except sotalol) are subject to hepatic metabolism and renal excretion in varying degree.
CHF = congestive heart failure; GI = gastrointestinal; AV = atrioventricular; SA = sinoatrial; RBB = right bundle branch block; LAHB = left anterior hemiblock. ↑ = increases

Table 7-4 B. Antiarrhythmic drugs used for chronic arrhythmias: Classes II, III, and IV

Drug	Dose (Oral)	Dose (IV)	Pharmacokinetics	Side Effects & Interactions	Precautions and Contraindications
CLASS II					
Propranolol β_1 β_2 blocker	80 mg × 2/day	0.5-1.0 mg/min total 1-6 mg	t½ 8-11 hrs	Exaggerated bradycardia, heart block, -ve inotropy.	Overt CHF, bradycardia Bronchospasm, asthma
Metoprolol β_1 selective	50-400 mg/day 1 or 2 doses	5 mg × 3 at 2 min intervals	t½ 3-7 hrs	Synergism with drugs with above actions.	Peripheral vascular disease, depression
Acebutolol β_1 selective	400-1200 mg/day 1 dose	—	t½ 8-13 hrs	Smooth muscle spasm, bronchospasm, cold extremities	
Timolol β_1 β_2 blocker	10-30 mg × 2/day	—	t½ 4-5 hrs		
CLASS III					
Sotalol*	80-320 mg × 2/day	100 mg. Over 5 min	t½ 15-17 hrs	β blockade ↓ LV Function, AV block	Sick sinus syndrome, overt CHF, Bronchospastic states
Amiodarone*	Loading 1200-1600 mg/day, maintenance 200-400 mg/day	5 mg/kg over 20 min to 500-1000 mg over 24 hrs	t½ 25-110 days PL 1.0-2.5 µg/ml	Complex extracardiac, neuronal, ataxia, peripheral neuropathy, hyperhypothyroidysm, pulmonary fibrosis, liver cirrhosis, GI effects, photosensitivity	Synergism with Class IA & C, 2
CLASS IV					
Verapamil	80-120 mg × 3 day	5-10 mg over 3-5 min	t½ 3-7 hrs. Repeat after 30 min	Headache, constipation	Pre-existing AV nodal dysfunction. Digitalis toxicity
Diltiazem	40-120 mg × 3/day	0.25 mg/kg over 2 min. May be repeated	t½ 4-7 hrs	Headache, constipation	Pre-existing AV nodal dysfunction. Digitalis toxicity

* See footnote to table 7-4A

Contraindications. These include shock, heart block, severe renal failure and myasthenia gravis (procainamide inhibits muscarinic receptors).

Adverse Effects. Following intravenous administration, procainamide may cause hypotension from vasodilatation, especially if administration is rapid, i.e. > 25 mg/min. Heart block may develop or, if present, be increased. Adverse effects associated with chronic oral administration include systemic lupus erythematosus (most common in slow acetylators), rash, fever, arthralgia, agranulocytosis, hepatitis, vomiting and diarrhea, depression and psychosis. For these reasons chronic therapy with procainamide should not exceed six months.

Drug Interactions. Cimetidine inhibits renal clearance of procainamide, thereby prolonging its elimination half life.

Dosage and Administration — See Table 7-3.

Quinidine. Though quinidine (Table 7-4A) is the prototype Class IA drug, its use for conversion of atrial flutter/fibrillation to sinus rhythm has now been largely superseded by electrical cardioversion. The latter is more effective and lacks the many serious side effects of quinidine (Leon and Melino, 1993). These include prolongation of QT interval and consequent proarrhythmia, "quinidine syncope" and even sudden death. Though quinidine may help maintain postcardioversion sinus rhythm, there may be less long term survival (Coplen et al, 1990). For these reasons, its use in cardioversion has been superseded in practice by *flecainide* and *ibutilide*, albeit these also have problems. In the anesthetic management of patients on chronic quinidine medication, an important interaction is the potentiation of depolarizing and nondepolarizing muscle relaxants.

Disopyramide (Norpace, Dirythmin, Rythmodan). In contrast to other Class IA agents, disopyramide (Table 7-4A) has a significant dose dependent negative inotropic effect on the myocardium, an action thought to be based on interference with excitation-contraction coupling (Marcus and Opie, 1995). Vasoconstrictive properties increase afterload and oxygen consumption and so may contribute further to myocardial depression. It prolongs the QRS and QT intervals so invoking the risk of torsades de pointes, but unlike the other Class IA drugs, it does not inhibit AV nodal conduction.

Class IB agents

While inhibiting the fast Na^+ current these agents also shorten the action potential duration (APD) in non-diseased myocardium. Though the effective refractory period (ERP) itself is not changed, ERP/APD ratio is increased, so ensuring that the QT interval is not prolonged while the QTc interval is slightly shortened. Accordingly, these drugs do not provide a proarrhythmic environment. Class IB agents act selectively on ischemic or diseased myocardium (conditions associated with acidosis and high K^+ levels) so producing conduction block and thereby interrupting reentry circuits. With a particular binding affinity for inactivated Na^+ channels, these agents comprise the group of "fast"

Na$^+$ channel blockers with the shortest time constants for recovery from block (<300msec) (Langenveld et al, 1990). This property may explain the ineffectiveness of these agents in terminating atrial arrhythmias.

Lidocaine **(Xylocaine, Xylocard).** Lidocaine has become the standard intravenous agent for management of ventricular tachyarrhythmias in the setting of acute myocardial infarction, open heart surgery, anesthesia and digoxin toxicity. The drug has no role in the control of chronic recurrent ventricular arrhythmias. Lidocaine reduces the temporal and spatial dispersion of refractoriness. This follows from its hastening of the AP repolarization in Purkinje and ventricular fibers, an effect most apparent in fibers with the longest APD. However, in circumstances of abnormal conduction lidocaine may decrease or increase His-Purkinje and ventricular conduction time (Bigger and Hoffman, 1990). In ischemic tissue conduction time usually decreases substantially whereas in tissues depolarized by stretch or low extracellular K$^+$, conduction time is prolonged. Accordingly lidocaine (and other IB agents) can oppose ventricular reentry by two mechanisms, either by improvement in conduction eliminating an area of unidirectional block or conversely by converting an area of unidirectional- to bidirectional block.

Lidocaine at therapeutic levels does not affect sinus node automaticity in the absence of intrinsic dysfunction. However, the normal automaticity of the Purkinje fibers and depolarization-induced (abnormal) automaticity may be suppressed. Lidocaine and Class IB agents, other than phenytoin, have no important autonomic effects. In the absence of left ventricular dysfunction, lidocaine in conventional dosage also has little hemodynamic effect. In the presence of heart failure, however, it may aggravate myocardial depression and hypotension.

Pharmacokinetics. Administration of lidocaine is only by the intravenous route. Lidocaine kinetics follow a 2 compartment model with first order kinetics. Distribution and elimination half-lives are 8 minutes and 1.5-2 hours respectively. Plasma concentrations correlate well with antiarrhythmic activity, the therapeutic range being from 1.5-5 μg/ml. When used during cardiopulmonary bypass, factors such as hemodilution with consequent reduction in red cell mass and protein concentration, decreased blood viscosity, exclusion of the lung as a first pass organ, and hypothermia cause marked alterations in the drug's kinetics (Morrell and Harrison, 1983). In this setting an increase in the initial bolus is required to attain therapeutic concentrations of lidocaine. The drug undergoes extensive hepatic microsomal degradation with a clearance equivalent to the hepatic blood flow. Two major metabolites result which themselves have antiarrhythmic and central nervous system (CNS) toxic effects. These metabolites are excreted renally. Their elimination half-life increases after infusions of >24hrs duration.

Indications. Lidocaine is considered the standard intravenous agent for the rapid suppression of ventricular tachyarrhythmias in the perioperative setting as well as that following AMI. It has no place in the management of chronic recurrent ventricular arrhythmias or SVT. In the past, lidocaine was given as a routine prophylactic antiarrhythmic agent after AMI or before attempted defibrillation of ventricular fibrillation during open heart surgery. Opinion has turned against both uses (Teo et al, 1993; Singh, 1992; MacMahon et al, 1988).

Contraindications. Lidocaine should not be administered when there is bradycardia or bradycardia with ventricular arrhythmias. In these circumstances atropine or temporary electrical pacing are indicated.

Adverse effects. Lidocaine may cause severe bradycardia and heart block in patients who suffer from pre-existing sinus nodal dysfunction or impaired conduction. Occasionally there may be sinus arrest during coadministration of lidocaine with drugs that potentially depress nodal function. Toxic effects are basically a result of overdosage, i.e. infusion rates exceeding 50 $\mu g/kg/min$. Such toxicity manifests as central nervous excitation progressing to epileptiform convulsions followed by depression and cardiovascular collapse. Hypertension may accompany the excitatory phase. In the conscious patients such toxicity may be heralded by confusion, excitement, tremor and tinnitus. Treatment consists of discontinuance of the lidocaine, intravenous administration of an anti-convulsant agent and thereafter symptomatic resuscitative support until the short half life of lidocaine ensures such events terminate benignly.

Drug interactions. In patients receiving cimetidine or when beta-blockade depresses the cardiac output, the hepatic clearance of lidocaine may be reduced. Accordingly, the dose should be reduced, as also in the elderly.

Dosage and administration — see Table 7-3.

Phenytoin (**Dilantin, Epanutin**). Phenytoin is the antiarrhythmic agent of choice in two specific circumstances —

(1)   Arrhythmias resulting from digoxin toxicity. In this setting it preserves, even enhances, conduction, especially in the presence of hypokalemia. It also inhibits delayed afterdepolarizations (DADs) acting in part through a central decrease in sympathetic activity (Wit et al, 1975).

(2)   Control of the ventricular arrhythmias which occur during corrective surgery for congenital cardiac defects.

Pharmacokinetics. Following oral administration absorption of phenytoin is slow and unpredictable, whereas after intravenous infusion distribution is rapid. The drug is highly protein bound and subject to hepatic microsomal biotransformation. This process (zero order kinetics) is slow ($t \frac{1}{2} \beta$ 16-24/hrs) and is little affected by liver blood flow. Thus, small increases in dose can lead to substantial rises in the plasma concentration. Therapeutic concentrations are 10-20 $\mu g/ml$.

Adverse effects. As with lidocaine, CNS excitation is the commonest adverse effect. Relatively common also are nausea, epigastric pain and anorexia. Chronic administration may produce the serious adverse effects of systemic lupus erythmatosus, pulmonary infiltrates, gingivitis, microcytic anemia and peripheral neuropathy.

Dosage and administration — see Table 7-3.

Other class IB agents

Tocainide (Tonocard) and *mexilitine* (Mexitil) are registered in the USA for oral use only although intravenous preparations of both are available in Europe and the United Kingdom (Table 7-4A). In common with lidocaine both display little or no proarrhythmic potential, nor do they produce any severe hemodynamic depression and so may be used after acute myocardial infarction. However neither can challenge the primacy of lidocaine in the perioperative period. Their incidence of toxic effects is high and mexilitine's therapeutic/toxicity margin is narrow (Marcus and Opie, 1995).

Class IC agents

Class IC agents (Table 7-4A), all potent antiarrhythmics, are used to control ventricular tachyarrhythmias resistant to other drugs. The IC group of antiarrhythmic drugs comprises 3 agents, (1) *flecainide (Tambocor)*, (2) *propafenone (Rythmol)*, and (3) *moricizine (Ethmozine)*. Efficacious also for the control of supraventricular tachycardia (SVT) especially recurrent atrial fibrillation/flutter, proarrhythmic effects limit safe use of class IC agents to patients without structural heart disease (Falk, 1989). Of this group, flecainide alone is of perioperative use, confined to the management of SVT. Class IC agents have three major electrophysiological effects.

1) Of the Class I agents, they are the most powerful inhibitors of the fast Na^+ channel, causing a marked depression of upstroke of the action potential. In addition they exhibit the longest time constant for recovery from block (>1500msec) (GAMBIT members, 1994).

2) They exert a marked inhibitory effect on His-Purkinje conduction with widening of the QRS.

3) They shorten APD and ERP of Purkinje fibers markedly, while not affecting surrounding myocardium (Ikeda et al, 1985).

Their significant proarrhythmic effect may be explained by the markedly depressant effect on conduction, and electrical inhomogeneity which results from differential effects on the APD in Purkinje and ventricular fibers. Because of this, these agents have acquired a particularly bad reputation (CAST, 1989; CASH, 1993; CAST II, 1992). Long term suppression of ventricular arrhythmias with Class IC agents after myocardial infarction is associated with a 2-3 fold increase in mortality from arrhythmias compared with placebo treated controls (Roden, 1994; Epstein et al, 1993).

Class II antiarrhythmic agents

Class II antiarrhythmic drugs are the β-adrenoceptor blocking agents (Table 7-4B). The properties and wide spectrum of therapeutic application of this group of drugs in the management of cardiovascular disease are covered in Chapter 4. Attention here is confined to those drugs approved for antiarrhythmic use with particular attention to those of use in the perioperative period. β-blocking agents approved for antiarrhythmic use include *esmolol, propranolol, metoprolol, acebutolol, timolol* and *sotalol* — the latter's actions being a combination of Class II and Class III activity. Though the first four of these are available in intravenous formulation, only *esmolol's* kinetics and very short action render it truly suitable for acute perioperative use, especially during anesthesia itself.

Table 7-5. Intraoperative maneuvres associated with acute arrhythmogenic autonomic stimulation

---

AIRWAY MANIPULATION:

Pharyngeal stimulation: laryngoscopy; endotracheal intubation

SURGICAL MANIPULATION:

Oculocardiac reflex; Anal dilatation, cervical dilatation; Organ traction and manipulation; Sternotomy; Cardiotomy; Aortic dissection; Carotid sinus stimulation; Pheochromocytoma; Brainstem traction.

INADEQUATE ANESTHESIA:

Pain, Awareness.

Most of the above cause both sympathetic and vagal stimulation, with either one or the other predominating. Tachycardia = Sympathetic, treat with β-adrenoceptor blockade;
Bradycardia = Vagal, treat with Atropine.

Before using any of the Class II antiarrhythmic agents it must be remembered that pulmonary disease, especially asthma and bronchospasm, constitutes an absolute contraindication to non-cardioselective agents. If the presence or absence of such conditions has not been specifically established at pre-anaesthetic assessment, the patient's safety is best served by confining choice of agent to β_1 selective agents such as esmolol. An additional caveat is that cardioselectivity declines or is lost at high dosage. No β-blocker is completely safe in the presence of asthma. However, with caution, low dose β_1-cardioselective blockers can be used safely in patients with pulmonary disease.

During the perioperative period the principal indication for antiarrhythmic therapy with β-blockade is the control of supraventricular and ventricular tachyarrhythmias, provoked or aggravated by excess sympathetic adrenergic stimulation (Table 7-5). For this purpose esmolol is the drug of choice (Atlee, 1997). The other agents listed are principally utilized for the chronic control of tachyarrhythmias associated with cardiac pathology, most prominently post infarction ischemia. In this role they are, at present, the closest to the ideal antiarrhythmic agent because of their broad spectrum of activity and established record of safety (Table 7-4B).

Esmolol **(Brevibloc).** The cardiac actions of esmolol are typical of other cardioselective beta-adrenoceptor blockers (Fig 7-9) with negative chrono-, dromo- and inotropic effects. These produce a slowing of the sinus rate, an increase in SA refractoriness and AV conduction times as well as reduced cardiac contractility and output. The latter is associated with a decreased myocardial oxygen demand. These effects are most marked when the underlying sympathetic tone is high, as during anesthesia.

Pharmacokinetics. Esmolol has distribution half-life of 2 min. It is hydrolyzed by red cell esterases with an elimination half-life of 9 min. The resulting metabolites are inactive.

Indications. Treatment with esmolol comes into its own in circumstances in which rapid on/off control of β-blockade is desired as in SVT, non-compensatory sinus tachycardia and ventricular tachycardia associated with conditions of excessive adrenergic stimulation during the perioperative period (Table 7-5). Esmolol slows the rate of reentrant SVT and the ventricular response rate to atrial fibrillation and flutter (Schwartz et al, 1988) though it may not terminate these conditions. Esmolol also limits digoxin-induced tachyarrhythmias.

Contraindications and adverse effects. Esmolol should not be used in the presence of cardiac failure or decreased AV conduction such as may be associated with the administration of verapamil, diltiazem, digoxin and amiodarone. Further it produces additive effects with catecholamine depleting drugs. For the control of tachyarrhythmias and hypertension in the management of pheochromocytoma,

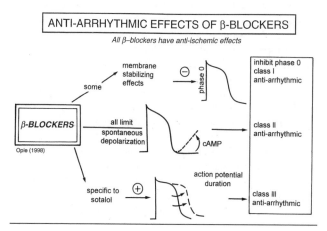

Fig 7-9. Antiarrhythmic properties of beta-blockers. Note that only sotalol has a Class III antiarrhythmic effect. It is questionable whether the membrane stabilizing effects of propranolol and related agents confer additional antiarrhythmic properties. (Fig. copyright © L H Opie, 1998)

esmolol must be preceded by pharmacologically induced vasodilation, failing which it may cause acute cardiac failure or even cardiac arrest. For this purpose use may be made of α-*adrenergic blockade, MgSO₄, sodium nitroprusside* or *nicardipine*. This same caveat applies to the use of esmolol for the control of severe reactive hypertension in the perioperative period (Table 7-6). Whenever the increase in BP is due mainly to increase in systemic vascular resistance

(SVR), then there is risk of cardiac arrest with esmolol. Furthermore, the success of resuscitation may be greatly jeopardized (Herschman et al, 1993).

Interactions. Esmolol has the potential to interact with inhalational anesthetics to cause bradycardia, AV block and to prolong non-depolarizing neuromuscular blockade. Esmolol may increase nodal inhibition caused by verapamil, diltiazem, and digoxin. Extravenous extravasation can lead to skin necrosis.

Dosage and administration — see Table 7-3.

Other antiarrhythmic β-blockers. Of the other β-blockers approved for antiarrhythmic use (Table 7-4B) *propranolol, metoprolol* and *atenolol* are available in intravenous formulation and may be used in the perioperative setting. However, their unfavorable kinetics compared with those of esmolol, i.e. slower onset and longer duration of action, have resulted in their replacement by the latter. *Metoprolol* premedication of high risk ischemic heart disease patients reduces the incidence of perioperative ischemia and arrhythmias, myocardial infarction and possible death (ACC/AHA Task Force Report 1996). In the field of cardiac surgery two meta-analyses assessing the prevention of postoperative atrial tachyarrhythmias have shown β-blockers to have a protective effect (Kowey et al, 1992; Andrews et al, 1991). Further, discontinuance of established β-blocker therapy preoperatively was associated with a higher incidence of postoperative atrial tachyarrhythmia (Abel et al, 1983).

Overdosage with β-blockers. The kinetics of esmolol allow it to be titrated to the desired effect. Any overstepping of the mark is managed simply by reducing or briefly discontinuing its infusion. Should this fail or in the circumstance that perioperative therapy with beta-blockers of less favorable kinetics may have resulted in overdosage, the following management is suggested. Bradycardia may be countered with intravenous atropine 1-2 mg. Should this be insufficient an intravenous infusion of glucagon (2.5-7.5 µg/hr) is the logical choice for this drug stimulates cyclic AMP production by direct activation of adenyl cyclase, a mechanism which bypasses the blocked beta receptor. Alternatively dobutamine may be infused at a dosage high enough (15 µg/kg/min) to overcome the competitive β-blockade. In patients not suffering from ischemic heart disease, isoproterenol is an acceptable alternative (Table 3-1).

Class III antiarrhythmic agents

Block of the delayed rectifier K^+ channel characterizes Class III agents. This prolongs the APD and hence refractoriness and is manifest as QT prolongation. By acting only on this repolarization phase of the action potential, Class III agents should leave conduction unchanged. However, three of the four drugs in this group currently approved for use have additional properties which modify conduction and may render them proarrhythmic.

These are: —

(1)   *Bretylium* — α- and β-adrenoceptor agonist and antagonist effects.

(2)   *Sotalol* — potent β-adrenoceptor blockade and Class IB and IC effects.

(3)   *Amiodarone* — a broad spectrum of actions of all classes of antiarrhythmic agents, with blockade of Na^+ and Ca^{++} channels as well as α- and β-adrenoceptors, and with many extra-cardiac adverse and side effects.

(4)   *Ibutilide* — the latest addition to this group is categorized as the first 'pure' class III agent.

Bretylium (Bretylol). Bretylium is selectively concentrated in sympathetic ganglia and post ganglionic adrenergic nerve terminals. Here, following an initial action causing release of stored norepinephrine, it inhibits further norepinephrine release by depression of sympathetic nerve terminal excitability, producing a "chemical sympathectomy". Bretylium's principal action is to increase the APD and ERP without change in the ERP/APD ratio or conduction velocity. It reduces APD disparity. This action prevents reentry and increases the ventricular fibrillation threshold. It has no effect on QRS duration, but does prolong the QT interval. After the response to initial norepinephrine release — increase in heart rate, contractility and blood pressure — bretylium can cause severe hypotension.

Pharmacokinetics. After intravenous administration bretylium it is widely distributed to the various tissues and is thereafter excreted renally with a very variable elimination half life of 7-9 hrs or more. There is no hepatic metabolism.

Indications. While not very effective for the treatment of SVT, bretylium has an impressive record when used for control of life-threatening ventricular tachyarrhythmias for which conventional therapy (correction of physiological deficits, lidocaine, procainamide) has failed. It may have special use in patients subject to defibrillation and external cardiac massage (Marcus and Opie, 1995) even leading to spontaneous conversion to sinus rhythm on occasion.

Side and adverse effects. Initial norepinephrine release may lead to transient aggravation of arrhythmias, tachycardias and hypertension. Profound hypotension is bretylium's major adverse effect. This is especially so in patients with depressed LV function, hypovalemia or sympathetic blockade such as accompanies spinal and epidural anesthesia, or the depressive hemodynamic effects of general anesthetic agents. This hypotension can be treated by intravenous administration of vasopressor catecholamines or protryptyline (5 mg/6hrly). The latter antagonises the hypotensive effects. *Dosage and administration* — see Table 7-3.

Sotalol (Betapace; Sotacor). Sotalol is a non-cardioselective beta blocker with prominent Class III activity. It prolongs APD and refractoriness in all fast response fibers by blocking K^+ repolarization currents and slows conduction in atrioventricular (accessory pathways) in both directions. It causes reverse use dependance QTc prolongation, i.e. more prolonged at slower rates, a property associated with the possible initiation of torsades de pointes (Hondeghem and Snyders, 1990).

Sotalol (intravenous bolus) terminates about 33% of episodes of atrial flutter and a somewhat lower proportion of episodes of atrial fibrillation, its efficacy increasing with continuous infusion (Teo et al, 1985). Sotalol may be used to prevent recurrences of atrial fibrillation and reentry tachycardias involving the AV node with or without accessory pathways. (Hohnloser and Woosley, 1994). This agent is effective too in the prevention of recurrences of symptomatic ventricular arrhythmias. In the cardiac surgical setting, oral sotalol (40 mg/6hrly) compared to placebo halved the incidence of atrial flutter/fibrillation in the first six postoperative days (Suttorp et al, 1991; Weber et al, 1996). However, its administration is associated with the risk of proarrhythmia (Ruffy, 1993). As therapy for postoperative atrial fibrillation and flutter, intravenous sotalol proved as efficacious as a combination of digitalis and disopyramide but acted significantly faster. Serious hypotension proved to be a major drawback (Campbell et al, 1985). For adverse reactions and dosage, see Table 7-4B.

Amiodarone (**Cordarone**). The product of a systematic search for coronary vasodilators, amiodarone is a unique "wide spectrum" antiarrhythmic which has actions that encompass those of all four classes of antiarrhythmic agents (Zipes, 1997; Bigger and Hoffman, 1991; Murray et al, 1994). However, its antiarrhythmic benefits need to be balanced against its slow and ponderous kinetics, a number of serious drug interractions which predispose to torsades de pointes and a wide spectrum of serious extra cardiac adverse side effects in patients on chronic oral medication (Table 7-4B). These include pulmonary fibrosis from which the resulting respiratory insufficiency is of particular concern to the anesthesiologist.

The electrophysiological effects of amiodarone include an increase in the APD and refractoriness of all cardiac tissues, lengthening the ERP without any effect on the resting membrane potential (RMP). It inhibits abnormal and normal automaticity of the sinus node and latent pacemakers. Amiodarone causes use-dependent Na^+ channel block coupled with an increased conduction time in all fast response fibers. Sinus rate is slowed and AV conduction time prolonged. ECG changes include increased QRS and QT intervals as well as T and U wave changes. These actions become more pronounced at faster heart rates. A peripheral and coronary vasodilator, amiodarone does not reduce LV ejection fraction.

Indications. Oral amiodarone is generally regarded as one of the most effective agents for the control of life-threatening ventricular arrhythmias (Nattel et al, 1992). Amiodarone also prevents recurrences of paroxysmal atrial fibrillation and flutter (Gosselink et al, 1992; Middelkauff et al, 1992), paroxysmal SVT and the tachyarrhythmias of the WPW syndrome (Markus and Opie, 1995). Because of the high incidence of serious adverse reactions its oral use is often indicated only when "all else has failed" although chronic use of low doses may prevent recurrent arrhythmias with relatively few side effects (Middelkauff et al, 1992). A disadvantage is that following oral administration, full activity takes days, even weeks, to develop. This may be overcome now by use of the intravenous preparation (Scheinman et al, 1995) when therapeutic activity may be achieved within 1-30 minutes (Martindale, 1996) (Table 7-3). Following intravenous administration amiodarone displays significantly different antiarrhythmic effects as well as a different profile of side effects to those evoked by its oral administration. Having high lipophilicity, amiodarone exhibits a large volume of distribution. Following intravenous administration, plasma concentration of the drug can decline to 10% of peak values within 30-45 minutes of cessation of infusion. Because the incidence of side effects increases over time — possibly related to the amount of drug accumulated — side effects are thought to be minimal in the setting of short term intravenous therapy (Desai et al, 1997).

The use of intravenous amiodarone is finding increasing application for the suppression of the arrhythmias associated with cardiac surgery. Prophylactic postoperative intravenous amiodarone administration has been shown to reduce the incidence of both supraventricular and ventricular arrhythmias without detrimental effect, even in the presence of left ventricular dysfunction (Hohnloser et al, 1991). The postoperative incidence of atrial fibrillation has also been reduced by a 7 day preoperative program of oral administration of amiodarone continued through the postoperative period (Daoud et al, 1997).

The fast onset of clinical effect following the intravenous administration of amiodarone has led to its incorporation into protocols of "advanced cardiac life support" for the treatment of VF or haemodynamically unstable VT.

For the *suppression of highly malignant ventricular tachycardias* resistant to other measures, recent experience has demonstrated intravenous amiodarone to be as effective as bretylium, yet to be accompanied by a lower incidence of severe hypotension [Kowey et al, 1995; Kowey et al, 1997]. In VT/VF caused by acute myocardial infarction, the AHA/ACC guidelines recognize only intravenous lidocaine, intravenous procainamide and intravenous amiodarone as being effective (ACC/AHA Task Force on Practice Guidelines, 1996). Following intravenous administration of the latter, maximum effect is achieved within 1-30 minutes and persists for 1-3 hours (Martindale, 1996).

Drug interactions. These have particular relevance in the perioperative setting and include prolongation of prothrombin time (risk of bleeding), increase in plasma digoxin levels with consequent risk of toxic bradyarrhythmias, adverse synergism with β-blockers and calcium antagonists. When combined with any drugs or factors that prolong the QTc interval there is risk of torsades de pointes. Interaction with the modern volatile inhalational anesthetic agents as well as other negatively inotropic, chronotropic, and dromotropic adjuvant drugs may produce severe cardiovascular depression, bradycardia or AV block (Atlee, 1990; Atlee, 1997).

These risks as well as the circumstance that up to 20% of patients on chronic oral amiodarone therapy manifest severe adverse reactions may suggest discontinuance of the drug. However, this course of action carries with it serious risk. Because of the drug's ponderous pharmacokinetics (very prolonged elimination half-life ranging from 27 – 107 days), the long wash-out period may see the reappearance of life-threatening ventricular arrhythmias and/or adverse postwithdrawal interaction with the substitute antiarrhythmic drug. Therefore patients must be closely monitored during this wash-out period and extended hospitalization may be necessary.

Dosage and Administration — See tables 7-3 and 7-4B.

Ibutilide (**Corvert**). Ibutilide is a recently approved (USA) intravenous class III drug that prolongs repolarization by increasing the slow inward Na^+ current and by blocking the rapid component of the delayed rectifier K^+ current (1_{Kr}) (Murray, 1998). In contrast to other class III agents, it does not appear to slow conduction significantly (Roden, 1996).

Ibutilide increases atrial refractoriness and terminates both atrial flutter and fibrillation. In animal models it has been shown to lower ventricular defibrillation thresholds. The drug displays minimal hemodynamic effects in the presence of ischemic LV dysfunction.

Pharmacokinetics. Because of high first pass metabolism following oral administration, ibutilide administration must be intravenous. Its elimination half life varies from 2-12 hours with a mean of 6 hours. Coadministration of digoxin, calcium channel antagonists or β-blockers with ibutilide has no effect on its pharmacokinetics, safety or efficacy. Abnormal liver function, however, is likely to lead to reduced clearance and prolongation of its action (Murray, 1998).

Indications. Ibutilide is indicated for rapid conversion of atrial flutter or fibrillation of recent onset. In initial clinical trials of its efficacy for short term rapid termination of atrial flutter and atrial fibrillation (Ellengoben et al, 1996; Stambler et al, 1996), it terminated the arrhythmia in 47% of patients within 19-27 minutes. Efficacy was greater in cases of atrial flutter than atrial fibrillation — 63% for flutter vs 31% for fibrillation.

In studies which directly compared the efficacy of ibutilide to other therapies in terminating atrial flutter or fibrillation, the drug was found to be superior to both intravenous sotalol and procainamide (Murray, 1998).

Despite this, due to ibutilide's proarrhythmic potential (see below), its role in this clinical circumstance is not well defined at the present time. DC cardioversion is highly successful but it does require brief concomitant anesthesia or sedation. In circumstances in which anesthesia is undesirable, the use of ibutilide can be considered. The use of ibutilide in the perioperative period still requires further evaluation.

Adverse effects. No significant hypotension, conduction block or bradycardia occur after ibutilide but this drug is proarrhythmic. Polymorphic   ventricular   tachycardia occurred in 3.6% of patients after a single dose and 8.3% after a second dose. This ventricular tachycardia was not sustained in just over half, the remainder requiring direct current cardioversion (Ellenbogen et al, 1996; Stambler et al, 1996).

Dosage and Administration — see Table 7-3.

Class IV antiarrhythmic agents

Class IV antiarrhythmic agents comprise the calcium channel antagonists (CCAs) *verapamil* (Isoptin, Calan, Verelan) and *diltiazem* (Cardizem, Dilacor, Tildiem). The dihydropyridine CCAs are not of use as antiarrhythmics (see Chapter 5). Binding to individual specific sites on the "slow current" L type Ca^{2+} channels, class IV agents directly inhibit Ca^{2+} entry into effector cells (Terrar, 1993; Opie et al, 1995). Consequent pharmacological effects are:

(i)   negative inotropic effect on the myocardium.

(ii) negative chrono- and dromotropic effects on the SA and AV nodes.

(iii) vasodilation — an effect more marked on arteriolar than venular vessels and which includes the coronary vasculature.

While prolonging the PR interval, verapamil and diltiazem have no effect on QRS duration or QT interval and consequently are not proarrhythmic. Normal automaticity of the SA node and latent pacemakers is slowed as also is abnormal automaticity in partially depolarised fast response fibres. AV nodal conduction time and refractoriness are increased and the action potential plateau amplitude and duration are reduced in fast response fibres. Conduction time and refractoriness in fast response fibres and those in AV bypass (accessory) pathways is not affected.

Pharmacokinetics. Verapamil and diltiazem are metabolized in the liver. After intravenous administration, AV nodal conduction is slowed, within 1-2 min, this effect lasting up to 6 hrs. Clinical management with these agents is facilitated by the fact that the AV nodal depression induced long outlasts the adverse hemodynamic effects (Singh et al, 1980). After oral administration, absorption is good but extensive first pass hepatic metabolism limits the bioavailability to 20-30%. Verapamil's elimination half life is 3-7 hrs, whilst that of norverapamil, its major active metabolite, is 8-10 hrs. Metabolites of diltiazem are not known to be active.

Indications. Until the advent of adenosine, verapamil and diltiazem were considered to be the drugs of choice (after vagal-stimulating maneuvers) in the management of paroxysmal reentry supraventricular tachycardias including the AV reciprocating tachycardia of the WPW syndrome. Success in the latter condition depends on the fact that although these drugs do not affect the refractoriness of the accessory bypass conduction pathways, one limb of the reentrant circuit goes through the slow fibers of the AV node, wherein conduction is slowed. However, chronic use of calcium antagonists in this condition is not appropriate because anterograde conduction along the accessory pathways is not depressed (it may even be facilitated by reflex sympathetic tone), so creating the risk of ventricular tachycardia or fibrillation. Verapamil and diltiazem also slow the ventricular rate in atrial flutter or fibrillation.

In the case of recurrent or sustained ventricular tachycardia, verapamil and diltiazem not only lack effect, but may cause fatal myocardial depression because of their negative inotropic effects. It is crucial therefore, that before such treatment the ECG of SVT (narrow complex QRS) be distinguished clearly from that of ventricular tachycardia (wide complex QRS). When confusion may exist because of SVT with aberrant conduction, administration of *adenosine* provides a therapeutic diagnostic test (Fig 7-11).

Strangely, *verapamil* and *diltiazem* as well as *adenosine* are effective against right ventricular outflow tract (RVOT) tachycardia. This is an unusual idiopathic type of VT thought to be a 'primary electrical disease'. The arrhythmia is exercise or stress induced in patients without structural heart disease (Markowitz et al, 1997). But again, verapamil and diltiazem can only be used safely when there is a certainty of diagnosis.

Contraindications and drug interactions. The negative chrono-, dromo- and inotropic effects of these compounds can worsen the similar actions of drugs such as β-blockers, digoxin, amiodarone and the volatile anesthetic agents. Bradycardia, heart block, severe hypotension and sudden LV failure may result. Administration to patients suffering sinus node dysfunction will have similar results. For the same reasons, the depression of myocardial function and AV nodal conduction inherently associated with hypothermic anesthetic techniques contraindicate use of these drugs for the treatment of the commonly associated atrial fibrillation.

Strategies for the management of these adverse reactions include the following:

i) Atropine for bradycardia and milder degrees of heart block;

ii) calcium chloride as a bolus;

iii) catecholamine (eg dobutamine) infusion. This may have limited efficacy in the face of heavily blocked Ca^{2+} channels;

iv) glucagon or phosphodiesterase inhibitors (e.g. amrinone), which increase intracellular Ca^{2+}. When available, management by temporary AV sequential pacing is preferred to that by drugs, especially during cardiac surgery.

Dosage and administration. (Table 7-3)

Class IV-like drugs

Adenosine (Adenocard). This drug has indirect calcium-blocking effects (Camm and Garrett, 1991). Three mechanisms are responsible (Fig 7-10):

(1) Stimulation of the myocardial A_1 receptors with consequent opening of the adenosine sensitive K^+ chan-

nels in AV and sinus nodes. This causes hyperpolarization of these cells, effectively inhibiting the voltage-dependent opening of the nodal Ca^{2+} channels.

(2) Reduced generation of myocardial cyclic AMP. This lessens phosphorylation of the Ca^{2+} channels so reducing their open state probability and attenuating catecholamine-stimulated Ca^{2+} fluxes. Cardiac sympathetic norepinephrine release is also decreased.

(3) Stimulation of vascular smooth muscle A_2 receptors increases cyclic AMP production at this site. Vascular contraction is inhibited with consequent general vasodilatation, decrease in SVR and systemic hypotension. This effect is predominantly arteriolar and includes the coronary vasculature.

Following from the above, SA nodal and latent pacemaker automaticity is decreased and AV nodal conduction time is increased. These events render adenosine highly effective in terminating paroxysmal SVT. The very same effects may cause transient heart block of varying degrees. Initial sinus bradycardia may be followed by a transient but longer-lasting reflex sinus tachycardia (Biaggioni et al, 1987). Adenosine has little effect on conduction or refrac-

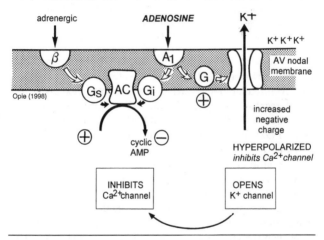

Fig 7-10. Adenosine and ion channels. *Role of adenosine in regulating the adenosine-sensitive potassium channel and indirectly regulating calcium channel opening. Note dual mode of action of adenosine. (Fig. copyright © L H Opie)*

β = beta-adrenoreceptor	G_s = stimulatory G protein
G = G protein, non-specific	AC = adenylate cyclase
A_1 = adenosine$_1$ receptor	G_i = inhibitory G protein

toriness in normal atrial or ventricular myocardium or the His-Purkinje system. It opposes catecholamine-induced triggered activity and ventricular automaticity (Murray et al, 1994).

Pharmacokinetics. Adenosine is metabolized extremely rapidly to AMP or deaminated to inosine by erythrocytes and vascular endothelium. With an elimination half-life of 10 sec (Faulds et al, 1991) the effect of exogenous adenosine terminates within minutes of administration. Sequential bolus doses are non-accumulative.

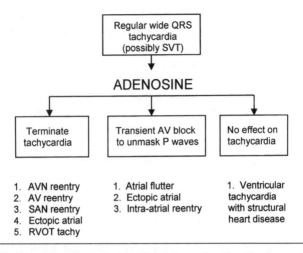

Fig 7-11. Adenosine and wide-QRS tachycardia. Algorithm for use of adenosine in treatment or differential diagnosis of regular wide-QRS tachycardia. If, after careful analysis of the patient's history, surrounding circumstances and the 12-lead ECG (if practical), wide-QRS tachycardia could be SVT with ventricular aberration, or findings are still inconclusive for VT, then adenosine can be administered for differential diagnosis provided the tachycardia is reasonably well tolerated and there is no immediate danger of hemodynamic collapse. AVN, atrioventricular node; SAN, sinoatrial node; RVOT, right ventricular outflow tract; tachy, tachycardia. (From J L Atlee's 'Arrhythmias and Pacemakers', WB Saunders Company, Philadelphia, 1996, with permission)

Indications. Adenosine has displaced the conventional CCAs and esmolol for initial treatment of paroxysmal supraventricular tachycardia, narrow complex SVT, AV nodal reentrant tachycardia and AV reciprocating tachyarrhythmias in WPW syndrome (Di Marco et al, 1990, Rankin et al, 1992). It has no effect on atrial flutter/fibrillation or that due to ectopic foci. Adenosine has a particularly valuable application in the differential diagnosis of supraventricular versus ventricular origin of regular wide complex tachycardias (Fig 7-11).

An exception to adenosine's ineffectiveness against ventricular VT is provided by exercise or stress induced right ventricular outflow tract (RVOT) tachycardia. This arrhythmia which is unassociated with structural heart disease is characteristically terminated by adenosine (Markowitz et al, 1997).

Adverse effects. Adenosine administration may be followed by transient AV block or transient new arrhythmias appearing at the time of chemical cardioversion. The conscious patient may experience headache, chest pain and flushing. In asthmatics there may be bronchoconstriction. However, adverse effects are extremely transient, disappearing within 2 minutes, except for bronchospasm which in asthmatic patients may persist for 30 minutes (Camm and Garrett, 1991).

Contraindications. Asthma or a history thereof, any degree of AV nodal block and sinus dysfunction, e.g. sick sinus syndrome.

Drug interactions. Dipyridamole inhibits the breakdown of adenosine, requiring much reduction of dose. Methylxanthines, on the other hand, competitively block adenosine receptors, necessitating an increase in dose (Marcus and Opie, 1995).

Dosage and administration (Table 7-3).

Magnesium Sulfate. When administered to patients to achieve a state of hypermagnesemia (plasma concentration 2-4 mM/L), magnesium evokes a core of cardiovascular pharmacological actions which mirror those of the conventional calcium antagonists, enjoying at the same time the advantage of easy controllability because of its short half life (James, 1992). The major effects are: —

(1)   Antiarrhythmic actions;
(2)   Negative inotropy; and
(3)   Peripheral vasodilation.

Pharmacokinetics. The kidney is the main regulator of magnesium plasma levels, its excretion being controlled by filtration and variable tubular reabsorption. The amount excreted responds directly to the load presented (Arsenian 1993). With normal renal function, excess magnesium is excreted within 4-8 hrs (Quamme and Dirks, 1986). Pharmacological effects require a circulating blood magnesium concentration of 2-4 mM/L (physiological level 0.7-1.0 mM/L).

Adverse effects and drug interactions. The hypotensive action of magnesium synergizes with the similar actions of the calcium antagonists, beta-blockers and the modern volatile anesthetic agents. Too rapid administration of excessively high doses of magnesium may cause sinus bradycardia or AV block and cardiac arrest (Mudge and Weiner, 1990). An action of particular relevance during anesthesia is magnesium's potentiation of the action of non-polarizing neuromuscular blocking agents.

Indications. Magnesium is effective against a variety of ventricular and supraventricular arrhythmias, especially those that are catecholamine-induced (Mayer et al, 1989). It is of particular value for termination of torsades de pointes and in countering the tachyarrhythmias engendered by digoxin toxicity.

Magnesium's anti-catecholamine and peripheral vasodilatory actions provide the rationale for the use of magnesium sulfate infusions as part of the anesthetic management of patients undergoing resection of pheochromocytoma (James, 1992). In these circumstances it is protective both against the episodes of extreme hypertension that accompany induction of anesthesia, intubation of the trachea, surgical stimulation or handling of the tumor, as well as the accompanying catecholamine-induced arrhythmias.

Dosage and administration (Table 7-3).

PERIOPERATIVE ARRHYTHMOGENIC ENVIRONMENT

Most perioperative arrhythmias are transient occurrences, precipitated by potentially correctable or reversible events. These should be identified and corrected before any definitive drug treatment is instituted (Fig 7-12). This, of itself, may often be sufficient to control the arrhythmia, so removing the need for antiarrhythmic drug therapy with its possible proarrhythmic or depressive haemodynamic potential. Failing which, it will improve the safety and success of subsequent drug therapy.

Table 7-6. Factors predisposing to arrhythmias in the perioperative period

1.	Excessive autonomic stimulation (Table 7-5).
2.	Pathophysiological conditions — iatrogenic and/or disease related.
3.	Drug interactions, toxicity, overdose, hypersensitivity or idiosyncrasy.
4.	Equipment or device (e.g. pacemakers) malfunction or microshock.

There are four major categories of causes for perioperative arrhythmias (Table 7-6). Firstly there are the maneuvers and manipulations related to both anesthetic and surgical technique which cause excessive autonomic stimulation (Table 7-5). Autonomic reactions to the maneuvres listed, while often transient and hemodynamically trivial, may have profound and serious effects if not controlled. On the one hand vagal-induced bradycardia, possibly associated with atrioventricular junctional rhythm, may result in a marked drop in cardiac output and so systemic hypotension and its sequelae (a particular problem in patients on β-blockers). On the other hand, sympathetically induced non-compensatory sinus tachycardia may precipitate supraventricular or ventricular tachycardia, especially in the presence of ischemic heart disease.

Stimulation of the autonomic nervous system (Table 7-5) is integral to the planned anesthetic technique and operative procedures. Autonomic effects therefore can either be prevented, e.g. by prophylactic atropine, or managed immediately if they become threatening. Furthermore, with cooperation between anesthesiologist and surgeon, causative organ traction can be discontinued immediately until pharmacological control is established.

The second group includes those pathophysiological conditions both iatrogenic and/or disease induced which alter the "milieu interior" of cardiac myocytes. Control of the patient's physiological homeostasis by the anesthesiologist is, in a sense, an ongoing process of "remedial intervention". Failure in the control of physiological homeostasis results in potential arrhythmogenic physiological imbalance. The latter includes such states as hypoxia, acid/base and electrolyte disturbance and temperature extremes.

Hypoxia provokes abnormal automaticity in depressed fast response fibers and when severe, conduction abnormalities and bradycardia predisposing to VF.

Acid/base and electrolyte disturbances. In general terms respiratory acidosis evokes a sympathetic catecholamine response and a lowering of the VF threshold, whereas the arrhythmogenesis of alkalosis is mediated through associated hypokalemia and hypomagnesemia. Failure of K^+ homeostasis manifests the major arrhythmogenic potential in this group, rapid change being of particular import. The anesthesiologist's control of the patient's respiratory home-ostasis has relevance here in the light of the reciprocal rela-tionship between acid/base status and plasma K^+ levels. Hypokalemia is a very arrhythmogenic state especially when associated with alkalosis and hypomagnesemia. Repolarization abnormalities and loss of membrane poten-tial effect conduction and refractoriness, so being conducive to re-entrant arrhythmias and disturbed automaticity or triggered activity. Thus the spectrum of hypokalemic arrhythmias resembles that of digitalis toxicity.

Moderate hyperkalemia, by contrast, is anti-arrhythmic, being associated with reduced automaticity of ectopic pace-makers, altered AV conduction and refractoriness which together prevent re-entry and abolish supranormal conduc-tion and excitability. However, severe hyperkalemia (> 7.5 mM/L) results in progressive slowing of AV conduction and decreased excitability, terminating in asystole or VF.

Magnesium deficiency, often present in the chronically ill, greatly enhances the arrhythmogenicity of hypokalemia. It is particularly associated with torsades de pointes.

Temperature extremes. Hypothermia, in particular, is arrhythmogenic. In the elderly atrial fibrillation may occur with a drop in temperature to 33°C. At body core tempera-ture of 30°C and lower, ventricular fibrillation comes to the fore and is all but invariable by the time a temperature of 26°C is reached. Successful defibrillation in these circum-stances depends on initial rewarming. *Hyperthermia* causes sinus tachycardia correlated to temperature rise, i.e. 10 beats per minute increase per 1°C rise. At extremes this can degenerate into malignant ventricular tachyarrhythmias. In the case of the pharmacogenetic Malignant Hyperthermia Syndrome, sudden onset of an endogenous catecholamine-induced sinus tachycardia almost invariably accompanies the onset of the syndrome, even before any change in body core temperature. Later when the temperature has risen, hyperkalemia and myocardial hypoxia complicate matters (Harrison, 1989).

The third group of arrhythmogenic factors embraces those due to *drug interactions, toxicity or overdosage.* It is not feasible to detail here all the possibilities for anaesthetic or adjuvant drug interactions in the causation of arrhythmia, but the following general observations are apposite. While their detailed cardiovascular pharmacodynamic profiles are varied, all the modern volatile anaesthetic agents — halothane, enflurane, isoflurane, sevoflurane and desflurane — display a central core of actions which are similar to those of calcium antagonists (Forrest, 1989; Hartman et al, 1992; Terrar, 1993). These actions, which stem from their effects on Ca^{2+} fluxes across cellular and organelle mem-branes (Franks and Lieb, 1994; Wide et al, 1993; Lee, 1994) are:

1) Negative inotropic effect.
2) Varying depressive chrono- and dromotropic effects on SA and AV nodes.
3) Reduction in systemic vascular resistance secondary to vasodilatation.

In general, drugs which reduce SA nodal automaticity or prolong AV nodal conduction time may cause or worsen bradycardias and escape arrhythmias in patients with sinus node dysfunction or impaired AV conduction. Drugs with negative inotropic effects are also likely to depress sinus node function and AV conduction. Drugs that cause hypotension following reduction in SVR may lead to reflex tachycardia. Those that impair myocardial perfusion either by coronary vasoconstriction or coronary steal, may invoke ischemic arrhythmias.

While not directly arrhythmogenic, certain anesthetics and/or adjuncts can sensitize the myocardium to catecholamine induced arrhythmias by lowering their catecholamine response threshold. While most volatile agents that do this have long since been withdrawn from practice, halothane is an example still with us. Should an arrhythmia occur during administration of this drug, change to a less arrhythmogenic agent e.g. enflurane/isoflurane or an opiod technique, is very often curative.

Technical equipment failure is the least common cause of arrhythmogenesis, and is usually preventable by adequate preoperative equipment checks. However, there is substantial potential for arrhythmias in patients with implanted pacemakers or defibrillators, especially with electrosurgery, electroshockwave lithotripsy, nuclear magnetic resonance imaging scanners, therapeutic radiation and the like (Atlee, 1996; Altee, 1998).

Management of perioperative arrhythmias

Specific treatment is required for an arrhythmia when it becomes hemodynamically significant, compromises myocardial oxygenation, is associated with sustained AV dyssynchrony or has the potential to lead to more life-threatening rhythm disturbances (Table 7-7, Fig 7-12).

While the occurrence of *extrasystoles* should always alert the anesthesiologist to check the patient's physiological homeostasis and correct deficiencies, the question arises as to when active drug intervention is required. In general, atrial extrasystoles are usually benign and do not require more active management. In the case of ventricular extrasystole (VES), distinction needs to be made as to whether

Table 7-7. Hemodynamically significant arrhythmias requiring specific treatment

---

Urgent treatment needed if the arrhythmia will:

1) **Compromise myocardial oxygenation**
   Any sustained tachycardia
   Tachyarrhythmia in patient with LV hypertrophy
   Ischemic heart disease

2) **Progress to life threatening arrhythmia**
   Frequent or multifocal ventricular extrasystoles
      (especially with ischemia)
   Ventricular tachycardia/fibrillation
   Persistent supraventricular tachycardia
   Heart block — advanced 2nd or 3rd degree.

3) **Progress to sustained AV dyssynchrony**
   Heart block with dropped beats
   AV junctional rhythm/tachycardia

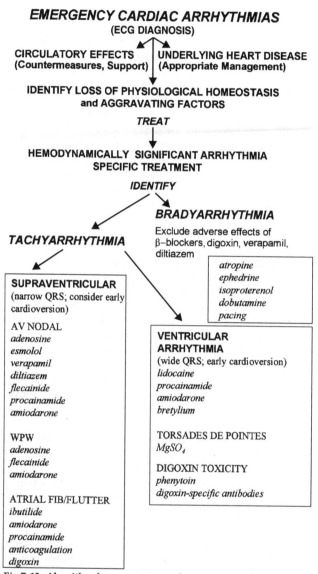

EMERGENCY CARDIAC ARRHYTHMIAS
(ECG DIAGNOSIS)

CIRCULATORY EFFECTS | UNDERLYING HEART DISEASE
(Countermeasures, Support) | (Appropriate Management)

IDENTIFY LOSS OF PHYSIOLOGICAL HOMEOSTASIS
and AGGRAVATING FACTORS

TREAT

HEMODYNAMICALLY SIGNIFICANT ARRHYTHMIA
SPECIFIC TREATMENT

IDENTIFY

BRADYARRHYTHMIA

Exclude adverse effects of
β–blockers, digoxin, verapamil, diltiazem

TACHYARRHYTHMIA

atropine
ephedrine
isoproterenol
dobutamine
pacing

SUPRAVENTRICULAR
(narrow QRS; consider early cardioversion)

AV NODAL
adenosine
esmolol
verapamil
diltiazem
flecainide
procainamide
amiodarone

WPW
adenosine
flecainide
amiodarone

ATRIAL FIB/FLUTTER
ibutilide
amiodarone
procainamide
anticoagulation
digoxin

**VENTRICULAR
ARRHYTHMIA**
(wide QRS; early cardioversion)
lidocaine
procainamide
amiodarone
bretylium

TORSADES DE POINTES
MgSO₄

DIGOXIN TOXICITY
phenytoin
digoxin-specific antibodies

Fig 7-12. Algorithm for management of perioperative arrhythmias.
WPW = Wolff-Parkinson-White; Fib = Fibrillation

they are uni- or multiform. If uniform and infrequent, and especially if similar beats had been manifest preanaesthetic, no further treatment is necessary. If their frequency increases significantly, treatment is indicated. On the other hand, consideration should be given to immediate treatment of multiform VES, especially if a new occurrence or in the setting of myocardial ischemia.

In dealing with *tachyarrhythmias* the most important distinction to be made is that between SVT (narrow QRS) and VT (wide QRS). This becomes difficult when the ventricular rate is excessive or in the case of SVT with aberrant conduction. In this circumstance the administration of adenosine may be both therapeutic and diagnostic (Fig 7-11).

Supraventricular tachyarrhythmias, in turn, must be differentiated into those of AV nodal re-entrant/reciprocating type or the atrial tachyarrhythmias, fibrillation or flutter.

Distinguishing atrial fibrillation or flutter from other supraventricular tachyarrhythmias is the very serious risk of thromboembolism and stroke accompanying the former (if sustained). Atrial tachyarrhythmias may occur in the early postoperative period, being especially common after cardiothoracic surgery, occurring in 11-40% of patients following coronary artery bypass grafting and in excess of 50% of patients after valve surgery. An independent factor most strongly associated with the development of atrial flutter/fibrillation is age — one third of patients over the age of 70 years developing it in comparison with less than 5% of those under 40 years of age (Ommen et al, 1997).

The principles of treatment of both types of supraventricular tachyarrhythmia are similar, viz. control of the ventricular rate, conversion to sinus rhythm and in the case of atrial flutter/fibrillation prevention of thrombogenesis by anticoagulation. For the latter, the risk of postoperative bleeding must be factored into its application.

While a number of drugs may be equally well used to control ventricular rate and induce cardioversion (Fig 7-12), the use of adenosine is more specific. *Adenosine*, the drug of choice for the control of AV nodal tachyarrhythmias, has no therapeutic effect on atrial fibrillation/flutter. *Esmolol* and the class IV antiarrhythmic agents are very effective for the control of the ventricular response rate but such control may be accompanied by hypotension especially in patients suffering LV dysfunction. With LV dysfunction, the positive inotropic effects of *digoxin* favour its use for slowing the ventricular response rate.

Ibutilide should be considered for the control of atrial tachyarrhythmias, especially atrial flutter (Ellenbogen et al, 1996; Stambler et al, 1996). It is also fairly effective for the pharmacological cardioversion of recent onset atrial fibrillation. However, there are, as yet, no published data on its perioperative use.

In general, with an etiology embracing such temporarily acting factors as pericardial inflammation and excess catecholamine production, postoperative supraventricular tachyarrhythmias are usually transient and respond to pharmacological cardioversion. However, with hemodynamic compromise, immediate electrical cardioversion is required.

For *ventricular tachyarrhythmias*, lidocaine remains the drug of first choice, unless digoxin is causative, in which case phenytoin and/or $MgSO_4$ are preferred. For patients with tachyarrhythmias related to advanced digoxin toxicity, digoxin-specific Fab antibody fragments (Fab) are recommended. Fab binds to digoxin and enhances its renal excretion (Atlee, 1996, Atlee, 1997).

Should lidocaine prove ineffective, though *procainamide* can be an effective second choice, current opinion favours the use of *amiodarone*. For the suppression of highly malignant ventricular arrhythmias, recent trials have shown intravenous *amiodarone* to be not only as effective as *bretylium* but also to evoke a lower incidence of immediate cardiovascular adverse effects (Kowey et al, 1995; Kowey et al, 1997). Thereafter, for recurrent ventricular fibrillation, bretylium may be considered as a third therapeutic choice.

With regard to *bradyarrhythmias* it is important to exclude possible adverse effects of other drugs the patient may have been taking, eg. β-blockers, digoxin, CCAs and when appropriate to consider specific antidotes.

Autonomically invoked bradyarrhythmias can be controlled by anticholinergic agents. The definitive treatment of persistent hemodymically disadvantageous bradyarrhythmias is transvenous or transesophageal pacing (Atlee, 1996; Atlee, 1998). For the milder degrees of *heart block* use of β-adrenergic agonists — ephedrine, isoproterenol, dobutamine — will suffice, while for the more severe, these agents will serve as a temporary support measure before temporary transvenous pacing.

DEFIBRILLATION, CARDIOVERSION AND PACING

Defibrillation

The only consistently effective treatment for ventricular fibrillation (VF) is electrical defibrillation (Figs 7-13, 14). Of recent years its application has been considerably simplified by the abandonment of the use of many past adjuncts for

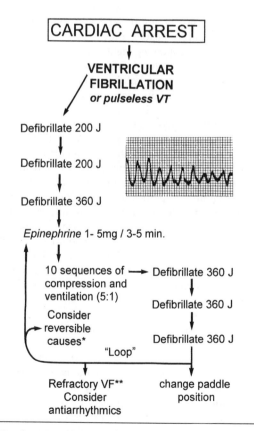

Fig 7-13. Algorithm for cardiopulmonary resuscitation, (CPR) when there is ventricular fibrillation. Epinephrine = adrenaline. Modified from European Resuscitation Council Working Party (1993).

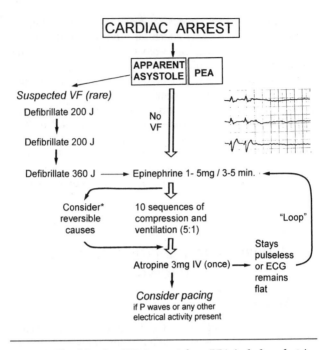

Fig 7-14. Algorithm for CPR in asystole or PEA (pulseless electrical activity) also called EMD (electromechanical dissociation) Epinephrine = adrenaline.

which no evidence of improvement in outcome has been forthcoming. Three factors only have been shown to improve outcome following defibrillation. These are duration of VF, efficacy of ventilation and cardiac compression, and administration of epinephrine (Atkins, 1986). The negative correlation of the duration of VF with the chance of successful defibrillation is the direct consequence of the high myocardial oxygen consumption and inadequate coronary perfusion with sustained VF. Ever-worsening ischemic damage correlates with its prolongation.

The efficacy of epinephrine administration in promoting success of defibrillation stems more from its α- rather than its β-agonist properties (Otto and Yakaitis, 1984). The former increases SVR, which in turn results in an increase in aortic diastolic pressure, hence coronary perfusion and blood flow. The optimum dose of epinephrine is still a matter of debate (Vincent, 1997). Human trials have failed to replicate animal studies which have demonstrated benefit from doses of epinephrine greatly in excess of those currently recommended for humans viz. 0.015-0.1 mg/kg/3-5 minutes (European Resuscitation Council, 1992; American Heart Association, 1992). As yet there is insufficient evidence to mandate any change from these. The use of pure β-*adrenergic agonists* (e.g. isoproterenol) in this context is now considered deleterious because the myocardial oxygen consumption is increased without any increase in SVR or in aortic diastolic pressure and coronary blood flow.

The administration of *sodium bicarbonate*, once a routine adjunct to CPR and defibrillation is also no longer recommended except in the presence of a severe pre-arrest metabolic acidosis. Not only is evidence lacking that sodium bicarbonate administration improves outcome from CPR but there is ample documentation of harmful complications (Vincent, 1997). During CPR, elimination of CO_2 is inefficient because of the combination of poor ventilation, reduced cardiac output and tissue perfusion. In these circumstances liberation of CO_2 from administered sodium bicarbonate can only worsen the intracellular acidosis with detrimental effect (Guerci et al, 1986). Further disturbance of the "milieu interior" follows from hypernatremia and hyperosmolarity consequent on sodium bicarbonate administration.

Discarded also is the routine administration of *calcium*. Because of the multiplicity of mechanisms by which elevated levels of cytosolic calcium can cause serious cell damage — summed up as "reperfusion injury" — not only is calcium administration now considered inappropriate but contrariwise the administration of CCAs has been suggested as beneficial (Otto, 1989). Lacking too is evidence in support for the routine use of lidocaine or bretylium prior to defibrillation, except for prevention of recurrences (Nieman, 1992; Vincent, 1997).

Cardioversion

Synchronised shock with cardioversion is effective in terminating reentrant tachyarrhythmias but ineffective for terminating automatic or triggered arrhythmias (Table 11-6). However, the tachyarrhythmia may recur if the abnormal conditions that provoked it initially are not corrected, and antiarrhythmic drugs may be needed to prevent recurrence. Arrhythmias effectively terminated by cardioversion include atrial fibrillation/flutter, paroxysmal SVT, tachyarrhythmias associated with the WPW syndrome and VT. Rarely cardioversion may cause VF. Therefore the practitioner should be prepared immediately to recharge the defibrillator to deliver a nonsynchronized shock.

Pacing

While electrical pacing of the heart is used primarily for the treatment of bradyarrhythmias due to SA node dysfunction and/or AV heart block, its use has been extended with success to the termination of the re-entry tachyarrhythmias (Atlee, 1998; Atlee, 1996; Deal, 1995; Wood, 1995). The several advantages over antiarrhythmic drug therapy claimed for pacing are (1) avoidance of adverse drug effects; (2) more prompt onset/offset of action; and (3) lessened requirements for precise identification of arrhythmia. The lack of simple, efficient, and cost-effective temporary cardiac pacemakers has been a barrier to more widespread use of pacing in the treatment of perioperative arrhythmias. In the future, the technique of transesophageal cardiac pacing may become important (Atlee, 1996, 1998).

SUMMARY

1. *Perioperative arrhythmias* are often transient occurrences precipitated by potentially correctable or reversible

events (arrhythmogenic environment). These include excessive autonomic stimulation, pathophysiological states induced by hypoxia, acid/base disturbances, electrolyte imbalance (especially hypokalemia), temperature extremes and drug interaction, toxicity or overdosage. In these circumstances the presence of structural heart disease serves as an additional aggravating factor. Such patients will manifest a lower tolerance of the arrhythmogenic environment than those with otherwise normal hearts.

2. The factors creating this *arrhythmogenic environment* must be identified and corrected before any definitive drug therapy is applied. Of itself, such action may often be, sufficient to control the arrhythmia, failing which it will improve the safety and success of subsequent therapy.

3. *Specific therapy* (Fig 7-12) is indicated when an arrhythmia becomes hemodynamically significant, compromises myocardial oxygenation, is associated with sustained AV dyssynchrony or has the potential to lead to a more life-threatening rhythm disturbance.

4. For hemodynamically disadvantageous, *life-threatening* arrhythmias, the most effective countermeasure is immediate electrical conversion (cardioversion/defibrillation) for tachyarrhythmias and transvenous or transesophageal pacing for bradyarrhythmias. When the arrhythmia is not considered immediately life-threatening or appropriate equipment for the above is not immediately available, drug therapy is indicated.

REFERENCES

Abel RM, van Gelder, Pores IH, Liguori J, Gilchinsky I, Parsonet V. Continued Propranolol administration following coronary bypass surgery: antiarrhythmic effects. *Arch Surg*, 1983; 118: 727-31.

ACC/AHA Task Force on Practice Guidelines. Guidelines for Perioperative Cardiovascular Evaluation for non-cardiac surgery. *Circulation*, 1996; 93: 1278-1317.

ACC/AHA Task Force on Practice Guidelines: Guidelines for the management of patients with acute myocardial infarction. *Circulation*, 1996; 94: 2341-50.

American Heart Association. Emergency Cardiac Committee. Guidelines for cardiopulmonary resuscitation and emergency cardiac care. *JAMA* 1992; 268: 2171-2295.

Andrews TC, Reimold SC, Berlin JA, Antman EM. Prevention of Supraventricular Arrhythmias after coronary bypass surgery: A meta analysis of randomised controlled trials. *Circulation*, 1991: 84 (Suppl III): III-236-III-243.

Anumonwo J, and Jalife J. Cellular and sub-cellular mechanisms of pacemaker activity, initiation and synchronization in the heart. In: *Cardiac Electrophysiology* Eds. Zipes D and Jalife J. W.B. Saunders Company, London, New York, 1995, 151-164.

Arsenian MA. Magnesium and cardiovascular disease. *Prog Cardiovasc Dis*, 1993; 33: 271-310.

Atkins JM. Emergency Medical Service Systems in acute cardiac care: State-of-the-Art. *Circulation,* 1986; 74 (Suppl 4): IV-4–IV-8.

Atlee JL. Perioperative cardiac dysrhythmias. 2nd Ed. *Yearbook Medical Publishers,* Chicago, 1990.

Atlee JL. Perioperative cardiac dysrhythmias. *Anesthesiology,* 1997; 86: 1397-1424.

Atlee JL. Cardiac Pacing and Electroversion. In: *Cardiac Anesthesia,* 4th Edition. (Ed) Kaplan J, W.B. Saunders Company, Philadelphia, 1998 (In press).

Atlee JL. In: *Arrhythmias and Pacemakers,* W.B. Saunders Company, Philadelphia, 1996.

Atlee JL. Temporary Cardiac Pacing: Practical aspects. In: *Arrhythmias and Pacemakers,* W.B. Saunders Company, Philadelphia, 1996, 247-292.

Baumgarten C and Fozzard H. Cardiac Resting and Pacemakers potentials. In: *The Heart and Cardiovascular System,* (Eds) Fozzard H, Haber E, Jennings R, Katz A, Raven Press, New York, 1992, 963-1001.

Biaggioni J, Olafsson B, Roberston R et al. Cardiovascular and respiratory effects of adenosine in conscious man: Evidence for chemoreceptor activation, *Circ Res,* 1987; 61: 779-786.

Bigger JJ and Hoffman B. Anti-arrhythmic drugs. In: The Pharmacological Basis of Therapeutics, Ed. Eds.Gilman A, Rall T, Nies A, Taylor P. Bergemann Press, New York. 1990; 840-873.

Bosnjak Z, and Lynch CI. Cardiac Electrophysiology. In: *Anesthesia: Biologic foundations,* Raven Press, New York, 1998, (in press).

Camm AJ and Garrett CJ. Adenosine and supraventricular tachycardia, *New Engl J Med.* 1991; 325: 1621-1629.

Campbell TJ, Gavaghan TP, Morgan JJ. Intravenous sotalol for the treatment of atrial fibrillation and flutter after cardiopulmonary bypass: comparison with disopyramide and digoxin in a randomised trial. *Br Heart J,* 1985; 54: 86-90.

CASH Study (Siebels J, Cappoto R, Ruppel R et al). Preliminary results of the cardiac arrest study, Hamburg, *Am J Cardiol,* 1993; 72: 109F-113F.

CAST Investigators (Cardiac Arrhythmia Supression Trial). Preliminary Report: Effect of encainide and flecainide on mortality in a randomised trial of arrhythmia suppression after myocardial infarction, *New Engl J Med,* 1989; 321: 406-412.

CAST Study II. (The Cardiac Arrhythmia Suppression Trial Investigation) Effect of the antiarrhythmic drug moricizine on survival after myocardial infarction, *New Engl J Med,* 1992; 327: 227-233.

Catterall W et al. Structure and modulation of voltage gated sodium channels. In: *Ion channels and the cardiovascular system,* (Eds) Spooner PN, Brown AM, Catterral WA, Strauss KGS and Strauss HC, Armonil, New York. Futura Publishing Company, 1994, 317-140.

Coplen SE, Antman EM, Berlin JA et al. Efficacy and safety of quinidine therapy for maintenance of sinus rhythm after cardioversion: a meta-analysis of randomised controlled trials, *Circulation,* 1990; 82: 1106-1116.

Curran ME, Splawski I, Timothy KW et al. A molecular basis for cardiac arrhythmias: HERG mutations cause long QT syndrome. *Cell,* 1995; 80: 795-803.

Daoud EG, Strickenberger SA, Man KC et al. Perioperative amiodarone as a prophylaxis against atrial fibrillation after heart surgery. *N Engl J Med,* 1997; 337: 1785-1791.

Deal B, Esophegal pacing. In: *Clinical Cardiac Pacing*. Ed. Ellenbogen K, Kay G, and Wilkoff B, W.B. Saunders Company, Philadelphia, 1990, 701-705.

Desai AD, Chun S, Sung J. The role of intravenous amiodarone in the management of Cardiac arrhythmias. *Ann Intern Med.* 1997; 127: 294-303.

Di Francesco D, Mangoni M et al. The Pacemaker Current in Cardiac Cells. In: *Cardiac Electrophysiology*, Eds. Zipes D and Jalife J. 2nd Ed. W.B. Saunders Company, Philadelphia, 1995, 96-103.

Di Marco JP, Miles W, Akhtar M et al. Adenosine for paroxysmal supraventricular tachycardia; dose ranging and comparison with verapamil. Assessment in placebo-controlled trials. *Ann Intern Med*, 1990; 113: 104-110.

Elharrar V and Zipes D, Voltage modulation of automaticity in purkinje fibers. In: *The Slow inward current and cardiac arrhythmias* Eds. Zipes D, Bailey J and Elharrar V. Martinus Nijhoff, The Hague, 1980, 357-373.

Ellenbogen KA, Stambler BS, Wood MA, Sager PT et al. Efficacy of intravenous ibutelide for rapid termination of atrial fibrillation and atrial flutter: a dose response study. *J Am Coll Cardiol*, 1996; 28: 130-136.

Emergency Cardiac Care Committee and Sub-Committees AHA. Guidelines for cardio-pulmonary resuscitation and emergency cardiac care. Part III. Adult advanced cardiac life support *JAMA*, 1992; 268: 2199-2241.

Epstein A, Hailstrom A, Rogers W, Mortality following ventricular arrhythmia suppression by encainide, flecainide and moricizine, *JAMA*, 1993; 270: 2451-2455.

European Resuscitation Council Working Party, Adult Advanced Life Support: The European Resuscitation Council Guidelines, 1992 (abridged) *Brit Med J*, 1993; 306: 1589-1593.

Falk RH. Flecainide induced ventricular tachycardia and fibrillation in patients treated for atrial fibrillation. *Ann Intern Med*, 1989; 111: 107-111.

Faulds D, Crisp P, Buckley MMT, Adenosine: An evaluation of its use in cardiac procedures in the treatment of paroxysmal supraventricular tachycardia. *Drugs*, 1991; 41: 596-624.

Forest JB, Comparative pharmacology of inhalational anesthetics. In: *General Anesthesia*, 5th Ed, Eds, Nun JF, Utting JE, Brown BR, Butterworth, London, 1989, 60-72.

Forest JB, Cahalan MK, Rehder K et al. Multicenter study of general anesthesia, II Results. *Anesthesiology*, 1990; 72: 262-268.

Forest JB, Cahalan MK, Rehder K et al. Multicenter study of general anesthesia, III Predictors of severe peri-operative adverse outcomes, *Anesthesiology*, 1992; 76: 3-15.

Fozzard H and Arnsdorf M, Cardiac Electrophysiology. In: *The Heart and Cardiovascular Systems*, Ed. Fozzard H, Haber E, Jennings R, Katz A and Morgan H. Raven Press, New York, 1992, 63-98.

Franks NP and Lieb, WR. Molecular and cellular mechanisms of anesthesia, *Nature*, 1994; 367: 607-614.

GAMBIT Members. In: *Antiarrhythmic Therapy*: A pathophysiological approach, Armunk, New York, Futura Publishing Company, 1994.

Gossalink ATM, Crijns HJM, Van Helde IC et al. Low dose amiodorone for maintenance of sinus rhythm after cardioversion of atrial fibrillation or flutter, *JAMA*, 1992; 267: 3289-3293.

Guerci AD, Chandra N, Johnson E, Rayburn B et al. Failure of sodium bicarbonate to improve resuscitation from ventricular fibrillation in dogs, *Circulation*, 1986; 74 (Suppl 4): IV-75–IV-79.

Harrison GG. Malignant Hyperthermia. In: General Anesthesia 5th. Ed. Eds. Nunn JF, Utting JE, Brown BR. Butterworth, London 1989; 655-667.

Hartmann JC, Bagel PS, Procter LT, Kampine JP et al. Influence of desflurane, isoflurance and halothane on regional tissue perfusion in dogs. *Canad J Anaes*, 1992; 39: 877-887.

Herschman Z, Dimich I, and Singh P. Sudden death in a young post-operative patient given esmolol. *Critical Care Medicine*, 1993; 21: 1975-1976.

Hoffmann B and Rosen M. Cellular mechanisms for cardiac arrhythmias, *Circ Res*, 1981; 49: 1-15.

Hohnloser SH, Meinertz T, Dam M, Bacher T et al. Electrocardiographic and antiarrhythmic effects of intravenous amiodarone: results of a prospective placebo controlled study. *Am Heart J*, 1991; 121: 89-95

Hohnloser S, and Woosley R. Sotalol, *New Engl J Med*, 1994; 33: 31-38.

Hondeghem LM, Snyders DJ. Class III antiarrhythmic agents have a lot of potential but a long way to go: reduced effectiveness and dangers of reverse use dependence. Circulation 1990; 81: 686-690.

Ikeda N, Singh BN, Davis LD, Hauswirth O. Effects of flecainide on electrophysiological properties of isolated canine and rabbit myocardial fibres, *J Am Coll Cardiol*, 1985; 5: 303-310.

Irisawa H, Brown H, Cardiac pacemaking in sinoatrial node, *Phys Rev*, 1993; 73: 197-227.

James MFM, Clinical use of magnesium infusions in anesthesia, *Anes Analg*, 1992; 74: 129-136.

Janse M, Reentrant arrhythmias. In: *The Heart and Cardiovascular System*, Eds Fozzard H, Haber E, Jennings R, Katz A and Morgan H, Raven Press, New York, 1992, 2055-2094.

Janse M and Wit A. Electrophysiological mechanisms of ventricular arrhythmias resulting from myocardial ischaemia and Infarction, *Phys Rev* 1989; 69: 1049-1169.

Keener J and Panfilov A. Three dimensional propagation in the heart: The effects of geometry and fibre orientation on propagation in the myocardium. In: *Cardiac electrophysiology*, Eds Zipes D and Jalife J, W.B. Saunders Company, Philadelphia, 1995, 335-347.

Kowey PR, Taylor JE, Rials SJ, Marinchak A. Meta-analysis of the effectiveness of prophylactic drug therapy in preventing supraventricular arrhythmia early after coronary bypass grafting. *Am J Cardiol*, 1992; 69: 963-965.

Kowey PR, Levine JH, Herre JM et al. Randomized double blind comparison of intravenous amiodarone and bretylium in the treatment of patients with recurrent hemodynamically destabilising ventricular tachycardia or fibrillation. *Circulation*. 1995; 92: 3255-3263.

Kowey PR, Roger A, Marinchak A, Rials SJ, Filart RA. Intravenous Amiodarone. *J Am Coll Cardiol*, 1997; 29: 1190-1198.

Langenfeld H, Weirich J, Kohler C, Kochier K. Comparative analysis of the action of Class I anti-arrhythmic drugs (lidocaine, quinidine and prajmaline) In rabbit atrial and ventricular myocardium, *J Cardiovasc Pharmacol*, 1990; 15: 338-345.

Lazzara R. Twisting of the points. *J Am Coll Cardiol*, 1997; 29: 843-845.

Lee DL, Zhang J, and Blanck JJ. Effects of halothane on voltage dependent calcium channels in isolated Langendorff perfused rat hearts, *Anesthesiology* 1994; 81: 1212.

Leon AR and Milino JD. Quinidine: its value and dangers. *Heart Dis and Stroke*, 1993; 2: 407-413.

MacMahon S, Collins R, Peter R et al. Effects of lidocaine in suspected acute myocardial infarction, *JAMA*, 1988; 260: 1910-1916.

Marcus FI and Opie LH. Antiarrhythmic drugs. In: *Drugs for the Heart*, 4th edition, Ed Opie LH, W.B. Saunders Company, Philadelphia, London, 1995, 207-247.

Markowitz SM, Litvak BL, Ramirez de Arellano EA et al. Adenosine-sensitive ventricular tachycardia: right ventricular abnormalities delineated by magnetic resonance imaging. *Circulation*, 1997: 96: 1192-1200.

Martindale. The Extrapharmacopoeia. 31st ed. Ed. Reynolds JEF. *Royal Pharmaceutical Society*, 1996, 817-819.

Mayer DB, Miletich DJ, Feid JM and Albrecht RF. The effects of magnesium sulphate on the duration of epinephrine induced ventricular tachyarrhymias in the anesthetised rat, *Anesthesiology*, 1989; 71: 23-28.

Middelkauff HR, Wiener I, Savon LA and Stevens OWG. Low dose amiodorone for atrial fibrillation. Time for a prospective study, *Ann Intern Med*, 1992; 116: 1017-1020.

Morrell DF and Harrison GG. Lignocaine kinetics during cardiopulmonary bypass, *Brit J Anaesth*, 1983; 35: 1173-1177.

Murray K. Ibutilide. *Circulation*, 1998; 97: 493-7.

Murray K, Ramo B, Hurwitz J. Clinical pharmacology and use of antiarrhythmic drugs, In: *Cardiac Arrhythmias*, 2nd Ed. Eds. Waugh R, Ramo B, Wagner G, Gilber M, F.A. Davis, Philadelphia, 1994, 347-391.

Mudge G, and Weiner I. Agents affecting volume and composition of body fluids. In: *The pharmacological basis of therapeutics*, 8th Ed. Eds, Goodman A, Rall T, Nies A and Taylor P, Bergemann Press, New York, 1996, 682-707.

Nattel S, Taljic M, Fermini B, Roy D. Amiodarone: Pharmacologic clinical actions and relationship between them, *J Cardiovasc Electrophysiol*, 1992; 3: 266-280.

Niemann JT. Cardiopulmonary resuscitation, *New Engl J Med*, 1992; 327: 1075-1080.

Ommen SR, Odell JA, Stanton MS. Atrial arrhythmias after cardiothoracic surgery. *N Engl J Med*, 1997; 336: 1429-1434.

Opie LH, Frishmann WH and Thadani U. Calcium Channel Antagonists. In: *Drugs for the Heart*, 4th Ed. Ed. Opie LH, W.B. Saunders Company, Philadelphia, London, 1995, 50-82.

Otto CW. Cardiopulmonary resuscitation of the adult. In: *General Anesthesia*, 5th ed. Eds. Nunn JF, Utting, JE and Brown BB, Butterworth, London, Boston, Sydney, 1989, 1331-1348.

Otto CW and Yakaitis RW. Role of epinephrine in cardiopulmonary resuscitation: A re-appraisal. *Ann Emerg Med*, 1984; 13: 840-843.

Pong SP. Molecular Biology of voltage dependent potassium channels, *Physiol Revs*, 1992; 72: 569-588.

Pressler M, Munster P et al. Gap junction distribution in the heart; functional relevance. In: *Cardiac Electrophysiology*, Ed Zipes D and Jalife J, W.B. Saunders Company, Philadelphia, Boston, London, 1995, 144-151.

Quamme GA and Dirks JH. The physiology of renal magnesium handling. *Renal Physiol*, 1986; 9: 257-269.

Rankin AC, Brooks R, Ruskin JN, McGovern BA. Adenosine and the treatment of supraventricular tachycardia, *Am J Med*, 1992; 92: 655-664,

Roden D. Risks and benefits of antiarrhythmic therapy, *New Engl J Med*, 1994; 331: 785-791.

Roden DM. Ibutelide and the treatment of atrial arrhythmias, *Circulation*, 1996; 94: 1499-1502.

Ruffy R. Sotalol, *J Cardiovasc Electrophysiol*, 1993; 4: 81-98.

Scheinman MM, Levine JH, Cannom DS, Friesling T et al. Dose ranging study of intravenous amiodarone in patients with life-threatening ventricular arrhythmias tachycardias, *Circulation*, 1995; 92: 3264-3272.

Schwartz M, Michelson EL, Swain HS, MacVaugh H. Esmolol: safety and efficacy in postoperative cardiothoracic patients with supraventricular tachyarrhythmias. *Chest*. 1988; 93: 705-11.

Singh BN. Routine prophylactic lidocaine administration in acute myocardial infarction; an idea whose time has all but gone? *Circulation*, 1992; 26: 1033-1035.

Singh BN, Collette JT, Chew CYC. New perspectives in the pharmacological therapy of cardiac arrhythmias, *Prog Cardiovasc Dis*, 1980; 22: 243-301.

Spach M. Microscopic basis of anisotropic propagation in the heart. In: *Cardiac Electrophysiology*. Eds. Zipes D and Jaliffe J. W.B. Saunders Company, Philadelphia, Boston, London, 1995, 204-213.

Sperelakis N. Origin of the cardiac resting potential. In: *Handbook of Physiology Section 2, Cardiovascular System*, Eds Berne R, Bethesda MD, Am Physiological Society (The Heart) 1979, 187-267.

Stambler BS, Wood MA, Ellenbogen KA, Perry KT et al. Efficacy and safety of repeated intravenous doses of ibutilide for rapid conversion of atrial flutter or fibrillation, *Circulation* 1996; 94: 1613-1621.

Suttorp M, Kingma J, Peels H et al. Effectiveness of sotalol in preventing supraventricular tachyarrhythmias shortly after coronary artery bypass grafting, *Am J Cardiol*, 1991; 68: 1163-1164.

Taskforce of the Working Group on Arrhythmias of the European Society of Cardiology. The Sicilian Gambit: A New approach to the classification of antiarrhythmic drugs based on their actions on antiarrhythmic mechanisms, *Circulation*, 1991; 84: 1831-1851.

Teo K. Heart EM, Horgan J. Sotalol infusion in the treatment of supraventricular tachyarrhythmias, *Chest* 1985; 87: 113-118.

Teo K, Yusuf F, Furberg D. Effects of prophylactic antiarrhythmic drug therapy in acute myocardial infarction. An overview of results from randomised controlled trials. *JAMA* 1993; 270: 1589-1595.

Terrar EA. Structure and function of calcium channel and the actions of anaesthetics, *Brit J Anaes*, 1993; 71: 39-46.

Vaughan-Williams EA. A classification of anti-arrhythmic actions reassessed after a decade of new drugs, *J Clin Pharmacol*, 1984; 24: 129-147.

Vincent R. Drugs in modern resuscitation. *Brit J Anaesth*. 1997; 79: 188-197.

Wang Q, Curran ME, Splawski I et al. Positional cloning of a novel potassium channel gene: KVLQT1 causes cardiac arrhythmias, *Nature Genet*, 1996; 12: 17-23.

Weber UK, Pfisterer M, Osswald S, Huber M, Buser P, Stulz P. Low dose sotalol to prevent supraventricular arrhythmias after CABG surgery and its effects on hospital stay. *J Am Coll Cardiol.* 1996; 27 Suppl. A: 309A (Abstract).

Wide DW, Davidson BA, Smith MD, Knight PR. Effects of isoflurane and enflurane on intracellular calcium mobilization, *Anesthesiology,* 1993; 79: 73-82.

Wit A and Janse M. *The ventricular arrhythmias of ischemia and infarction,* Futura Publishing Company, New York, 1993,

Wit A and Rosen M. After depolarizations and triggered activity: Distinction from automaticity as an arrythmogenic mechanism. In: *The Heart and Cardiovascular System,* 2nd Ed; Eds. Fozzard H, Haber, Jennings R, Katz A, Morgan H. Raven Press, New York, 1992, 2113-2163.

Wit AL, Rosen MR, Hoffman BF. Electrophysiology and pharmacology of cardiac arrhythmias. VIII: Cardiac effects of diphenyl hydantoin. *Am Heart J,* 1975; 90: 397-404.

Wood M. Temporary Cardiac pacing. In: *Clinical Cardiac Pacing,* Eds. Ellenbogen K, Kay G and Wilkoff B. W B Saunders Company, Philadelphia, Boston, London, 1995, 687-703.

Zipes D. Genesis of cardiac arrhythmias: Electrophysiological considerations. In: *Heart Disease,* 5th Ed. Ed. Braunwald E, W.B. Saunders Company, Philadelphia,1997, 548-592.

Zipes D. Management of Cardiac Arrhythmias: Pharmacological Electrical and Surgical techniques. In: *Heart Disease,* 5th Ed, Ed. Braunwald E, W.B. Saunders Company, Philadelphia, 1997, 593-639.

CHAPTER 8

Arterial Hypertension

Pierre Foëx, Simon J. Howell, Lionel H. Opie

This chapter will consider the principles of treatment of arterial hypertension as a medical condition, and the implications of hypertension in surgical patients, including the interaction between antihypertensive medication and anesthesia and the approach to the anesthetic management of hypertensive patients. Special attention will be given to the problem of peri-operative severe hypertension and its management.

PATHOPHYSIOLOGY OF HYPERTENSION

Hypertension is not a disease but a chronic elevation of blood pressure (BP) above certain arbitrary levels, which appear to be falling all the time. If sufficiently high BP levels prevail for sufficiently long, then end-organ damage results in increased morbidity and mortality.

The basic equation for control of BP is:

$$BP = CO \times SVR$$

where CO = cardiac output, and SVR = systemic vascular resistance.

Patients with arterial hypertension may therefore have either an increased cardiac output or an increased systemic vascular resistance, or both (Fig 8-1). There are many body systems influencing the BP (Fig 8-2). The increased load on the left ventricle associated with the elevated peripheral vascular resistance eventually induces left ventricular hypertrophy (LVH) and left ventricular dysfunction (Frohlich, 1991). In younger hypertensives, the cardiac output is more often elevated, whereas in the older age groups, the peripheral resistance is high. An increase in vascular tone results from enhanced α-adrenergic catecholamine input, or peptides such as angiotensin or endothelin, the final pathway being an increased cytosolic calcium concentration. An increase in vascular muscle mass, *vascular remodeling*, results from a chronic increase in arterial pressure and/or the effects of several growth factors, including angiotensin (Dzau and Gibbons, 1991).

The distribution of *body fluids* is altered in essential

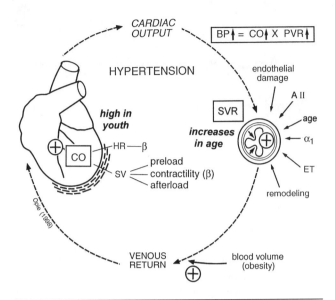

Fig 8-1. Basic mechanisms in hypertension. In younger hypertensive patients, the cardiac output (CO) is generally increased, whereas in older hypertensive patients, it is the systemic vascular resistance (SVR) that is increased. SV = stroke volume; HR = heart rate; α_1 = α_1-adrenergic; ET = endothelin; AII = angiotensin II. (Fig. copyright © LH Opie, 1998)

hypertension with a decrease in intravascular fluid volume, and an increase in interstitial fluid volume, so that there is an inverse relationship between the height of arterial pressure and the circulating volume (Tarazi et al, 1970). Conversely, in forms of hypertension associated with fluid retention such as renal failure, steroids, or obesity, both blood volume and BP rise.

The *autonomic nervous system* plays an important role in the normal control of blood pressure. In hypertensive patients, increased release of, and enhanced peripheral sensitivity to norepinephrine may be found, which could explain increased vasoconstriction. Responsiveness to catecholamines and to stressful stimuli is increased in hypertensive patients. There must also be impaired baroreceptor sensitivity because normally functioning baroreflexes keep

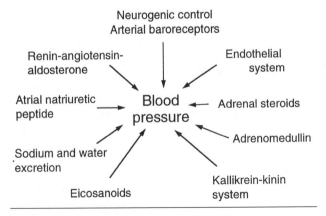

Fig 8-2. Diagrammatic representation of the major body systems involved in the control of blood pressure.

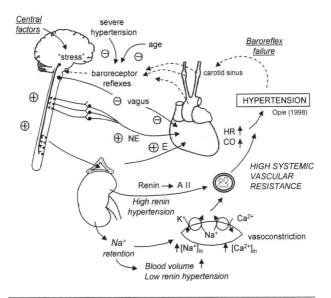

Fig 8-3. The mutifactorial origins of hypertension. (Fig. copyright © LH Opie, 1998)

the BP within normal limits despite changes in the SVR. A neural defect is suggested by orthostatic hypertension and diastolic overshoot during the Valsalva maneuver (Ferrario et al, 1991).

The *renin-angiotensin system* is clearly involved in some forms of hypertension, e.g. renovascular hypertension, and is suppressed in hyperaldosteronism. Some groups of patients tend to have low-renin hypertension, such as the elderly or black patients, and other (the minority) tend to have high renin levels. Those in the latter group are more likely to develop complications such as myocardial infarction (Alderman et al, 1991).

The various systems involved in the control of blood pressure are summarized in Figs 8-2 and 8-3, the latter also showing the role of the baroreflexes. These systems are involved in the development of essential hypertension. They may also be deranged in the small proportion of patients suffering from secondary hypertension, the immediate cause of which are listed in Table 8-1.

Complications of Hypertension

Complications include both those that are pressure related and those resulting from vascular disease (Table 8-2).

Left ventricular hypertrophy (LVH) is a major cardiac adaptation to chronic pressure overload. Concentric hypertrophy, with an increase in muscle mass and thickness but not in ventricular volume, provides the force necessary to overcome the excessive peripheral vascular resistance (Frohlich et al, 1992). LVH is an independent risk factor for cardiovascular disease, especially for sudden death. Left ventricular hypertrophy impairs diastolic function (Fig 8-4), as shown echocardiographically by a decreased E/A ratio (early phase filling rate compared with atrial filling). An atrial gallop rhythm (fourth heart sound), when present,

Table 8-1. Causes of secondary hypertension

1. Renal diseases
   — acute nephritis
   — chronic pyelonephritis
   — pyelonephritis
   — interstitial nephritis
   — renal arterial disease
   — polycystic kidney
   — connective tissue disease
       polyarteritis nodosa
       disseminated lupus erythematosus

2. Coarction of the aorta

3. Pheochromocytoma

4. Cushing syndrome

5. Primary aldosteronism (Conn's syndrome)

6. Toxemia of pregnancy

7. Disorders of the autonomic nervous system

Table 8-2. Manifestations of target-organ disease

Cardiac	Clinical, ECG, radiographic evidence of coronary artery disease, LVH with diastolic dysfunction, LV, systolic failure, congestive heart failure.
Cerebrovascular	Stroke, transient ischemic attacks.
Renal	Elevated serum creatinine, proteinuria, proteinuria
Ocular	Hemorrhages, exudates

reflects the increased force of atrial systole. Left atrial enlargement is often detected electrocardiographically as abnormalities of the P wave. Especially in the elderly, left ventricular failure may occur solely because of the diastolic dysfunction while systolic function is still maintained.

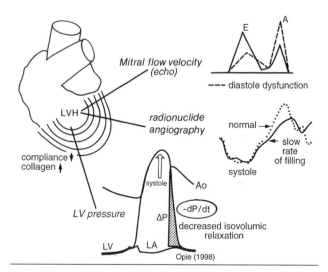

Fig 8-4. Concentric hypertrophy in hypertension. (Fig. copyright © LH Opie, 1998)

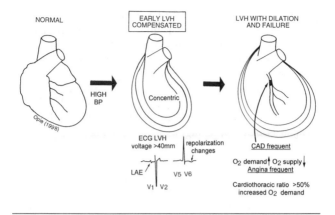

Fig 8-5. Hypothetical evolution of hypertensive heart disease. (Fig. copyright © LH Opie, 1998)

Heart failure may start as diastolic dysfunction and then progress to overt systolic failure with congestive signs (Fig 8-5).

Coronary artery disease is associated with and accelerated by chronic hypertension (MacMahon et al, 1990), possibly the result of endothelial damage. Myocardial ischemia and myocardial infarction are, therefore, major complications of hypertension. The ischemia may not be clinically evident; silent ischemia is detected by continuous electrocardiographic monitoring. Two main factors may be responsible for myocardial ischemia: an increased myocardial demand (excessive wall stress) and a decrease in coronary blood supply because of the associated atherosclerosis (Fig. 8-6). In addition, the coronary vascular reserve is reduced in hypertension.

Aortic disease with development of plaques may be a source of cerebral embolism. Especially with age, stiffening of the aorta leads to loss of its buffer function and the development of systolic hypertension. Dissection of aneurysms of the thoracic or abdominal aorta is now an infrequent complication of hypertension, probably because of increasingly effective antihypertensive therapy.

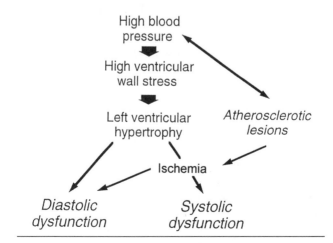

Fig 8-6. Effects of arterial hypertension on the heart.

Malignant and accelerated hypertension have also become less common. However, if untreated, mortality remains high. A major feature is the fibrinoid deposition in the glomeruli with a decrease in renal blood flow, resulting in intense renin-angiotensin stimulation.

Renal disease is initially manifest as microalbuminuria, and may take many years to become clinically evident. Established renal disease may result from renal and glomerular arteriolar thickening, and may eventually lead to end-stage renal failure. Conversely, hypertension is frequently a complication of renal diseases.

Strokes have always been recognized as major complications of hypertension. Cerebral hemorrhage is pressure-related, while thromboembolism is on the basis of associated carotid or aortic arch disease, or left atrial enlargement. The advent of antihypertensive therapy has substantially reduced the risk of cerebrovascular accidents, which nevertheless remain as serious complications.

LONG-TERM TREATMENT OF ARTERIAL HYPERTENSION

As blood pressure is the product of cardiac output and peripheral vascular resistance, all antihypertensive drugs must act either by reducing the cardiac output or the peripheral vascular resistance. The classes of drugs used in the treatment of hypertension include the diuretics, beta-blockers, angiotensin converting enzyme (ACE) inhibitors, calcium antagonists, alpha-blockers, combined alpha- and beta-blockers, some direct vasodilators, and some centrally active drugs (Fig 8-7).

The treatment of hypertension reduces overall cardiovascular mortality mostly by reducing stroke (Collins et al, 1990). The complications of coronary artery disease are not convincingly reduced by the treatment of hypertension. This may be because lipid-lowering is not undertaken as often as it should be. Other possibilities include coronary hypo-perfusion from overtreatment, too short a duration of treatment, inadequate control of blood pressure, or metabolic side-effects of drug such as beta-blockers or high dose diuretics. Any or all of these factors may explain the disappointing effect of the antihypertensive therapy in not reducing the incidence of coronary events as much as expected.

Life-style modification, the first step in general clinical practice, includes moderate sodium restriction, weight reduction in the obese, decreased alcohol intake, and an increase in aerobic exercise. Drugs are normally reserved for patients who remain hypertensive despite this regime, or those who have seriously high BP levels to start with. The level of blood pressure reduction to be aimed at is a function of the associated risk factors such as high blood cholesterol, smoking, diabetes, and coronary artery disease. While it is customary to treat hypertension as a function of the diastolic blood pressure (Swales, 1993), the level of systolic blood pressure is very important especially in the

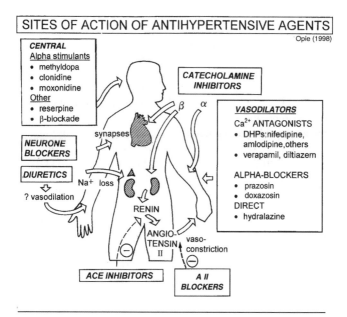

SITES OF ACTION OF ANTIHYPERTENSIVE AGENTS
Opie (1998)

CENTRAL
Alpha stimulants
- methyldopa
- clonidine
- moxonidine
Other
- reserpine
- β-blockade

NEURONE BLOCKERS

DIURETICS
Na⁺ loss
? vasodilation

synapses

CATECHOLAMINE INHIBITORS

β   α

VASODILATORS
Ca²⁺ ANTAGONISTS
- DHPs:nifedipine, amlodipine,others
- verapamil, diltiazem

ALPHA-BLOCKERS
- prazosin
- doxazosin
DIRECT
- hydralazine

RENIN

ANGIO-TENSIN II   vaso-constriction

ACE INHIBITORS   **A II BLOCKERS**

Fig 8-7. Different types of antihypertensive agents act as different sites. Because hypertension is frequently multifactorial in origin, it may be difficult to find the ideal drug for a given patient and drug combinations are often used. DHPs = dihydropyridines. (Fig. copyright © LH Opie, 1998)

elderly. *Systolic hypertension*, with a systolic BP consistently exceeding 160 mmHg, and a diastolic BP below 90 mm Hg, is now a recognized reason for diuretic-based treatment in the elderly (SHEP, 1991).

Choice of first drug

A diuretic is generally advocated as first line drug treatment. American and British practice recognizes a beta-blocker as an alternate (JNC VI, 1997), whereas the International Society of Hypertension and the World Health Organization (Zanchetti, 1995) allow for a choice among four types of agents: diuretics, beta-blockers, calcium antagonists, and ACE inhibitors. It is often feared that beta-blockers and high-dose diuretics impair insulin sensitivity, with the risk of patients developing overt diabetes and/or disorder of lipid metabolism. By contrast ACE inhibitors and alpha-blockers may improve insulin sensitivity, with calcium antagonists being neutral. Thus, the first line drug may be selected as a function of the patient's condition. For example, patients with diabetes or renal disease or high circulating renin values, should benefit from ACE inhibitor therapy. Conversely, in patients with overt coronary artery disease, there is a stronger case for using beta-blockers or calcium antagonists, and in those with high renin levels, ACE inhibitors are indicated. Recently, strong emphasis has been laid on the requirement for evidence based choices, and both the calcium antagonists and the ACE inhibitors have been criticized for lack of beneficial outcome studies, with only one available for calcium antagonists (Syst-Eur, 1997) and none for ACE inhibitors.

Diuretics

Low dose diuretic therapy is often effective, especially when associated with a low sodium diet. Low dose diuretics reduce stroke, coronary heart disease, congestive heart failure and cardiovascular and total mortality (JNC VI, 1997). Hydrochlorothiazide, chlorthalidone, benzofluazide, indapamine and others are used successfully with minimal metabolic side-effects. Loop diuretics may also be used. It is claimed that torsemide is anti-hypertensive in sub-diuretic doses, yet in the USA the minimum approved antihypertensive dose is also diuretic. Potassium-sparing diuretics have the advantage of lessening diuretic-induced hypokalemia and hypomagnesemia when combined with a standard diuretic. Even very small doses of diuretics may be effective when given together with another drug category such as beta-blockers, or ACE inhibitors (Frishman et al, 1994, Canter et al, 1994). Whether there is added antihypertensive effect when diuretics are added to calcium antagonists remains controversial. Whether even low doses of diuretics may decrease plasma potassium, impair glucose tolerance, increase uric acid, and increase blood LDL (low density lipoprotein) levels, is also still controversial. However in the TOHM study, the metabolic changes induced by a low dose diuretic over 4 years were minimal (TOHM, 1992).

Recently a case control study (Hoes et al, 1995) has shown that the risk of sudden cardiac death in hypertensive patients is greater when non-potassium sparing diuretics are used, especially in patients younger than 75 years. This is also true when non-potassium sparing diuretics are used together with beta-blockers. The adverse effect of non-potassium sparing diuretics appears to relate to the their dosage (Siscovick, 1994), with a thiazide dose of 25 mg in a potassium-retaining combination apparently safe when compared with beta-blockade.

Beta-blockers

Beta-blockers may be preferentially chosen in patients with high sympathetic activity, angina, or after myocardial infarction. A low dose has the advantage of minimizing the risk of fatigue, and in the elderly of excess bradycardia. There is little antihypertensive advantage in using large doses of beta-blockers as combination therapy is more effective. This can be achieved by adding a low-dose diuretic. Thus the majority of elderly patients successfully treated in the STOP study and 21% of those in the SHEP study (STOP, 1991; SHEP, 1991), were receiving combined diuretic with beta-blocker therapy. Dihydropyridines (DHPs) such as long acting nifedipine or amlodipine may also be combined with a beta-blocker. DHPs provide powerful afterload reduction, which via baroreflexes, minimizes the risk of bradycardia. However, this combination receives no support from outcome studies.

The triple combination of a diuretic plus a beta-blocker plus a calcium antagonist is often efficacious in severe or refractory hypertension (Heagerty et al, 1988).

Calcium antagonists

Pharmacologically, the calcium antagonists may be divided into two main groups, the dihydropyridines (DHPs; prototype: nifedipine), and the non-DHPs, represented by verapamil and diltiazem. For both groups, the main site of action is vascular at the level of the arterioles. Both groups rapidly reduce peripheral vascular resistance to decrease blood pressure even in patients otherwise refractory. With short-acting DHPs (nifedipine capsules and similar agents), rapid vasodilation is associated with reflex adrenergic activation with tachycardia that can precipitate ischemia. With such agents, which are vascular selective, there is no negative inotropy in patients with normal left ventricular function. Both plasma catecholamines and renin activity tend to increase. Long acting DHPs, such as amlodipine and truly long acting preparations of nifedipine, are slower in onset of action and correspondingly cause less sympathetic activation. Nonetheless, as a group, even long-acting DHPs cause some sympathetic activation in contrast to the decrease found with long-acting non-DHPs (Grossman and Messerli, 1997).

Non-DHPs such as verapamil act on the heart in addition to the arterioles. Thus besides reducing blood pressure, they decrease the heart rate, and have a more prominent negative inotropic effect than the DHPs. These properties may explain why verapamil confers post-myocardial protection against re-infarction. Calcium antagonists as a group are effective in elderly patients and may be selected as monotherapy particularly in patients who also have angina pectoris, Raynaud's phenomenon, or peripheral vascular disease. In the latter two groups beta-blockers may worsen peripheral ischemia. The absence of metabolic disturbances (potassium, glucose, uric acid, lipid metabolism) is an advantage of calcium antagonists when compared with diuretics and beta-blockers. Calcium antagonists can be used safely in asthmatics and in patients with peripheral vascular disease. They are contraindicated in the presence of heart failure, except for amlodipine which may be used for hypertensive heart failure in patients who are otherwise fully treated by diuretics, an ACE inhibitor, and digoxin (Packer et al, 1996). *In diabetic hypertensives*, however, DHP calcium antagonists have more cardiovascular complications than ACE inhibitors (Estacio et al, 1998; Tatti et al, 1997). On the other hand, the non-DHP verapamil was better at slowing diabetic renal disease than the β-blocker, atenolol (Bakris et al, 1996).

Nifedipine is one of the most effective drugs in severe hypertension and often used in capsular form, frequently without due care for the risk of excess hypotension or other adverse effects (Grossman and Messerli, 1997). Amlodipine is another DHP calcium antagonists with, however, slow onset of action and a very long half life, that is well tolerated (TOMH study, 1991). One of the most vascular specific of the dihydropyridine calcium antagonists, nisoldipine, has a high affinity for vascular smooth muscle, especially in the coronary arteries, and a low affinity for the myocardium (Godfraind, 1994). Nisoldipine has a higher affinity for calcium channels inactivated by prolonged depolarisation, so that it may be more effective in ischemic tissue (Knorr, 1995). This aspect still needs clinical confirmation.

The combination of DHP calcium antagonists and beta-blockers is hemodynamically sound. The addition of a diuretic to a calcium antagonist has demonstrable benefits in the case of verapamil (Holzgreve et al, 1989) or diltiazem, but not so clearly in the case of DHPs such as nifedipine, which seem to have a diuretic action in their own right.

The combination of calcium antagonists and ACE inhibitors has also been advocated (Singer et al, 1987), especially verapamil with an ACE inhibitor in patients with early renal disease (Bakris et al, 1992). However, long-term outcome studies are still awaited.

ACE inhibitors

Initially, ACE inhibitors were reserved for refractory hypertension, especially of renal origin. More recently, they have started to be used as first line drugs in hypertension. With the exception of cough, they have relatively few side-effects, and have no contra-indications except for bilateral renal artery stenosis and pregnancy. There are few differences between the drugs currently available except in terms of plasma half-life. Not all patients respond to ACE inhibitor monotherapy, maybe because of the importance of moderate dietary salt restriction (World Hypertension League, 1993).

In renovascular hypertension, the hypotensive response to ACE inhibitors may be very dramatic with risk of renal failure, so that the initial dose should be very low. Blood flow to a single stenotic kidney may remain depressed by ACE inhibitors with the risk of ischemic atrophy (Postma et al, 1989). Thus, angioplasty or surgery is preferable to long-term medical therapy. In case of bilateral renal artery stenosis, the risk of renal failure has been well documented and extreme caution is required if ACE inhibitors are given at all.

In diabetic hypertensives, ACE inhibitors are agents of first choice. They offer some protection against progressive glomerulosclerosis. Captopril reduces albuminuria. In hypertensive renal failure in type 1 diabetics, ACE inhibitors slow the progression of the disease when compared with beta-blockers (Lewis et al, 1993). In type 2 diabetes, ACE inhibitors give better results than a DHP calcium antagonist, as judged by hard cardiovascular endpoints (Estacio et al, 1998; Tatti et al, 1997).

In hypertension with heart failure, ACE inhibitors are the first choice drugs. They are often combined with diuretics. However, there is a risk of hyperkalemia when they are used in combination with potassium-retaining diuretics.

The association with non-DHP calcium antagonists may have advantages in terms of renal protection.

ACE inhibitors can increase vasoconstrictor requirements after cardiopulmonary bypass as shown in a large study involving over 4,000 adult patients. Logistic regression analysis showed pre-operative use of ACE inhibitors to be one of the significant determinants of vasoconstrictor requirements (Tuman et al, 1995). In practical terms, the dose of the ACE inhibitor due on the morning of the operation should be omitted, and the anesthesiologist should be prepared to sustain the blood volume or to give vasopressors as needed.

Angiotensin II receptor blockers

Angiotensin stimulates both AT_1 and AT_2 angiotensin receptors. The effects of AT_1 stimulation are to cause vasoconstriction and the synthesis and release of aldosterone, whereas the functions of the AT_2 receptor are largely related to fetal growth. Angiotensin is one of the mediators in the control of blood pressure and it contributes to the increased blood pressure in patients with essential hypertension, renal hypertension, or renin-secreting tumors.

Losartan, a benzyl substituted imidazole, is a specific competitive antagonist at the AT_1 receptors. It is the forerunner of a host of other AT_1 receptor blockers, now entering the market, and all ending in "-artan". Examples are valsartan and candesartan. In the liver, losartan is partially converted into an alpha-carboxylic acid, which is a noncompetitive AT_1 antagonist. Once daily dosing (in doses equal to or greater than 50 mg) is effective in reducing blood pressure (Weber et al, 199). When added to a thiazide diuretic, losartan causes a further reduction of diastolic pressure (Soffer et al, 1995). Hyperkalemia occurs in approximately 1.5% of patients; this is similar to the incidence of hyperkalemia with ACE inhibitors. Therefore, losartan (like an ACE inhibitor) should not be taken with a potassium sparing diuretic (Dahlof et al, 1995). Cough is much less of a problem than with ACE inhibitors (Lacourciere et al, 1994). No outcome studies are available in hypertensive patients. These drugs could put the patient at risk of operative hypotension, as in the case of the ACE inhibitors.

Although now widely used in hypertension, AT-receptor blockers have not yet achieved registration for heart failure. Hypothetically, ACE inhibitors might be superior for heart failure because they generate increased amounts of protective bradykinin. Conversely, AT-blockers might be superior because ACE inhibitors do not block those pathways that generate angiotensin independently of the converting enzyme, such as chymase.

Alpha-1 adrenergic blockers

These drugs are free from metabolic side-effects, reduce blood cholesterol, and are effective in reducing the peripheral vascular resistance. Examples are prazosin and the long acting agents doxazosin and terazosin. In elderly males, alpha-1 blockers have the added advantage of helping to decrease functional prostatic obstruction. Side-effects such as drowsiness, postural hypotension and occasionally tachycardia can be troublesome. Fluid retention may require the addition of a diuretic. The combinations with diuretics or beta-blockers are logical, while added calcium antagonists may cause excess vasodilatation. No outcome studies are available.

Direct vasodilators

Hydralazine and minoxidil are direct vasodilators which are no longer widely used because of the fear of lupus with hydralazine, and hirsutism with minoxidil. Other hazards of minoxidil are fluid retention, pericarditis, and left ventricular hypertrophy. The use of minoxidil is therefore limited to men with severe hypertension that is genuinely refractory to all the many other agents available.

Central adrenergic inhibitors

These include reserpine, methyldopa, clonidine, guanabenz and guanafacine. *Methyldopa* is still frequently used, despite costs and unfavorable central side-effects which give a poor quality of life (Croog et al, 1986) It acts on central alpha$_2$-receptors. Hepatic and hematologic side-effects are rare but serious. *Clonidine* is a very effective drug, and gave the best BP reduction in a large American study that encompassed both older and younger patients, and black and Caucasian patients (Materson et al, 1993). The disadvantage was that drug intolerance was also the most common with this agent, afflicting 11% of subjects.

For the anesthesiologist, the main concern about clonidine is the risk of withdrawal of the drug during the perioperative period as severe rebound hypertension may occur (Kaukinen et al, 1978). The earlier recommendation was that clonidine should be replaced by other antihypertensive agents in patients presenting for elective surgery. More recently, it has become clear that alpha$_2$-adrenoceptor agonists can minimize the release of catecholamines during surgery, thereby making the circulation more stable (Quintin et al, 1991). Clonidine also decreases opioid requirements and the MAC (minimal alveolar concentration) values of inhalational anesthetics.

Moxonidine is representative of a new class of central antihypertensive agents, acting on I_1 (imidazoline $_1$) receptors, that is claimed to have fewer central side-effects. This selective imidazoline agonist, is effective in the management of hypertension. Its main effect is reduction of sympathetic activity with a fall in peripheral vascular resistance, without any reflex tachycardia or change in cardiac output (Ernsberger et al, 1994).

Long-term Aims of Antihypertensive Therapy

The first aim of therapy is BP reduction, without which the risk of end-organ complications cannot be avoided. A second and even more important aim that is increasingly emphasized is the need to lessen morbidity and mortality. Thus far only diuretic drugs have achieved both of these ends with beta-blockers lessening morbidity but not mortality (JNC VI, 1997). All of these, with the exception of the management of acute complications such as left ventricular failure and severe hypertension, are long-term goals and not the main concerns of the anesthesiologist.

Prevention of stroke

Stroke reduction is the most consistent effect of antihypertensive therapy by diuretics and beta-blockers and the expected but thus far unproved benefit of therapy by ACE inhibitors or alpha$_1$-blockers. In the case of calcium antagonists, one randomized but unblinded study showed a striking reduction in stroke in elderly Chinese males treated by nifedipine tablets (Gong et al, 1996). In a well-designed trial in systolic hypertension of the elderly, nitrendipine tablets reduced stroke by 42% compared with placebo (Syst-Eur, 1997), so that long acting DHPs are now recommended as second choice for systolic hypertension after diuretics (JNC VI, 1997).

Prevention of coronary artery disease and acute myocardial infarction

This has been an elusive aim, thus far only achieved by low dose diuretics (JNC VI, 1997). Hypothetically, agents such as diuretics and beta-blockers have adverse metabolic effects such as insulin resistance that may predispose to coronary disease. Usually, in most trials, blood lipids have not been well monitored or well controlled. From the practical point of view, the anesthesiologist needs to consider that extensive coronary disease can be present even in patients with well-controlled BP values.

Regression of left ventricular hypertrophy (LVH)

Left ventricular hypertrophy is another important adverse complication of hypertension that causes diastolic dysfunction with exertional dyspnea or even overt "backward" failure with congestive signs. In achieving regression, it is often thought that ACE inhibitors are most effective, with diuretics least so. Several prospective studies have shown that calcium antagonists are as good as ACE inhibitors. Furthermore, in the long run diuretics are surprisingly effective, so that the issue of the drug of choice is not settled (Gottdiener et al, 1997). Because LVH is a response to prolonged excess mechanical stress on the left ventricular wall, logical therapy is to control the BP as well as possible over 24 hours, using combination therapy as needed according to ambulatory monitoring.

Prevention of early morning rise in blood pressure

The largest proportion of sudden death, acute myocardial infarction and stroke occur in the early morning hours. This is also the time at which adrenergic activity and blood pressure may be at its highest. Thus, drug management should blunt the early morning rise in blood pressure as should be accomplished by agents that act over 24 hours. However, no studies have specifically targeted this aim.

First Line Treatment Revisited

Recently, it has been suggested from case control and cohort studies that antihypertensive treatment may carry with it some unexpected risks which have been best publicized in the case of the calcium antagonists but also found with beta-blockers, alpha blockers, and high dose diuretics. The new demand is that a drug should not only reduce the BP, but do so safely and effectively over 24 hours, with a reduction in outcome endpoints such as stroke, coronary disease, and heart failure. Case control and cohort studies can not provide irrefutable evidence of harm because it is never clear why a given drug was chosen to start with. For example, short acting nifedipine, the culprit in several studies, may have been chosen because the patients were more ill and deemed worthy of more powerful antihypertensive therapy. Thus it is not surprising that case control and cohort studies have yielded conflicting evidence about the safety of calcium antagonist drugs (McMurray and Murdoch, 1997). There are several major outcome studies presently underway with calcium channel blockers versus other agents. Logically, short acting nifedipine and similar rapidly acting DHPs should be avoided whenever possible because 1) the BP control over 24 hours is erratic and not smooth and 2) each episode of hypotension evokes a brisk reactive catecholamine response with an increased heart rate that is undesirable in patients with associated ischemic heart disease. A recent case control study has demonstrated that short-acting calcium channel blockers increase the risk of cardiovascular events when compared with long-acting calcium channel blockers or beta-blockers (Alderman et al, 1997). In general, low dose diuretics remain first line therapy to which a variety of long acting agents can then be added.

SPECIAL PATIENT GROUPS

Hypertension in the elderly

In several trials, better protection against strokes and congestive heart failure has been obtained in elderly than in middle-aged patients (JNC VI, 1997). Furthermore, cardiovascular mortality may be reduced (STOP study, 1991). Thus, treatment of hypertension in the elderly is amply justified, and isolated systolic hypertension should be actively treated (SHEP, 1991; Syst-Eur, 1997). However, it is essential to avoid excess reductions in diastolic pressure in patients over the age of 75, and specifically powerful agents such as short acting nifedipine should not be given to those with initial BP levels below 160/90 mmHg (Pahor, 1995). In the elderly, low-dose diuretics are first choice because they have been used in most of the large drug trials. On the basis of the Syst-Eur study, the recent report of the American Joint National Committee (JNC VI, 1997) also recommends the use of long-acting DHPs in systolic hypertension in the elderly, as a second choice after a diuretic has been considered. Beta-blockers, although often used, have risk of excess sinus or AV node inhibition and decreased cardiac output, and in the MRC study (MRC Working Party, 1992), atenolol was no better than placebo and might have increased cardiovascular mortality. The combination of low-dose diuretic and a beta-blocker does seem effective from the indirect evidence supplied by the SHEP and STOP studies. ACE inhibitors are increasingly popular, yet there is no proof of reduction of adverse outcome.

Black patients

In black patients over and above consideration of associated disorders, monotherapy with a diuretic or a calcium antagonist is more effective than with an ACE inhibitor or beta-blocker. These restrictions apply especially to elderly black patients in whom captopril was no more effective than placebo (Materson et al, 1993).

Hypertensive Disease in Surgical Patients

Arterial hypertension is regarded as a risk factor for cardio-vascular complications of anesthesia and surgery (Dagnino and Prys-Roberts, 1989). There is concern that the long term consequences of arterial hypertension, such as coronary artery disease, cerebrovascular disease, left ventricular hypertrophy and impaired renal functions render the patient less fit for anesthesia and surgery. Indeed, hypertension, in a multivariate analysis of risk factors in man, was found to increase the odds ratio when compared with nor-motensives for postoperative death to 3.8, while severe limitation of physical activity had an odds ratio of 9.7, and a creatinine clearance of less than 50 ml/min conferred an odds ratio of 6.8 (Browner and Mangano, 1992).

During the perioperative period, patients with arterial hypertension are at risk of developing stroke, myocardial infarction or even death. Much more frequently they may develop exaggerated hypotension at induction of anesthesia, excessive pressor responses to laryngoscopy, endotracheal intubation or extubation, as well as hypertensive crises during the perioperative period (Prys-Roberts et al, 1971a). Hypertensive episodes may be associated with arrhythmias and/or myocardial ischemia. Acute cerebrovascular accidents may result from excess hypertension or hypotension. The instability of the blood pressure in hypertensive patients is caused by exaggerated vascular responsiveness to changes in autonomic activity (Folkow, 1987). In untreated hypertensive patients, there is an enhanced tendency to peripheral vasoconstriction, so that the effect of a unit change in vascular smooth muscle tone is a larger increase in vascular resistance than in normotensive patients. Long-term treatment of hypertension returns vascular reactivity to more normal levels and may increase the stability of patients during the perioperative period (at least in theory).

Pre-operative hypertension: Ideal vs empirical approaches

Studies in the early seventies have shown that treated hypertensive patients exhibited more stable responses to anesthesia and awakening than their untreated counterparts (Prys-Roberts et al, 1971b). Those receiving beta-adrenoceptor blockers had reduced responses to laryngoscopy and intubation and suffered less from arrhythmias and myocardial ischemia in the immediate perioperative period (Prys-Roberts et al, 1973). These studies led to a generally agreed policy that (1) treatment of hypertension should be continued up until the morning of surgery and that (2) untreated hypertensive patients should be treated before elective surgery, in the hope that hemodynamic stability would improve and the cardiovascular risks of anesthesia and surgery would be reduced. Yet if the policy of first initiating long-term treatment in all untreated hypertensive patients were to be adopted, there would be a large number of cancellations or deferments of elective operations, as many hypertensives are either untreated or poorly controlled, or may have a temporary "stress" reaction with apparent hypertension in those otherwise normotensive ("white coat hypertension").

In contrast to the work of Browner and Mangano (1992), several other studies of risk factors for cardiovascular complications of anesthesia and surgery have failed to identify hypertension (Goldman et al, 1977; Detsky et al, 1986). Thus a more widely agreed approach has developed empirically on the basis of the severity of the hypertension (Table 8-3). Patients with *severe arterial hypertension*, here defined as a diastolic pressure consistently greater than 110–115 mmHg, should be treated before elective surgery as the risk of devastating hypertensive crises is clearly high and these may cause intracranial hemorrhages, acute left ventricular failure, life-threatening ventricular arrhythmias, or precipitate renal failure. For patients with *moderate hypertension* (diastolic pressure between 100 and 110 mmHg) treatment is recommended for those with target organ involvement (coronary artery disease, impaired renal functions, cerebrovascular disease). For those with *mild hypertension* (diastolic BP below 100 mmHg, no clinical end-organ damage), treatment is considered to be optional. This pragmatic approach reduces the number of operations delayed or cancelled because of hypertension.

The major problem in establishing guidelines for the management of hypertensive patients in the perioperative period is that no study has as yet conclusively shown that treatment of hypertension brings about a significant improvement in outcome (Goldman and Caldera, 1979). Most studies addressing the question of hypertension in

Table 8-3. Classification of blood pressure*

Category	Systolic (mmHg)	Diastolic (mmHg)
Normal	<130	<85
High normal	130–139	85–89
Hypertension		
Stage 1 (mild)	140–159	90–99
Stage 2 (moderate)	160–179	100–109
Stage 3 (severe)	≥180	≥110

* See JNC VI, 1997

surgical patients have examined the association between hypertension and outcome without paying any attention to the presence or absence of treatment. As a result of the inclusion of treated and untreated hypertensive patients in the same group, differences, if any, are necessarily blurred. No study has tried to stratify the risk of adverse outcome as a function of the actual level of hypertension. Furthermore, no study has allowed for "white coat" hypertension.

Two recent studies provide some guidelines. First, a case control study has shown that a history of hypertension was present in 43% of patients who died within a month of surgery, and only in 19% of matched patients who survived the operation (Howell et al, 1996a); hypertension was identified as a significant predictor of death even after other factors such as myocardial infarction had been taken into consideration. Nonetheless at the time of operation, the blood pressures in the two groups (those with and those without a history of hypertension) were similar, suggesting that it was the long history of hypertension with its vascular complications such as coronary disease that predisposed to postoperative complications, rather than the actual blood pressure at the time of the operation. These findings support the pragmatic approach to control of blood pressure, as outlined above. In a second study, perioperative silent myocardial ischemia was more common in poorly controlled hypertensive than in normotensive patients (Howell et al, 1996b; Muir et al, 1991; Allman et al, 1994). Therefore in those clinically suspected of myocardial ischemia, increased blood pressure levels may increase the risk of ischemia. The hypertension should therefore be as tightly controlled as possible, preferably with the aid of a beta-blocking drug (See Chapter 9). However, there are as yet no prospective studies showing that control of perioperative silent myocardial ischemia improves the outcome.

PREOPERATIVE EVALUATION OF HYPERTENSION

Three questions need answering:

1. *Is hypertension primary or secondary?* Although secondary hypertension is relatively rare, recognition of the possibility of pheochromocytoma, renovascular hypertension, renal parenchymal hypertension, or hyperaldosteronism is important because of the need to avoid preventable morbidity and mortality related to the primary cause of hypertension. This is especially true of pheochromocytoma because of the risk of life-threatening hypertensive crises in the peri-operative period.

2. *Is the hypertension severe?* To establish the severity of hypertension requires multiple blood pressure readings both supine and standing. High admission blood pressure with subsequent normalization should not be discounted as it is a predictor of perioperative blood pressure lability (Bedford and Feinstein, 1980).

3. *Are target organs involved?* Presence of coronary heart
    disease or of risk factors for coronary heart disease is
    of major concern. Equally important is the presence of
    cerebrovascular disease including transient ischemic
    attacks. Assessment of renal function is essential. Signs
    of left ventricular hypertrophy (ECG, chest X-ray, echo-
    cardiography) when present indicate reduced left ven-
    tricular compliance. Presence of heart failure is an
    ominous sign and every effort should be made to com-
    pensate the patients before surgery.

In addition, the very frequent use of diuretics in the
management of arterial hypertension may cause problems
as prolonged use results in hypokalemia unless adequate
potassium supplements or retainers or ACE inhibitors are
administered. Recent evidence suggests that potassium
sparing diuretics may be superior to non-sparing diuretics
(Hoes et al, 1995). If chronic hypokalemia is present, the
question of preoperative potassium supplementation
remains controversial. Rapid normalization of plasma
potassium concentration may worsen the transmembrane
potassium gradient, thereby increasing rather than decreasing the risk of arrhythmias, as chronic diuretic therapy
without potassium supplements decreases the intracellular
potassium concentration (Wong et al, 1993). The absence of
arrhythmias, absence of U waves, and normal T waves
probably indicate that the transmembrane potassium gradient is within an acceptable range, i.e. a 35 fold difference. If
correction of hypokalemia is thought to be indicated it
should be done slowly. Intravenous supplementation may
correct the kalemia but worsen the transmembrane gradient, and is therefore unhelpful.

Hemodynamic Response to Anesthesia and Surgery

An important question is the influence of medical treatment
of hypertension on the hemodynamic response to anesthesia and surgery. Early studies had shown that beta-adrenoceptor blockers were well tolerated and improved
hemodynamic stability (Prys-Roberts et al, 1973). Later studies established that administration of beta-adrenoceptor
blockers as a single dose with the premedication prevented
immediate perioperative myocardial ischemia (Stone et al,
1988) and that this protection extended to the first 12 hours
of surgery (Dodds et al, 1994). The benefits of beta-adrenoceptor blockade extend to the whole of the perioperative
period if their administration is continued (Wallace et al,
1998; Mangano et al, 1996).

Do other antihypertensive agents such as calcium channel blockers, ACE inhibitors, alpha-adrenoceptor blockers,
or central α_2-adrenoceptor agonists, have possible interactions with anesthesia? In patients with mild hypertension,
on single drug medication (diuretics, beta-adrenoceptor
blockers, calcium channel blockers, or ACE inhibitors), a
comparison of the hemodynamic responses to induction of
anesthesia, laryngoscopy and intubation revealed no differ-

ence, except for the slower heart rate in those on beta-adrenoceptor blockers (Sear et al, 1994). No group had exaggerated hypotensive responses to induction of anesthesia.

Nonetheless, there may be *adverse effects of ACE inhibitors or angiotensin II receptor blockers* in surgical patients. More patients who had received captopril or enalapril on the morning of surgery developed hypotension by comparison with those in whom treatment had been stopped the night before (Coriat et al, 1994). In patients undergoing cardiopulmonary bypass, ACE inhibitors were the only cardiovascular drugs to be associated with a significantly increased need for vasopressor therapy (Myles et al, 1993). Thus stopping the administration of ACE inhibitors the day before surgery must be considered.

Premedication by Clonidine and Related Agents

Clonidine, a central alpha$_2$-agonist, inhibits sympathoadrenal activity (Quintin et al, 1991). The anxiolysis, sedation, and hemodynamic stability associated with oral clonidine given as premedicant have been documented in adults and in children (Nishina et al, 1994). The dose of induction agents and of inhalation anesthetics are reduced by the use of clonidine.

Similarly, the quality of regional anesthesia is improved. Thus, clonidine is now advocated as a premedicant drug in both normotensive and hypertensive patients, in the hope that hypertensive episodes and tachycardia could be minimized, thereby making anesthesia safer. In addition, intravenous clonidine attenuates the hemodynamic and adrenergic reactions to stress (Kulka et al, 1995). Other benefits of clonidine include reduction in shivering, minimal increases in oxygen consumption and in CO_2 production (Delaunay et al, 1991) as well as a smoother hemodynamic profile during emergence from anesthesia (Bernard et al, 1991). In coronary artery surgery, however, the beneficial effects of clonidine have not been confirmed. Rather, clonidine increased the need for vasoactive and inotropic support (Abi-Jaoude, 1993). *Dexmedetomidine*, a more selective alpha$_2$-agonist, has some of the advantages of clonidine in that hemodynamic stability is greater. As expected, dexmedetomidine attenuates both hemodynamic and stress hormone response to surgery (Aho et al, 1992). The price to be paid is a greater need for intraoperative pharmacological interventions. Post-operatively, dexmedetomidine minimizes tachycardia (Talke et al, 1995), at the risk of an unacceptable degree of bradycardia (Erkola et al, 1994).

PERIOPERATIVE RISKS AND THEIR MANAGEMENT

In hypertensive patients, induction of anesthesia is often associated with exaggerated reductions in blood pressure because of their enhanced vascular responsiveness to changes in sympathetic tone. The fall in blood pressure may precipitate myocardial ischemia because of the reduced diastolic (and hence coronary perfusion) pressure. Similarly, cerebral hypoperfusion may cause a stroke. The hemodynamic response to induction of anesthesia was more pronounced in untreated than in well controlled hypertensive patients (Prys-Roberts et al, 1971b). However, in a more recent study (Sear et al, 1994), moderately hypertensive patients had similar changes in blood pressure following induction of anesthesia whether they were untreated or on monotherapy (diuretic, beta-blocker, calcium antagonist or ACE inhibitor). The differences between these studies is likely to reflect the better tolerance of newer anesthetic agents and the lesser severity of hypertension in the more recent study. Whenever possible induction of anesthesia should rely on an opioid and the smallest effective dose of the selected induction agent. Fluid loading and/or small doses of ephedrine may be required to maintain an acceptable blood pressure.

The second phase of instability occurs with laryngoscopy and intubation. Laryngeal spraying with local anesthetics is ineffective in preventing hypertensive responses to laryngoscopy. In the past, beta-adrenoceptor blockade has been shown to be effective, preventing both hypertension and tachycardia (Prys-Roberts et al, 1973). Protection was obvious in patients given beta-blocker intravenously before intubation and in those started on a beta-blocker three days before surgery. Many studies have shown that beta-adrenoceptor blockers have no major deleterious interactions with the majority of anesthetic drugs and procedures so that there is now consensus that beta-adrenoceptor blockade should be maintained before and during surgery in patients with hypertensive and/or coronary disease. It must be emphasized that maintenance of beta-blockade post-operatively is important, as withdrawal symptoms may be exaggerated by post-operative stress. Interventions that prevent hypertensive responses to laryngoscopy and endotracheal intubation include intravenous esmolol, phentolamine, glyceryl trinitrate, sodium nitroprusside and labetalol. The reason for preventing such hypertensive episodes is that hypertension and the associated tachycardia may cause myocardial ischemia and/or ventricular arrhythmias. While halothane potentiates the arrhythmogenic effect of sympathetic overactivity, the more recent inhalation anesthetics, appear to be less arrhythmogenic than halothane. These newer agents are, however, not necessarily devoid of adverse features. Desflurane increases sympathetic activity, heart rate and arterial pressure (Ebert and Muzi, 1993). These effects have been noted at the induction of anesthesia, and when its concentration is rapidly increased from 1.0 to 1.5 MAC (minimal alveolar concentration). Caution should therefore be exercised when desflurane is administered to patients with hypertensive and/or coronary heart disease.

Monitoring of Blood Pressure

While preoperative control of blood pressure decreases the risk of adverse outcome, the hypertensive patient is still likely to be less stable than normotensive subjects. This instability cannot be left unchecked and a rather aggressive approach to the perioperative control of blood pressure is justified. In order for such a policy to succeed, information is needed. While for relatively minor procedures non-invasive measurement of blood pressure may be adequate, for major surgery, especially in patients whose blood pressure is poorly controlled, *invasive measurement* of blood pressure is necessary as large changes in blood pressure are detected immediately and can be corrected more rapidly and with greater safety. Extent, type and duration of surgery as well as blood pressure level, presence or absence of target organ involvement are major factors for decisions about invasive monitoring of arterial pressure. When non-invasive monitoring of blood pressure is used, it is critical that the size of the cuff be appropriate for the size of the arm upon which pressure is measured. There is, overall, a good correlation between pressure readings obtained from automatic or semi-automatic oscillometric monitors and intra-arterial pressure measurements. However, auscultatory and oscillometric methods are known to underestimate systolic pressure and overestimate diastolic pressure (Hutton et al, 1984; Gourdeau et al, 1986), and differences between non-invasive and invasive pressure measurements of the order of 40 mmHg are not exceptional.

Monitoring of the ECG is essential and whenever blood loss or fluid disturbances are expected, measurement of the central venous pressure is indicated. In patients with severe hypertension, left ventricular hypertrophy and strain, measurement of the pulmonary capillary wedge pressure is very useful in view of the increase in left ventricular stiffness. In such patients excessive fluid loading can easily cause pulmonary edema whilst uncorrected hypovolemia can cause severe reductions in cardiac output.

Severe Peri-operative Hypertension

Whether the hypertensive response needs to be prevented or treated is an unsettled question. So long as blood pressure does not increase above the level observed prior to induction of anesthesia, it seems unnecessary to intervene. However, marked pressure overshoots should be avoided or treated if they occur. In practice, most anesthesiologists are uncomfortable with blood pressure rises in excess of about 20% of the preoperative value, and intervene to stabilize the pressure.

During anesthesia and surgery, hypertensive patients may continue to exhibit exaggerated pressure responses resulting from the "unmatching" of depth of anesthesia and intensity of the surgical stimulus. Close attention should be paid to matching to avoid "alpine anesthesia" (Longnecker, 1987).

The consequences of peri-operative hypertension include bleeding from vascular suture lines, cerebrovascular hemorrhages and myocardial ischemia. Mortality rate of such accidents may be as high as 50% (Leslie, 1993). The primary etiology of peri-operative hypertension is an increase in peripheral vascular resistance caused by elevated levels of circulating catecholamines. Correction or prevention of the increase in peripheral vascular resistance are the most appropriate therapy. However, no single agent appears to be ideal for all hypertensive episodes. The many agents available include sodium nitroprusside, alpha-blockers, calcium channel blockers (nifedipine), the combined alpha- and beta-blocker labetalol, and others including the short-acting beta-blocker esmolol; all appear to be effective (Table 8-4).

Some principles of choice may be proposed although it must be emphasized that there are no studies to show which drug among these many candidates is optimal for any given patient. First, when acute urgent reduction of BP is required, sodium nitroprusside is often the agent of choice simply because the majority of anesthesiologists have had the widest experience with this agent and because it works. Next, we propose that the presence or absence of cardiac complications should be a decider. When there is ischemia, with or without poor left ventricular function, then a nitroglycerin infusion is used. When there is ischemia with good LV function, then esmolol is logical as a bolus but prolonged infusion is expensive so that labetalol may be chosen instead. When there is heart failure, an ACE inhibitor is preferred provided the patient is not pregnant. When there are no cardiac complications, an agent that invokes a reflex tachycardia such as phentolamine, hydralazine, nifedipine or nicardipine is acceptable. When there is renal dysfunction, then fenoldopam helps to induce a sodium diuresis. When there is a pheochromocytoma, then the alpha-blocker phentolamine or the combined alpha-beta-blocker labetalol may be used, whereas straight beta-blockade is contraindicated.

In the face of severe hypertensive episodes, *sodium nitroprusside* at an initial infusion rate of 0.3–0.5 µg/kg/min, titrated as needed up to 2 µg/kg/min, is a very effective treatment. If more than 2 µg/kg/min is needed, however, additional drugs need to be used to reduce the risk of toxicity (Friederich et al, 1995). It is light sensitive and a special infusion kit is needed. Tachycardia may also be a problem, requiring added beta-blockade. The administration of sodium nitroprusside implies careful clinical attention and the availability of intra-arterial pressure monitoring. (For more details see page 294.)

Though *nitroglycerin* is often advocated in the management of hypertension and is reported to reduce the risk of myocardial ischemia, it does not always prevent the development of ischemia in patients undergoing non-cardiac surgery, particularly at the time of emergence from anesthesia (Dodds et al, 1993). Perhaps the associated tachycardia counteracts some of the benefit.

Esmolol is a short-acting cardioselective beta-adrenoceptor blocker that has gained wide acceptance in the control of tachycardia and hypertension in surgical patients. It has a half life of only about ten minutes, because it is rapidly metabolized by the erythrocyte esterases. Esmolol can be used as a 100 mg bolus to protect against the effects of sympatho-adrenergic responses to intubation or extubation

Table 8-4. Drugs used in perioperative hypertensive urgencies and emergencies

Clinical requirement	Mechanism of anti-hypertensive effect	Drug choice	Dose
Urgent reduction of severe acute hypertension	NO donor	Sodium nitroprusside infusion	0.3–2 µg/kg/min (careful monitoring)
Hypertension plus ischemia (poor LV)	NO donor	Nitroglycerin infusion	0.25–5 µg/kg/min
Hypertension plus ischemia plus tachycardia	Beta-blocker (good LV)	Esmolol bolus or infusion	50–250 µg/kg/min
(as above)	Alpha-beta-blocker	Labetalol bolus infusion	2–10 mg 2.5–30 µg/kg/min
Hypertension plus heart failure	ACE inhibitor (avoid negative inotropic drugs)	Enalaprilat (iv) Captopril (s-l)	0.5–5 mg bolus 12.5–25 mg s-l
Hypertension without cardiac complications	Vasodilators including those that increase heart rate	Hydralazine (H) Phentolamine (P) Nifedipine (Nif) Nicardipine (Nic) bolus infusion	5–10 mg boluses 1–4 mg boluses 10 mg s-l 5–10 µg/kg/min 1–3 µg/kg/min
Hypertension plus poor renal function	Dopamine (DA-1 agonist)	Fenoldopam*	0.2–0.5 µg/kg/min
Hypertension plus pheochromocytoma	Alpha-blocker or combined alpha-beta blocker (avoid pure beta-blocker)	Phentolamine Labetalol bolus infusion	1–4 mg boluses 2–10 mg 2.5–30 µg/kg/min

LV = left ventricle, iv = intravenous, s-l = sublingual

* not licensed in the USA or UK.

(Schaffer et al, 1994) especially in hypertensive patients. If longer duration protection is desirable, esmolol can be given as a continuous infusion, which, however, is very expensive, compared with other agents. Esmolol may be particularly useful when doubts exist as to how patients may tolerate more conventional beta-blockade as the effect of esmolol is so short. Nonetheless, its negative inotropic effect can be powerful and the usual cautions and contra-indications applicable to beta-blockade remain in force.

Labetalol is a combined alpha-beta blocker that is well studied especially in the management of resection of pheo-chromocytoma (Sollazzi et al, 1994). In addition, labetalol is very effective in a wide spectrum of operative procedures, in the elderly (Singh et al, 1992) and in younger patients. The added alpha-blockade allows rapid peripheral vasodila-tion in contrast to standard beta-blockade by esmolol. Nonetheless, standard contra-indications to beta-blockade also apply to labetalol. *Carvedilol*, an orally active drug of similar properties, is registered for adjuvant use in heart failure in the USA, when commenced in very low doses and given to patients already fully treated by standard therapy.

Enalaprilat is an ACE inhibitor that is intravenously available and best suited for the combination of acute hypertension and heart failure. It is contraindicated in bilat-eral renal artery stenosis and in pregnancy. Sublingual cap-topril is relatively rapidly acting (within 30 min) with otherwise the same advantages and disadvantages of enala-prilat.

Intravenous hydralazine is an old "stand-by" that is still used, with however the disadvantage of causing a marked tachycardia and therefore not being suited for patients with myocardial ischemia. It is often used in obstetrical practice.

Phentolamine likewise is a well-tested agent, acting by combined alpha$_1$- and alpha$_2$-peripheral blockade, with the advantage of having no negative inotropic effect. Again, there is the risk of tachycardia.

Sublingual nifedipine is losing favor especially in the presence of ischemia, because of the tachycardia and the powerful blood pressure reduction are difficult to regulate with the sublingual route (Grossman et al, 1996). Nonethe-less it remains simple to use and often effective in restoring BP to normal. *Nicardipine* is a similar dihydropyridine com-pound that it available for intravenous use in the USA but not in the UK.

Intravenous fenoldopam is a relatively new agent that has been specifically tested in postoperative hypertension (Goldberg et al, 1993). It is a dopamine A-1 receptor agonist that seems similar to sodium nitroprusside in hypotensive potency, but induces a sodium diuresis whereas nitroprus-side causes sodium retention (Elliott et al, 1990). Unfortu-nately, like nitroprusside, it significantly elevates the heart rate (Goldberg et al, 1993). Nonetheless, it has been approved for use in severe hypertension in the USA (Mas-sie, 1997).

Most of the *interactions* between anti-hypertensive agents and anesthetic drugs are predictable, and easily managed. Though monoamine oxidase inhibitors (MAOI) are no longer used in the management of hypertension, it remains common practice that when given as antidepressants, they should be stopped two weeks before surgery and replaced by other drugs. Nonetheless, provided that pethidine is avoided, withdrawal of MAOI may not be required (Stack, et al, 1988).

Post-operative hypertension

At the end of surgery there is again a significant risk of hypertension when patients are starting to wake up and are still intubated. Esmolol is effective in blunting the hypertension and tachycardia that are often associated with emergence from anesthesia (O'Dwyer et al, 1993). Short acting vasodilators are also effective with however the disadvantage of tachycardia which can harm those with myocardial ischemia. But it is probably more important that the anesthesiologist should first ensure that the endotracheal tube is not left in place for longer than necessary. If intubation has to be maintained after the end of surgery, adequate sedation is necessary, particularly when patients have to be transported from the theatre suite to a recovery or intensive care unit. In the absence of adequate sedation, life-threatening hypertensive crises may occur even though antihypertensive drugs are given.

Regarding long term follow-up, all patients with a pre-anesthetic history of coronary disease or deemed to be at high risk (e.g. age over 65, hypertension) appear to benefit from the administration of a beta-blocker which protects against future heart attacks and improves mortality (Mangano et al, 1996).

CONCLUSIONS

Twenty-five years after the first detailed studies of the responses to anesthesia of hypertensive patients, specific evidence-based guidelines for management are still lacking. Progress has been made, however. For all patients, hypertensive or not, better anesthetic techniques, better monitoring, and better recovery facilities have decreased the risk of cardiovascular complications of anesthesia and surgery and allowed more extensive procedures to be carried out in compromised patients. Within this framework, improved assessment and care of hypertensive patients has made an important contribution.

Pre-operatively, a history of hypertension indicates a relatively poor prognosis, probably as result of long standing vascular complications. This observation would suggest that the tighter the BP control in the period leading up to the operation, the better. The exact blood pressure at the time of pre-operative assessment seems of lesser importance, so that a pragmatic policy can be pursued especially because there are no solid data linking the pre-operative blood pressure to the outcome. Pragmatically, severe hypertension with a diastolic BP consistently exceeding

115 mmHg, should be treated before elective surgery is undertaken. Values between 100 and 115 mmHg require treatment if there is end-organ damage, and treatment may be regarded as optional for mild hypertension with diastolic BP values of 90–100 mmHg.

The treatment of peri-operative hypertension is likewise pragmatic, with BP rises in excess of about 20% often taken as an indication for acute treatment. For acute severe hypertension, sodium nitroprusside is often regarded as the drug of choice, with intravenous nitroglycerin used especially if there is associated myocardial ischemia. Beta-blockade by esmolol or labetalol is the therapy of choice if there is an associated tachycardia in the absence of heart failure. In the presence of heart failure, an ACE inhibitor should be chosen. BP lowering can also be achieved by a variety of other agents such as hydralazine and phentolamine given either as repetitive boluses or by infusion or in the case of nifedipine, sublingually. Most of these agents cause a tachycardia, which is undesirable in patients suspected of myocardial ischemia. Such agents should therefore only be used when there is no heart disease. Beta-blockers, on the other hand, although ideal for ischemia, have negative inotropic properties, which the vasodilators as a group do not.

SUMMARY

1. *Arterial hypertension is a major cause of morbidity and mortality.* Advances in its treatment over the last decade have reduced its morbidity, and it has become clear that treatment of relatively moderate hypertension is beneficial. In treated hypertensive patients maintenance of medication throughout the perioperative period is standard practice with most antihypertensive drugs. However, caution should be exercised with ACE inhibitors and AT receptor blockers as excessive reductions of blood pressure may occur.

2. *The level of blood pressure above which surgery should be postponed is still unsettled,* even though there is evidence that hypertension per se is a risk factor for perioperative cardiovascular complications of anesthesia and surgery. Purely empirical guidelines suggest that severe hypertension (here defined as diastolic pressures greater than 110 mmHg) calls for postponement and treatment. Similarly, patients with moderate hypertension (diastolic pressure between 100 and 110 mmHg) and target organ involvement, should be treated before surgery. Finally, those with mild hypertension (diastolic pressure less than 100 mmHg) may benefit from treatment, but the problems associated with postponement may outweigh the reduction in morbidity. Long-term, however, all hypertensive patients benefit from the control of their blood pressure.

REFERENCES

Abi-Jaoude F, Brusset A, Ceddaha A, et al. Clonidine premedication for coronary artery bypass grafting under high-dose alfentanil anesthesia: intraoperative and postoperative hemodynamic study. *J Cardiothorac Vasc Anesth* 1993; 7: 35–40.

Aho M, Scheinin M, Lehtinen AM, et al. Intramuscularly administered dexmedetomidine attenuates the hemodynamic and stress hormone responses to gynecologic laparoscopy. *Anesth Analg* 1992; 75: 832–939.

Alderman MH, Cohen H, Roqué R and Madhavan S. Effect of long-acting and short-acting calcium antagonists on cardiovascular outcome in hypertensive patients. *Lancet* 1997; 349: 594–598.

Alderman MH, Madhavan S, Ooi WL, et al. Association of the renin sodium profile with the risk of myocardial infarction in patients with hypertension. *N Engl J Med* 1991: 324: 1098–1104.

Allman KG, Muir A, Howell SJ, et al. Resistant hypertension and preoperative silent myocardial ischemia in surgical patients. *Br J Anaesth* 1994; 73: 574–578.

Bakris GL, Barnhill BW and Sadler R. Treatment of arterial hypertension in diabetic humans: importance of therapeutic selection. *Kidney Int* 1992; 41: 912–919.

Bakris GL, Copley B, Vicknair N, et al. Calcium channel blockers versus other antihypertensive therapies on progression of NIDDM associated nephropathy. *Kidney Int* 1996; 50: 1641–1650.

Bedford RF and Feinstein B. Hospital admission blood pressure: a predictor for hypertension following endotracheal intubation. *Anesth Analg* 1980; 59: 367–370.

Bernard JM, Bourreli B, Hommeril JL and Pinaud M. Effects of oral clonidine premedication and postoperative i.v. infusion on hemodynamic and adrenergic responses during recovery from anesthesia. *Acta Anaesthesiol Scand* 1991; 35: 54–59.

Browner WS and Mangano DT. In-hospital and long-term mortality in male veterans following noncardiac surgery. The Study of Perioperative Ischemia Research Group. *JAMA* 1992; 268: 228–232.

Canter D, Frank GJ, Knapp LE et al. and the Quinapril Investigator Group. Quinapril and hydrochlorothiazide combination for control of hypertension: assessment by factorial design. *J Human Hypertension* 1994; 8: 155–162.

Collins R, Peto R, MacMahon S, et al. Blood pressure, stroke, and coronary heart disease. Part 2, Short-term reductions in blood pressure: overview of randomised drug trials in their epidemiological context. *Lancet* 1990; 335: 827–838.

Coriat P, Richer C, Douraki T, et al. Influence of chronic angiotensin-converting enzyme inhibition on anesthetic induction. *Anesthesiology* 1994; 81: 299–307.

Croog SH, Levine S, Testa MA, et al. The effects of antihypertensive therapy on the quality of life. *N Engl J Med* 1986; 314: 1657–1664.

Dagnino J and Preys-Roberts C. Strategy for patients with hypertensive heart disease. Bailliere's Clinical *Anesthesiology* 1989; 3/1: 261–289.

Dahlöf B, Keller SE, Makris L, et al. Efficacy and tolerability of losartan potassium and atenolol in patients with mild to moderate essential hypertension. *Am J Hypertens* 1995; 8: 578–583.

Delaunay L, Bonnet F and Duvaldestin P. Clonidine decreases postoperative oxygen consumption in patients recovering from general anaesthesia. *Br J Anaesth* 1991; 67: 397–401.

Detsky AS, Abrams HB, Forbath N, et al. Cardiac assessment for patients undergoing non-cardiac surgery: a multifactorial clinical risk index. *Arch Intern Med* 1986; 146: 2131–2134.

Dodds TM, Stone JG, Coromilas J, et al. Prophylactic nitroglycerin infusion during noncardiac surgery does not reduce perioperative ischemia. *Anesth Analg* 1993; 76: 705–713.

Dodds TM, Torkelson AT, Filliger MP and Tosteson A. Prophylactic beta-blockade reduces perioperative myocardial ischemia in high-risk patients undergoing noncardiac surgery. *Anesth Analg* 1994; 78: S92.

Dzau VJ and Gibbons GH. Endothelium and growth factors in vascular remodeling of hypertension. *Hypertension* 1991; 18 (III): 115–121.

Ebert TJ and Muzi M. Sympathetic hyperactivity during desflurane anesthesia in healthy volunteers. A comparison with isoflurane. *Anesthesiology* 1993; 79: 444–453.

Elliott WJ, Weber RR, Nelson KS, et al. Renal and hemodynamic effects of intravenous fenoldopam versus nitroprusside in severe hypertension. *Circulation* 1990; 81: 970–977.

Erkola O, Korttila K, Aho M, et al. Comparison of intramuscular dexmedetomidine and midazolam premedication for elective abdominal hysterectomy. *Anesth Analg* 1994; 79: 646–653.

Ernsberger P, Haxhiu M, Collins LA, et al. A novel mechanism of action for hypertension: moxonidine as a selective 1-imidazoline agonist. *Cardiovasc Drugs Ther* 1994; 8 (suppl 1): 27–41.

Estacio RO, Jeffers BW, Hiatt WH, et al. A randomized controlled trial of nisoldipine versus enalapril in hypertensive patients with non-insulin dependent mellitus (NIDDM): Effects on cardiovascular outcomes. ABCD Study. *New Engl J Med* 1998; 338: 645–652.

Ferrario CM and Averill DB. Do primary dysfunctions in neural control of arterial pressure contribute to hypertension? *Hypertension* 1991; 18: 38–51

Folkow B. Structure and function of the arteries in hypertension. *Am Heart J* 1987; 114: 938–948.

Friederich JA and Butterworth JF. Sodium nitroprusside: twenty years and counting. *Anesth Analg* 1995; 81: 152–162.

Frishman WH, Bryzinski BS, Coulson LR et al. A multifactorial trial design to assess combination therapy in hypertension: treatment with bisoprolol and hydrochlorothiazide. *Arch Intern Med* 1994; 154: 1461–1468.

Frohlich ED, Apstein C, Chobanian AV, et al. The heart in hypertension. *N Engl J Med* 1992; 327: 998–1008.

Frohlich ED. The heart in hypertension: a 1991 overview. *Hypertension* 1991; 18 (III): 62–68.

Godfraind T. Cardioselectivity of calcium antagonists. *Cardiovasc Drugs Ther* 1994; 8 (Suppl 2): 353–364.

Goldberg ME, Cantillo J, Nemiroff MS, et al. Fenoldopam infusion for the treatment of postoperative hypertension. *J Clin Anesth* 1993; 5: 386–391.

Goldman L, Caldera DL, Nussbaum SR, et al. Multifactorial index of cardiac risk in noncardiac surgical procedures. *N Engl J Med* 1977; 297: 845–850.

Goldman L and Caldera DL. Risks of general anesthesia and elective operation in the hypertensive patient. *Anesthesiology* 1979; 50:285–292.

Gong L, Zhang W, Zhu Y et al. Shanghai trial of nifedipine in the elderly (STONE). *J Hypertens* 1996; 14: 1237–1245.

Gottdiener JS. Reda DJ, Massie BM, et al. Effect of single-drug therapy on reduction of left ventricular mass in mild to moderate hypertension. Comparison of six antihypertensive agents. The Department of Veterans Affairs Cooperative Study Group on Antihypertensive Agents. *Circulation* 1997; 95: 2007–2014.

Gourdeau M, Martin R, Lamarche Y and Tetrault L. Oscillometry and direct blood pressure: a comparative clinical study during deliberate hypotension. *Can Anaesth Soc* 1986; 33: 300–307.

Grossman E, Messerli H, Grodzicki T and Kowey P. Should a moratorium be placed on sublingual nifedipine capsules given for hypertensive emergencies and pseudoemergencies? *JAMA* 1996; 276: 1328–331.

Grossman E and Messerli H. Effect of calcium antagonists on plasma norepinephrine levels, heart rate and blood pressure. *Am J Cardiol*, 1997; 80: 1453–1458.

Heagerty AM, Swales J, Baksi A, et al. Nifedipine and atenolol singly and combined for treatment of essential hypertension: comparative multicentre study in general practice in the United Kingdom. *Br Med J* 1988; 296: 468–472.

Hoes AW, Grobbee DE, Lubsen J, et al. Diuretics, β-blockers, and the risk for sudden cardiac death in hypertensive patients. *Ann Int Med* 1995; 123: 481–487.

Holzegreve H, Distler A, Michelis J et al. on behalf of the Verapamil versus Diuretic (VERDU) Trial Research Group. Verapamil versus hydrochlorothiazide in the treatment of hypertension: results of long-term double-blind comparative trial. *Br Med J* 1989; 299: 881–886.

Howell SJ, Hemming E, Allman KG, et al. Predictors of post-operative myocardial ischemia: the role of intercurrent arterial hypertension and other cardiovascular risk factors. *Anaesthesia* 1996a; 52: 107–111.

Howell SJ, Sear YM, Yeates D, et al. Hypertension, admission blood pressure and perioperative cardiovascular risk. *Anesthesia* 1996b; 51: 1000–1004.

Hutton P, Dye J and Prys-Roberts C. An assessment of the Dinamap 845. *Anesthesia* 1984; 39: 261–267.

Kaukinen S, Kaukinen L and Eerola R. Preoperative and postoperative use of clonidine and neurolept anesthesia. *Acta Anaesthesiol Scand* 1978; 23: 113–120.

Knorr AM. Why is nisoldipine a specific agent in ischemic left ventricular dysfunction? *Am J Cardiol* 1995; 75: 36E–40E.

Kulka PJ, Tryba M and Zenz M. Dose-response effects of intravenous clonidine on stress response during induction of anesthesia in coronary artery bypass graft patients. *Anesth Analg* 1995; 80: 263–268.

Lacourciere Y, Brunner H, Irwin R et al. Effects of modulators of the renin-angiotensin-aldosterone system on cough. *J Hypertens* 1994; 12: 1387–1393.

Leslie JB. Incidence and etiology of perioperative hypertension. *Acta Anaesth Scand* 1993; Suppl 99: 5–9.

Lewis EJ, Hunsicker LG, Bain RP and Rohde RD for the Collaborative Study Group. The effect of angiotensin-converting enzyme inhibition on diabetic nephropathy. *N Engl J Med* 1993; 329: 1456–1462.

Longnecker DE. Alpine anesthesia: can pretreatment with clonidine decrease the peaks and valleys. *Anesthesiology* 1987; 67, 1–2.

MacMahon S, Pero R, Cutler J, et al. Blood pressure, stroke, and coronary heart disease. Part I: Prolonged differences in blood pressure: prospective observational studies corrected for the regression dilution bias. *Lancet* 1990; 335: 765–774.

Mangano DT, Layug EL, Wallace A and Tateo I, for the Multicenter Study of Perioperative Ischemia Research Group. Effect of Atenolol on mortality and cardiovascular morbidity after noncardiac surgery. *N Engl J Med* 1996, 335: 1713–1720.

Massie, BM. Cardiovascular News. *Circulation* 1997; 96: 2483.

Materson BJ, Reda DJ, Cushman WC, et al. Single-drug therapy for hypertension in men. A comparison of six antihypertensive agents with placebo. The Department of Veterans Affairs Cooperative Study Group on Antihypertensive Agents. *N Engl J Med* 1993; 328: 914–921.

McMurray J and Murdoch D. Calcium-antagonist controversy: the long and short of it. *Lancet* 1997; 349: 585–586.

MRC Working Party. Medical Research Council trial of treatment of hypertension in older adults: principal results. *Br Med J* 1992; 304: 405–412.

Muir AD, Reeder MK, Foëx P, et al. Preoperative silent myocardial ischemia: Incidence and predictors in a general surgical population. *Br J Anaesth* 1991; 67: 373–377.

Myles PS, Olenikov I, Bujor MA and Davis BB. ACE-inhibitors, calcium antagonists and low systemic vascular resistance following cardiopulmonary bypass. A case-control study. *Med J Aust* 1993; 158: 675–677.

Nishina K, Mikawa K, Mekawa N, et al. Clonidine decreases the dose of thiamylal required to induce anesthesia in children. *Anesth Analg* 1994; 79: 766–768.

O'Dwyer JP, Yorukoglu D and Harris MN. The use of esmolol to attenuate the hemodynamic response when extubating patients following cardiac surgery — a double blind controlled study. *Eur Heart J* 1993; 14: 701–704.

Packer M, O'Connor CM, Ghali JK, et al. Effect of amlodipine on morbidity and mortality in severe chronic heart failure. Prospective Randomized Amlodipine Survival Evaluation Study Group. *N Engl J Med* 1996; 335: 1107–1114.

Pahor M, Guralnik JM, Corti MC, et al. Long-term survival and use of antihypertensive medications in older persons. *J Am Geriatr Soc* 1995; 43: 1191–1197.

Postma CT, Hoefnagels WHL, Barentsz JO, et al. Occlusion of unilateral stenosed renal arteriesrelation to medical treatment. *J Human Hypert* 1989; 3: 185–190.

Prys-Roberts C, Foëx P, Biro GP and Roberts JG. Studies of anaesthesia in relation to hypertension V. Adrenergic beta-receptor blockade. *Br J Anaesth* 1973; 45: 671–681.

Prys-Roberts C, Greene L, Meloche R and Foëx P. Studies of anaesthesia in relation to hypertension. II. Haemodynamic consequences of induction and endotracheal intubation. *Br J Anaesth* 1971a; 43: 531–547.

Prys-Roberts C, Meloche R and Foëx P. Studies of anaesthesia in relation to hypertension. I. Cardiovascular responses of treated and untreated patients. *Br J Anaesth* 1971b; 43: 122–137.

Psaty BM, Heckbert SR, Koepsell TD, et al. The risk of myocardial infarction associated with antihypertensive drug therapies. *JAMA* 1995; 274: 620–625.

Quintin L, Roudot F, Roux C, et al. Effect of clonidine on the circulation and vasoactive hormones after aortic surgery. *Br J Anaesth* 1991; 66: 108–115.

Schaffer J and Karg C, Piepenbrock S. Esmolol als Bolus zur Prophylaxe der sympathikoadrenergen Reaktion während der Narkoseausleistung. *Anaesthetist* 1994; 43: 723–729.

Sear JW, Jewkes C, Tellez J-C and Foëx P. Does the choice of antihypertensive therapy influence haemodynamic responses to induction, laryngoscopy and intubation. *Br J Anaesth* 1994; 73: 303–308.

SHEP Cooperative Research Group. Prevention of stroke by antihypertensive drug treatment in older persons with isolated systolic hypertension. Final results of the Systolic Hypertension in the Elderly Program (SHEP). JAMA 1991; 265: 3255–3264.

Singer DRJ, Markandu ND, Shore AC and MacGregor GA. Captopril and nifedipine in combination for moderate to severe essential hypertension. *Hypertension* 1987; 9: 629–633.

Singh PP, Dimich I, Sampson I and Sonnenklar N. A comparison of esmolol and labetalol for the treatment of perioperative hypertension in geriatric ambulatory surgical patients. *Can J Anaesth* 1992; 39: 559–562.

Siskovick DS, Raghunathan TE, Psaty BM, et al. Diuretic therapy for hypertension and the risk of primary cardiac arrest. *N Engl J Med* 1994; 330: 1852–1857.

Soffer BA, Wright JT, Pratt JH, et al. Effects of losartan on a background of hydrochlorothiazide in patients with hypertension. *Hypertension* 1995; 26: 112–117.

Sollazzi L, Perilli V, Crea MA, et al. Anaesthetic management of phaeochromocytoma in a long term hemodialyzed patient. *Acta Anaesthesiol Belg* 1994; 45: 13–17.

Stack CG, Rogers P and Linter SPK. Monoamine oxidase inhibitors and anaesthesia. A review. *Br J Anaesth* 1988; 60: 222–227.

Stone JG, Foëx P, Sear JW, et al. Myocardial ischemia in untreated hypertensive patients: effect of a single small oral dose of a beta-adrenergic blocking agent. *Anesthesiology* 1988; 68: 495–500.

STOP Study. Ekbom T, Dahlof B, Hansson L et al. Morbidity and mortality in the Swedish Trial in Old Patients with Hypertension (STOP-Hypertension). *Lancet* 1991; 338: 1281–1285.

Swales JD. Guidelines on guidelines. *J Hypertens* 1993; 11: 899–903.

Syst-Eur Trial, Staessen JA, Fagard R, Thijs L, et al. Randomised double-blind comparison of placebo and active treatment for older patients with isolated systolic hypertension (Syst-Eur Trial). *Lancet* 1997; 350:754–764.

Talke P, Li J, Jain U, Leung J, et al. Effect of perioperative dexmedetomidine infusion in patients undergoing vascular surgery. The Study of Perioperative Ischemia Research Group. *Anesthesiology* 1995; 82: 620–633.

Tarazi RC, Dustan HP, Frohlich ED, et al. Plasma volume and chronic hypertension. Relationship to arterial pressure level in different hypertensive diseases. *Arch Intern Med* 1970; 125: 835–842.

Tatti P, Pahor M, Byington RP, et al. Results of the Fosinopril Amlodipine Cardiovascular Events Trial (FACET) in hypertensive patients with non-Insulin dependent diabetes mellitus (NIDDM). (Abstract) *Circulation* 1997; 96 (Suppl D): 1–764.

TOMH study — Treatment of Mild Hypertension Research Group (TOMH). The treatment of mild hypertension study. A randomized, placebo-controlled trial of a nutritional-hygienic regimen along with various drug monotherapies. *Arch Intern Med* 1991; 151: 1413–1423.

Tuman KJ, McCarthy RJ, O'Connor CJ, et al. Angiotensin-converting enzyme inhibitors increase vasoconstrictor requirements after cardiopulmonary bypass. *Anesth Analg* 1995; 80: 473–479.

Wallace A, Layung E, Tateo I et al. McSpi Research group. Prophylatic atenolol reduces postoperative myocardial ischemia. *Anesthesiology* 1998; 88: 7–17.

Weber MA, Byyny RL, Pratt H et al. Blood pressure effects of the angiotensin II receptor blocker, losartan. *Arch Intern Med* 1995; 155: 405–411.

Wong KC, Schafer PG, Schultz JR. Hypokalemia and anesthetic implications. *Anesth Analg* 1993; 77: 1238–1260.

World Hypertension League. Nonpharmacological interventions as an adjunct to the pharmacological treatment of hypertension. *J Human Hypertens* 1993; 7: 159–164.

Zanchetti A. Guidelines for the management of hypertension: the World Health Organization/International Society of Hypertension view. World Health Organization. International Society of Hypertension. *J Hypertens* 1995; 13 (suppl): S119–22.

CHAPTER 9

Coronary Artery Disease and Myocardial Ischemia

Pierre Foëx

In the USA, UK and other westernized countries, a large proportion of adult patients presenting for surgery suffer from coronary artery disease. While the presence of coronary disease increases the risk of cardiovascular complications of anesthesia and surgery, there are some groups of patients in whom the risks are particularly high. These patients need to be identified at an early stage in order for their management to be optimized prior to anesthesia and surgery. This may include better medication, coronary angioplasty and stenting, or coronary bypass surgery. Identification of high risk patients is also important for the planning of their monitoring and management during the postoperative period (Table 9-1). The management of high risk patients rests on a sound understanding of the pathophysiology of coronary disease and its drug management. The risk of coronary events during the perioperative period must be considered, as well as the management of peri- and post-operative myocardial ischemia.

Table 9-1. Risk stratification.

Evaluation of all surgical patients by clinical indices

1. Low risk
Need no further evaluation before surgery

2. Intermediate risk
May benefit from noninvasive stress tests
Eg dobutamine stress echocardiography
(especially prior to vascular surgery)

3. High risk
Need optimal management of high risk problems
May need β-blockade
May need elective procedures canceled

For details, see Palda and Detsky (1997).

Pathophysiology
of Coronary Disease

Ischemia means reduced blood flow (literally, "to hold back blood"), and ischemic heart disease is the consequence of coronary atherosclerosis. The latter starts as a focal intimal disease with fatty streaks which evolves, with the increased production of collagen, into a raised fibrolipid plaque. Many plaques are situated eccentrically and there is a residual area of normal vessel opposite the plaque. Arteries may remodel themselves by increasing their external diameter so that the lumen is not compromised. However, the remodeling process may be insufficient and focal narrowing ensues. The plaque becomes angiographically visible and flow may be limited. Clinical symptoms may result from the reduction in diameter (and flow), from local thrombosis, or from altered vascular tone. In response to increased flow normal arteries dilate, whereas in atherosclerosis vasoconstriction may be elicited.

Endothelial dysfunction is thought to initiate coronary artery disease (CAD). Thus, many of the risk factors for CAD such as hypercholesterolemia, smoking, hypertension, and diabetes mellitus damage the endothelium to lessen the release of nitric oxide. These same factors are thought to promote the release of endothelin, which has opposite properties to those of nitric oxide. Nitric oxide, besides being vasodilatory, also inhibits the atherosclerotic process by lessening neutrophil adesion to the endothelium, by limiting platelet aggregation, and by inhibiting smooth muscle proliferation. Endothelin may act to promote atheroma formation.

Thrombosis may occur because the endothelium is damaged over the plaque or because the plaque has developed microfissures. As blood enters the plaque, its volume increases and this may facilitate thrombosis. In response to thrombi formation, there is incomplete spontaneous lysis. Thrombus that is not removed causes local smooth muscle proliferation and replacement by collagen tissue. Atheromatous plaques when unstable, have a high risk of further thrombosis. As lipid-rich plaques are more likely to be unstable, therapy that reduces blood lipids may lead to more solid fibrous plaques, which are less likely to undergo fissure and thrombosis.

The main *determinants of coronary blood flow* in normal coronary arteries are the aortic diastolic and left ventricular end-diastolic pressures, the duration of diastole, and the ability of the coronary arteries to dilate. Experimentally, myocardial ischemia can be induced in the absence of coronary artery stenoses by the combination of high left ventricular diastolic pressure, low aortic diastolic pressure and tachycardia. However, more frequently, ischemia develops because there are coronary artery stenoses. In effort angina, oxygen demand is increased. Coronary blood flow may increase but as its velocity increases across the stenosis, the pressure drop is accentuated (Brown et al, 1984), and subendocardial ischemia ensues.

Metabolic Effects of Ischemia

In the absence of oxygen, production of high energy phosphates depends upon the anaerobic glycolysis. When this is sufficiently rapid, enough "membrane-related" ATP is made to lessen potassium loss and to limit the rise in intracellular sodium as the sodium pump fails. During total ischemia, all the ATP must be derived from glycogen breakdown, which is protective until there is glycogen depletion with accumulation of metabolic end-products such as lactate and protons that are potentially harmful to the ischemic myocytes. Furthermore as intracellular sodium rises, there is an exchange with external calcium which also rises. Cytosolic calcium overload is, hypothetically, responsible at least in part for ischemic ventricular arrhythmias and ischemic cell death. Macromolecules are released into the circulation by severely injured cells, including cardiac enzymes such as creatine kinase (CK), troponin T, myoglobin and breakdown products of myosin. A substantial increase in plasma levels indicates myocardial cell death.

Potassium Loss, Current of Injury, and Ischemic Arrhythmias

Extracellular leakage of K^+ is one the earliest metabolic abnormalities of myocardial ischemia, and can be recorded by electrocardiographic changes that occur within a few beats of the onset of ischemia. The origin of this early K^+ loss into coronary venous blood is complex but represents in part opening of the ATP-sensitive K^+ channels as the ATP available at the level of the cell membrane falls. A later phase of K^+ loss results from impairment of energy-requiring ion pumps. Such ion leaks cause local membrane depolarization, which causes the current of injury which flows from injured to non-injured tissue during electrical diastole or repolarization, and from uninjured to injured tissue during electrical systole or depolarization. These currents are seen as ST-segment changes. Surface electrocardiography records ST-segment elevation when the injury current is coming towards the recording electrode, and ST-segment depression when the injury current travels away from it (i.e. subendocardial ischemia).

An important effect of the current of injury is the establishment of *re-entry circuits* at the boundaries between ischemic and non-ischemic myocardium leading to ventricular arrhythmias and ventricular fibrillation. The conduction delay in the ischemic area makes it possible for currents to re-enter recently repolarized myocardial fibers. The risk of ventricular fibrillation increases if the boundary between ischemic and non-ischemic area is large and if there is hypokalemia (low arterial K^+). The latter results from the adrenergic stress of anesthesia and surgery, with increased plasma catecholamine levels, which increase the transfer of potassium ions from blood to liver cells.

Mechanical Effects of Ischemia

Normally the left ventricular myocardium shortens and thickens by 15–20% of its resting length and thickness.

Regional myocardial ischemia causes lack of ATP and retention of metabolites such as inorganic phosphate, protons and carbon dioxide, which inhibit contraction. Successively hypokinesia (reduced systolic shortening/thickening), akinesia (absence of systolic shortening/thickening), and dyskinesia (paradoxical systolic lengthening/thinning) occur. A reduction of coronary flow by 10–20% is sufficient to reduce systolic shortening and thickening. Abolition of wall motion requires an 80% reduction of flow, and paradoxical wall motion (pure passive systolic lengthening and thinning) occurs when flow is reduced by 95% (Vatner et al, 1980). A specific type of dyskinesia termed post-systolic shortening (Lowenstein et al, 1981) is a marker of potential recovery of ischemic myocardium after reperfusion (Takayama et al, 1988).

Triggers for Acute Myocardial Infarction

Acute myocardial infarction (AMI) is the result of acute coronary thrombosis, which may be triggered by a number of events. For example, the early morning rise of BP, heart rate and circulating catecholamines may all account for the increase of AMI at this time. Following severe natural disasters such as an earthquake, the incidence of AMI rises, presumably the result of emotional stress. Likewise, the stress response to anesthesia and surgery is also likely to act as a trigger, especially in those with prior myocardial infarction. An enhanced adrenergic drive may also explain the development of angina for the first time in patients recently hospitalized, as when awaiting cardiac surgery.

New Ischemic Syndromes: Stunning and Hibernation

The success of thrombolytic therapy has brought reperfusion to the forefront. Thrombolysis reduces mortality and improves left ventricular function in survivors. However, reperfusion may not mean immediate recovery of function but may rather cause *myocardial stunning* which is the prolonged contractile dysfunction that persists after acute severe ischemia followed by reperfusion (Braunwald and Kloner, 1982). The recovery of contractile function post-thrombolysis may take several weeks or even months. This contractile dysfunction includes both decreased systolic function (systolic stunning) and increased myocardial stiffness (diastolic stunning). Stunning may result from injury caused by excess cytosolic calcium or by the formation of oxygen free radicals, either or both of which may cause inadequate excitation-contraction coupling (Schipke et al, 1996). The severity and duration of postischemic dysfunction vary considerably for apparently similar ischemic insults. Duration of ischemia, amount of collateral perfusion, and left ventricular end-diastolic pressure are significant determinants of postischemic contractile dysfunction and recovery.

Another important concept is that of *myocardial hibernation* (Rahimtoola, 1989). In this state, severe coronary artery disease is accompanied by a chronically hypocontractile myocardium. The proposed explanation is that chronic myocardial ischemia is compensated for by "downregulated" left ventricular function, so that the energy demands are reduced to the limits of the available blood supply. An alternate and current hypothesis is that repetitive episodes of ischemia could each be followed by stunning, and that the summation of the many episodes of stunning gives the appearance of hibernation which could therefore be termed pseudo-hibernation. This hypothesis would explain why the reduction of coronary blood flow found in association with hibernation may only be borderline or at the lower limit of normal.

It should be recalled that reductions of perfusion pressure do not impair ventricular function as long as they take place within the autoregulatory range. Where coronary blood flow is reduced below the autoregulatory range, function is reduced: perfusion and contraction are matched and the myocardium may be regarded as hibernating. Increased levels of interstitial adenosine, which inhibit myocardial contraction, may help to downregulate myocardial energy demands (Gao et al, 1995).

In anesthetic practice, the crucial aspect of myocardial hibernation is that chronic left ventricular dysfunction undergoes a significant recovery of function after revascularization. In surgical patients, the risks depend upon the extent of ventricular dysfunction (Lazor et al, 1988). If coronary revascularization allows some hibernating areas to function normally, the overall ventricular function increases and the risks of surgery decrease. Thus it is of practical importance to know whether a given patient with LV dysfunction, about to undergo revascularization, has reversible (hibernating) myocardial dysfunction or whether the myocardium is dead and therefore a much greater peri-operative hazard.

TREATMENT OF CORONARY ARTERY DISEASE

The major drugs used to bring symptomatic relief in the therapy of coronary artery disease are the beta-adrenergic blockers, the nitrates and the calcium channel antagonists (Fig 9-1). These agents are not well documented from the point of view of achieving outcome benefit in terms of increased longevity and decreased complications such as the need for revascularization or the development of myocardial infarction. A clear exception, however, is the reduction of post-infarction complications and decreased mortality in those given beta-blockers. This protective effect of beta-adrenergic blockers may also apply to the perioperative period (Mangano et al, 1996). To reduce the actual severity of coronary artery disease requires additional therapy by, at the least, aspirin, and usually by a specific lipid lowering agent such as a statin.

Nitrates

Nitrates provide an exogenous source of nitric oxide (NO) in the vascular smooth muscle, inducing coronary vasodila-

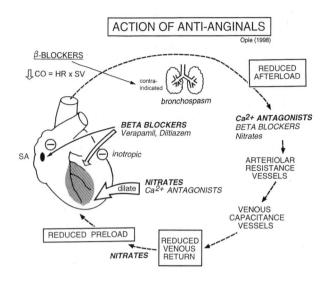

Fig 9-1. Principles of actions of antianginal drugs. CO = *cardiac output, HR = heart rate, SV = stroke volume (Fig copyright © 1998, LH Opie)*

tion. Nitrates dilate large coronary arteries and arterioles greater than 100 μm in diameter, to facilitate the distribution of flow along the collateral vessels and from epi- to endocardial regions. In addition, they induce venodilation thereby reducing the venous return and indirectly lessening the wall stress on the left ventricle. To a lesser extent, they cause peripheral arteriolar dilation to lessen the blood pressure and to reduce the afterload. Nitrates relieve symptomatic coronary spasm as in Prinzmetal's angina, and dynamic stenoses. In contrast, the more distally active vasodilators (dipyridamole) divert blood from the compromised areas with risk of coronary steal, and without relief of angina.

The cellular mechanisms of action of nitrates are not fully understood. An unidentified nitrate receptor is likely to be situated on the vascular myocyte. Thereafter, an intracellular enzyme system converts nitrates, after they have entered into the cell, into NO. The latter stimulates guanylate cyclase to produce cyclic GMP. This, in turn, reduces calcium levels in vascular smooth muscle cells either by minimizing calcium entry or enhancing calcium exit.

Nitroglycerin is readily absorbed from the skin and the oral mucosa, hence the popularity of ointments, patches, sprays and sublingual tablets. The onset of action of sublingual nitroglycerin occurs within 1–2 minutes and lasts for up to 1 hour. Nitroglycerin spray has the same pharmacokinetics as sublingual nitroglycerin. Extended release preparations have a more prolonged effect lasting 3 to 5 hours. Nitroglycerin ointment has a slow onset of action and its anti-anginal effect is sustained for up to 7 hours. Proof of efficacy during prolonged use is still missing. Nitroglycerin patches provide fairly constant plasma levels from 2 to 24 hours. The amount of nitroglycerin released varies with the surface of skin covered by the patch. To avoid nitrate tolerance, the patch should be removed at night when used for effort angina, and during the day when used for nocturnal angina.

Isosorbide dinitrate is absorbed from the oral mucosa and the gut. It has a slower onset of action than nitroglycerin and its effects last longer. Isosorbide dinitrate is metabolized by the liver into active mononitrate metabolites — the latter are excreted by the kidneys.

Mononitrates have a high bio-availability and a relatively long duration of action (6 to 8 hours) that can extend to 12 hours in the case of slow-release preparations. As with all nitrates, tolerance is a problem if inappropriate dosages are used. Drugs and doses recognized as lessening the risk of tolerance are (1) short acting mononitrate (Monoket or Ismo), 20 mg twice daily 7 hours apart; and (2) long acting mononitrate (Imdur) 120 or 240 mg once daily.

Side-effects of nitrates include headaches and hypotension. In addition, patients with chronic lung disease may exhibit worsening of their hypoxemia because of an increase in venous admixture. Prolonged administration of nitrates may cause methemoglobinemia.

Nitrate tolerance may be explained, in part, by depletion of vascular sulfhydryl groups as these are necessary for the intracellular formation of NO, the major mediator of vasodilatation. Acetylcysteine provides sulfhydryl groups that may protect against nitrate tolerance in veins but not in medium sized arteries (Boesgaard et al, 1994). Another explanation for nitrate tolerance is that nitrate-induced venodilation activates both the renin-angiotensin and adrenergic systems which oppose vasodilatation (Fung and Bauer, 1994). A new proposal is that nitrate tolerance is caused by production of free radicals from the endothelium (Parker and Parker, 1998). This could explain why Vitamin E and hydralazine may lessen tolerance. A further theory is that hypothetical nitrate receptors may be down-regulated. Prevention of nitrate tolerance includes interval-dosing as this causes seesaw blood levels (Thadani and Lipicky, 1994). Dose escalation may also be a short-term maneuver to overcome tolerance (Mehra et al, 1993). Co-therapy with either ACE-inhibitors or with hydralazine may lessen tolerance.

Beta-adrenoceptor Blockers

Beta-adrenergic receptor antagonists remain standard therapy for effort angina, mixed effort and rest angina, and unstable angina. They decrease mortality in the post-infarction phase, and at the time of operation in non-cardiac patients at risk of infarction when given acutely and for one week thereafter (Mangano, 1996).

Mechanism of action. The beta-adrenergic receptors link to the adenylate cyclase system which produces cyclic AMP, the intracellular messenger, from ATP. Beta-adrenoceptor stimulation increases the opening probability of L-type calcium channels (inotropic effect) and enhances the re-uptake of cytostolic calcium by the sarcoplasmic reticulum (lusitropic or relaxing effect). Beta-adrenergic agonists also increase the rate of discharge of the sinus node pacemaker (chronotropic effect), and accelerate conduction (dromotropic effect). Beta-adrenoceptor antagonists have the opposite effect, and reductions in the inotropic, chronotropic and dromotropic states depend upon the pre-existing level of beta-adrenoceptor stimulation.

Beta-adrenoceptor antagonists protect against ischemia mostly because they decrease heart rate and contractility, thus reducing myocardial oxygen consumption while increasing the duration of diastole. The longer diastolic filling time also leads to better diastolic myocardial perfusion. The reduction of the atrioventricular conduction is relevant to the efficacy of beta-blockers in supraventricular tachycardia, and in the control of the ventricular rate in atrial fibrillation.

Pharmacological properties of beta-adrenoceptor blockers. Some are relatively selective ("cardioselective") for the β_1-receptors, so that they are safer in chronic airways disease, while others such as propranolol are non-selective (Table 9-2). Such selectivity is lost at high doses, a point often forgotten. Yet other beta-adrenoceptor blockers cause peripheral vasodilation by additional α-adrenoceptor blocking properties or β_2-agonist properties. One such agent, with combined α-β blocking properties, *carvedilol*, has now been registered in the USA for use in congestive heart failure already fully treated by diuretic, ACE inhibition and digitalis. Finally, some beta-adrenoceptor blockers activate the receptors and are truly partial agonists (or are classified as exhibiting ISA or intrinsic sympathomimetic activity), but this quality has never been recognized by any registration authority as conferring specific benefit on patients. Some of the pharmacokinetic properties of the beta-blockers are displayed in Table 9-3.

Esmolol, an ultra-short acting cardioselective betablocker, has a half-life of 9 minutes because it is converted into inactive products by blood esterases. Full recovery from beta-blockade is expected within 30 minutes. This

Table 9-2. Types of beta-adrenoceptor blockers

Type	Pure antagonists	Partial agonists
Selective (β_1)	Atenolol Bisoprolol Esmolol Metoprolol	Acebutolol
Non-selective ($\beta_{1,2}$)	Propranolol Nadolol Timolol Sotalol*	Pindolol
With α blockade	Labetalol Carvedilol	
With α blockade and β_2 agonism	Celiprolol**	

* sotalol has class III antiarrhythmic properties
** not available in USA

Table 9-3. Absorption and bioavailability of β-blockers, with a comparison of oral and intravenous doses

	Absorption (% of dose)	Bioavailability (% of dose)	Oral dose (daily)	IV dose
Atenolol	≈50	≈40	50–100mg	150μg/kg
Labetalol	>90	≈33	100–800mg	50–200mg
Metoprolol	>90	≈50	50–300mg	2–15mg
Propranolol	>90	≈30	80–320mg	1–10mg
Sotalol	≈70	≈60	80–320mg	20–120mg
Timolol	>90	≈75	5–60mg	N/A

Acebutolol, bisoprolol, celiprolol, nadolol, pindolol and timolol are not available in intravenous formulation.

makes esmolol an extremely useful agent in the perioperative period as it has an almost immediate onset of action and, should adverse effects develop, its effects are very short lived.

Side-effects of beta-blockade include smooth muscle spasm, excessive cardiac effects (bradycardia, heart block, negative inotropy) and central nervous effects (insomnia, depression). The latter are more likely to happen with lipid soluble blockers such as propranolol.

Contra-indications to beta-blockers include asthma (an absolute contraindication even to cardioselective agents), severe bradycardia, high-degree heart block, overt untreated left ventricular failure, severe depressive states and, to a lesser extent, active peripheral vascular disease.

Down-regulation of the beta-adrenoceptors is known to occur after prolonged beta-adrenergic stimulation, either because of internalization of the receptors or because of lysosomal destruction. This occurs after administration of beta-adrenoceptor agonists and in chronic heart failure in association with long-term sympathetic overactivity. Up-regulation represents an increase in the number of beta-adrenoceptors, as during the prolonged administration of beta-adrenoceptor blockers. Ischemic events may be precipitated by the abrupt withdrawal of beta-blockers (*withdrawal syndrome*). Therefore in patients receiving pre-operative beta-blockade, a change from oral to intravenous administration may be needed to cover the peri-operative period.

Calcium Antagonists

As more fully discussed in Chapter 5, these agents possess anti-ischemic properties by virtue of coronary vasodilation especially during exercise, by afterload reduction, and (in the case of verapamil and diltiazem, but not the nifedipine-like agents) by reduction of heart rate and by a negative inotropic effect. They also relieve Prinzmetal's vasospastic angina, a rather rare cause of unstable angina. They are metabolically neutral, not altering blood lipid levels nor insulin resistance in diabetes. Recent concerns about their safety focus on the short-acting but not the long-acting agents (Alderman et al, 1997), and particularly on short-acting nifedipine which induces a vigorous abrupt peripheral arteriolar vasodilation with a reflex tachycardia, making it unsafe for use in unstable ischemic syndromes. On present evidence, this drug is unsafe, especially in high doses such as 80 mg per day, for any patient with myocardial ischemia that is not caused by coronary vasospasm. Because there is no fear of a withdrawal syndrome with these agents, oral dosage can be stopped at the time of the operation, which can then be covered by intravenous nitroglycerin as needed. Post-operatively, the calcium antagonist is then restarted.

Newer Anti-anginal Agents

Molsidomine and pirisidomine are nitric oxide donors; the former is widely used in Germany but not in the USA or UK. Molsidomine has been shown to increase the exercise tolerance in patients with stable angina and to reduce the extent of ST-segment depression (Messin et al, 1995). In patients with myocardial infarction, however, molsidomine and its active metabolite linsidomine, a nitric oxide donor, did not improve mortality when compared with placebo in 4,017 patients with acute myocardial infarction (ESPRIM trial, 1994).

    Nicorandil is a nicotinamide nitrate, widely used in the UK and Japan, but not licensed in the USA. It acts both as a nitrate and as an activator of ATP dependent potassium channels (Richter et al, 1990). Nicorandil causes vascular smooth muscle relaxation, particularly in veins, and so reduces ventricular filling. It also dilates the coronary arteries. Opening of the potassium channels hyperpolarizes the cell membrane and inhibits calcium entry. This causes vasodilatation. The effect of nicorandil on ATP-dependent potassium channels is also observed in ischemic myocardium. This is associated with limitation of experimental infarct size and enhanced recovery of stunned myocardium (Warltier et al, 1993). The hemodynamic effects of nicorandil resemble those of a combination of a nitrate and a longer-acting dihydropyridine calcium-channel blocker (slow-release nifedipine or amlodipine). Doses of 10–30 mg twice daily reduce filling pressure, systemic vascular resistance, blood pressure and cardiac work without effect on heart rate. In patients with congestive heart failure, cardiac output usually increases. A number of relatively small placebo-controlled and of double-blind trials have shown nicorandil to be effective in stable angina, yet no more effective than more conventional therapy. However, a recent USA study showed that it was not superior to placebo in stable effort angina.

Statins

Patients with coronary artery disease will increasingly be receiving statins, even if their blood cholesterol levels are not particularly high, because of the very promising results of recent trials. These showed a mortality reduction (especially in high cholesterol patients), fewer interventions, and a lessened risk of first infarction. Because statins take months to act, they will not be started acutely in the perioperative period. They can safely be discontinued over the operation. Of importance is that they can be combined with anti-ischemic drugs such as beta-blockers without fear of interaction, and, as far as is known, they do not interact with anesthetic agents.

TREATMENT OF SPECIFIC CLINICAL SYNDROMES

Stable Angina

In angina, short acting nitrates give symptomatic relief. The problem with long acting nitrates has been the development of tolerance, but dosages for the mononitrates lessen tolerance and help to prevent angina. Nitrates are often combined with beta-blockers or calcium antagonists, which have a different mechanism of antianginal action, and sometimes the triple combination is used. Because nitrates tend to increase the heart rate, logical combinations are with beta-blockade or with the heart rate slowing calcium antagonists, such as verapamil or diltiazem. Nonetheless in practice nitrates are often combined with dihydropyridine calcium antagonists, such as nifedipine.

Regarding *beta-adrenergic antagonists,* about 80% of patients respond while about 20% do not, which may be because of very severe obstructive coronary disease (very low level exertion). Alternatively, excessive left ventricular end-diastolic pressures caused by the negative inotropy of the beta-blocker with an increase in left ventricular size, could increase myocardial oxygen demand. High end-diastolic pressures also compromise subendocardial blood flow. The addition of an ACE inhibitor should minimize these risks.

Beta-adrenoceptor blockers are often combined with nitrates and calcium antagonists. While dihydropyridines such as nifedipine, amlodipine and felodipine are relatively easy to combine with beta-blockers, the combination of these agents with verapamil or diltiazem is potentially hazardous. The potential problem is excess nodal inhibition with extreme bradycardia or atrio-ventricular block, besides additive negative inotropy.

Calcium antagonists are often used as first line agents (instead of beta-blockers) with nitrates. Arguments for their use become most compelling when beta-blockade induces side-effects such as fatigue or depression or impotence, or when there is respiratory disease or metabolic disorders such as a raised blood cholesterol or insulin-requiring diabetes mellitus. There is no place for short acting nifedipine in patients with symptomatic myocardial ischemia in the absence of documented coronary spasm. In general, short acting calcium antagonists should be avoided where possible.

Silent Myocardial Ischemia

In silent myocardial ischemia, even modest increases in heart rate are important, and beta-blockade has been shown to reduce both the number and duration of ischemic episodes. This is true in the immediate perioperative period

(Prys-Roberts et al, 1973; Stone et al, 1988; Dodds et al, 1994), extending up to the first week (Wallace et al, 1998).

Unstable Angina

In unstable angina, i.e. increasingly severe and prolonged pain, with threat of myocardial infarction, the basic patho-physiology involves plaque fissure and partial coronary thrombosis. This requires urgent *anti-thrombotic therapy* by heparin plus aspirin. New platelet receptor inhibitors such as abciximab are increasingly used.

Anti-ischemic therapy by beta-blockade is useful espe-cially when heart rate and blood pressure are elevated. Further symptomatic benefits appear to accrue from the addition of a calcium antagonist. Nifedipine alone is contra-indicated, as probably are all the dihydropyridines. The rapid onset of action makes nitroglycerin an effective drug in the management of pain in patients with unstable angina. Doses ranging between 0.3 mg/hr and 6 mg/hr (on occasion up to 30 mg/hr) have been used for this indica-tion. Similarly, intravenous isosorbide dinitrate (not in the USA) can be used in doses ranging between 1.25 and 5 mg/hr. These doses are also applicable in the treatment of peri-operative myocardial ischemia.

From the point of view of outcome studies on anti-ischemic drugs, there are only two of note: one showed benefits for intravenous diltiazem versus nitroglycerin (Gobel, et al, 1995), and the other for metoprolol versus short acting nifedipine (HINT study, 1986).

Once the acute phase of unstable angina is controlled, coronary angiography is indicated and is likely to demon-strate the need for coronary bypass graft or angioplasty and/or coronary stenting.

In Prinzmetal's variant angina coronary artery spasm may be exacerbated by beta-adrenoceptor blockade. Cal-cium antagonists, including nifedipine, are effective. During anesthetic hypocapnea, a coronary vasoconstrictive stimulus should be avoided (Coetzee et al, 1984).

Acute Myocardial Infarction and Follow-up

Intravenous beta-blockade given for early acute myocardial infarction, decreases the risk of ventricular fibrillation, espe-cially within the first 4 hours (Yusuf et al, 1980). The bene-fit, as estimated in the first ISIS trial, results in one life saved for 150 patients treated (ISIS-1 trial, 1986). However, the widespread use of thrombolytic agents has decreased the perceived benefits of early beta-blockade. The TIMI-II study showed that metoprolol added to thrombolysis improved early but not late outcome (Borzak and Gheor-ghiade, 1993). *Calcium antagonists* are contraindicated for early phase myocardial infarction, because of fear of nega-tive inotropic effects.

Nitrates do not improve outcome when combined with thrombolysis and aspirin, as shown in recent large trials (ISIS-4, 1995; GISSI-3, 1994). Possibly the dosage of nitrates was not optimal. Nitrates are probably useful when there is on-going anginal pain, or elevated left ventricular end-diastolic pressure (i.e. large anterior infarcts) or severe hypertension. Low dose intravenous nitroglycerin is used initially and titrated against the blood pressure. Nitrates may be combined with ACE inhibitors, with a large reduction in early mortality (17%) in GISSI-3 (1994), and a lower late benefit.

Post-infarction beta-blockade, given prophylactically, reduces sudden death and re-infarction by approximately 25%, and additive benefits appear to result from the combination of ACE inhibitors and beta-blockers (Pfeffer et al, 1992). Therefore, beta-blockade should be given whenever possible. If contraindicated or not tolerated, verapamil is the agent of choice. (See Ch 5.)

Congestive Heart Failure

Basic therapy is by diuretics and ACE inhibitors. Digoxin has modest benefits, which do not include a reduction in mortality. *Nitrates* serve as unloading agents both in acute and chronic heart failure. Nitroglycerin is effective both sublingually and intravenously especially in patients with acute pulmonary edema. However, there is a risk of hypotension. In the long-term treatment of congestive heart failure, nitrates combined with hydralazine (the latter possibly helping to reduce nitrate tolerance) are useful but inferior to ACE inhibitors in decreasing mortality. In otherwise fully treated patients (diuretics, ACE inhibitor, digoxin) cautiously added beta-blockade lessens mortality (Ch 10). In patients with heart failure and angina, therapy may be by carvedilol, the vasodilating *beta-blocker* recently approved for heart failure but not for this combination, or by the *calcium antagonist* amlodipine which showed promising results in a sub-group analysis of the PRAISE study (Packer et al, 1996). In general calcium antagonists remain contraindicated in heart failure.

CORONARY RISK FACTORS IN SURGICAL PATIENTS

While it is recognized that coronary artery disease increases the risk of complications of anesthesia and surgery, some groups of patients must be identified because they are particularly at risk (Table 9-4).

Previous Myocardial Infarction

In such patients, the risk of peri-operative infarction is increased 10–20 fold. For many years the delay between previous infarction and surgery was regarded as the major determinant of the incidence of reinfarction (Table 9-5). Reinfarction rates of approximately 30% were quoted for delays of less than three months (Steen et al, 1978). More recent studies suggest that even within the first three months after infarction the incidence of reinfarction may be much smaller than twenty years ago. This change could result from better management of myocardial infarction and greatly improved monitoring and anesthetic management

Table 9-4. Clinical predictors of perioperative cardiovascular events*

Minor predictors

Advanced age
Abnormal electrocardiogram
Arrhythmias, non-serious
Exercise intolerance
Past stroke
Systemic hypertension (see Chapter 8)

Intermediate predicators

Mild angina pectoris
Prior myocardial infarction
Mild congestive heart failure
Diabetes mellitus

Major predictors

Unstable coronary syndromes
Acute myocardial infarction
Moderate or severe congestive heart failure
Serious arrhythmias
Severe valvular disease

* Modified from the guidelines of the American College of Cardiology and the American Heart Association (ACC/AHA, 1996)

of patients with known coronary artery disease (Rao et al, 1983; Shah et al, 1990). However, a cautious approach is still recommended. Elective surgery should generally be delayed for three months after acute myocardial infarction.

The *risk of reinfarction,* irrespective of the delay between surgery and previous infarction is known to be highest after vascular surgery, prolonged operations, intra-abdominal and intra-thoracic surgery, and much less after body surface surgery. Another major risk factor is the presence of left ventricular failure, or simply of reduced left ventricular function. Though the patient may not exhibit signs of heart failure at the time of pre-operative assessment, the clinical history of an episode of heart failure is strongly associated with adverse outcome (Dirksen and Kjoller, 1990; Palda and Detsky, 1997).

Table 9-5. Risk of postoperative reinfarction in relation to time after previous infarction

Time after previous infarction	Steen et al 1978	Rao et al 1983	Shah et 1990
< 3 months	27%	6%	4%
3–6 months	11%	2%	0%
> 6 months	4%	1.5%	6%

Unstable or Disabling Angina Prior to Surgery

It is not too uncommon to discover that surgical patients have exhibited their first ever episode of angina very shortly before admission to hospital, or have experienced a substantial worsening of previously stable angina. If patients have not been previously investigated, this is the time for coronary angiography followed by coronary angioplasty, coronary stenting or coronary artery bypass graft, as perioperative mortality is very high in such patients unless their coronary circulation has been improved. If patients cannot benefit from coronary artery surgery or angioplasty, then medical treatment must be optimized in order to render them more stable.

Major Vascular Surgery in those with Severe Coronary Artery Disease

The question of coronary artery interventions before major surgery has been extensively debated, especially for those presenting for surgery of the abdominal aorta and its branches, and carotid endarterectomy. Because of the strong association between peripheral vascular disease and coronary artery disease, this is a common problem. The prevalence of serious angiographic coronary artery disease ranges from 37% to 78% in patients undergoing peripheral vascular surgery, while the prevalence of clinical evidence of coronary disease ranges from 22% to 70% in individual series. Even among patients without clinical indications of coronary disease, the incidence of significant angiographically demonstrable surgical coronary disease may be as high as 14% (Hertzer et al, 1984). The presence of coronary artery disease is associated with an increased risk of adverse outcome. In patients suspected of coronary disease perioperative mortality is approximately four times higher than in those without coronary disease (Gersh et al, 1991b). Irrespective of the underlying peripheral vascular disease, late mortality is cardiac related in 40% to 60% of cases. After surgery of abdominal aortic aneurysms, the long-term prognosis of survivors is much better for those without than for those with coronary artery disease, as the cumulative incidence of cardiac events at 8 years is quoted at 15% and 61% respectively (Roger et al, 1989).

Prophylactic coronary artery bypass surgery must be considered because of the high risk of cardiac events in patients with coronary artery disease undergoing non-cardiac surgery, especially vascular surgery. Randomized trials and data base studies show that the relative benefits of coronary artery surgery are greater in the patients with severe ischemia, left ventricular dysfunction, and multiple vessel disease. The European Coronary Surgery Study (1982) has shown that the relative improvement in survival rate was substantially greater in patients when vascular disease was present (85% vs 52%) than in patients without vascular disease (90% vs 81%). Not surprisingly, non-randomized studies have shown that the risk of non-cardiac surgery is low after prior coronary artery bypass, being similar to the risk in those without significant coronary disease (Foster et al, 1986; Gersh et al, 1991b). In the more specific setting of vascular surgery, the mortality rate was 1.5% among patients with prior coronary artery bypass surgery, 1.3% among those without overt coronary artery disease as opposed to

6.8% in those with suspected coronary disease (Hertzer et al, 1987). Similarly, the long-term mortality is less in those who have undergone coronary artery bypass surgery prior to vascular surgery (20% 5-year mortality), than in those with overt but uncorrected coronary artery disease (41% 5-year mortality).

Such benefits of coronary bypass surgery must be put into perspective. As patients undergoing vascular surgery are usually elderly, mortality of coronary surgery can be expected to be higher than in younger patients, and the late mortality after coronary surgery is worse in patients with peripheral vascular disease than in those without (European Coronary Surgery Study, 1982).

Prophylactic angioplasty has been undertaken in too few studies to draw firm conclusions regarding its value. However, a small study suggests that in patients with severe coronary artery disease treated by angioplasty, non-cardiac operations (at a mean of nine days later) were followed by a lower than anticipated event rate (Huber et al, 1990).

PREOPERATIVE MYOCARDIAL ISCHEMIA

An abnormal *12-lead ECG* has been found to be an independent predictor of postoperative events (Carliner et al, 1985). However, functional cardiac testing is necessary for adequate risk stratification. Presence of a clearly abnormal exercise test is associated with a high incidence of perioperative myocardial infarction: 16% in the study of Cutler and colleagues (1981). Similarly, the quality of the resting left ventricular function is important. An inverse relationship exists between the ejection fraction and the risk of perioperative myocardial infarction (Table 9-6). However, in subsequent studies the striking association between low ejection fraction and high risk has not always been confirmed, except that an ejection fraction of less than 35% remains a predictor of poor outcome.

Dipyridamole-thallium scintigraphy has been used extensively. The cumulative experience with dipyridamole is that redistribution of blood flow away from the potentially ischemic area is predictive of perioperative cardiac events (essentially myocardial infarction and unstable angina). However, some studies have failed to identify a reversible defect as a significant determinant of adverse outcome. It may be that it is in patients with intermediate risk that the presence of a reversible defect is the most useful indicator of risk, whereas in low and high risk groups (based on other criteria) presence of redistribution is not significant (Gersh et al,

Table 9-6. Ejection fraction and postoperative myocardial infarction

Ejection Fraction	Postoperative myocardial infarction
>56%	0%
36–55%	19%
<36%	75%

(After Pasternak et al, 1985)

1991a). *Dobutamine stress echocardiography* may be a useful alternative test (Palda and Detsky, 1997).

Silent myocardial ischemia occurs very frequently during the perioperative period as demonstrated by ambulatory ECG monitoring for several days before and after surgery. Early studies have shown a strong association between pre-operative silent myocardial ischemia and perioperative cardiac events (Raby et al, 1989). Later studies have shown postoperative silent myocardial ischemia to be an even stronger predictor of post-operative cardiac events (Raby et al, 1992), and of the long-term prognosis (Mangano et al, 1992).

A number of therapies have been proposed to decrease myocardial ischemia and adverse outcome. These include the administration of beta-blockers (Stone et al, 1986; Mangano et al, 1996), the adenosine modulator *acadesine* (Menasche et al, 1995), and the central alpha-agonists, *dexmedetomidine* and *mivazerol* (Talke et al, 1995). Of these, evidence is strongest for *beta-adrenoceptor blockade* (Mangano et al, 1996). In a trial still unpublished, mivazerol reduced mortality in high-risk vascular patients. In a meta-analysis on 4 043 patients, acadesine decreased perioperative myocardial infarction and cardiac death, with however the confidence intervals being just short of unity, so that now the search is for subgroups with the best response (Mangano, 1997).

MANAGEMENT OF PERIOPERATIVE ISCHEMIA

Rapid treatment of ischemia (evidenced by ST-segment depression) is essential as perioperative ischemia is associated with adverse cardiac events, and followed by myocardial stunning (Smith et al, 1985; Coriat et al, 1985). Hemodynamic stability is an important goal of anesthesia and postoperative management that helps to protect the oxygen balance. Though myocardial ischemia may occur without hemodynamic changes, several studies have shown a lower incidence of perioperative ischemia and infarction when hemodynamic values were controlled throughout the operative period (Wells and Kaplan, 1981; Rao et al, 1983; Goehner et al, 1988).

Ischemia during anesthesia and surgery may result from inadequate depth of anesthesia. The resulting hypertension and tachycardia may cause myocardial ischemia; both are easily controlled by deepening the anesthesia. Tachycardia and ischemia may reflect an underlying hypovolemia likely to respond to fluid replacement. When such maneuvers have failed to control the tachycardia, a small dose of a beta-blocker is indicated. When ischemia occurs in the context of hypotension, withdrawal of inhalational anesthetics and fluid replacement may fully reverse the ST-segment changes.

If ischemia occurs in the absence of any hemodynamic aberrations, nitroglycerin and/or calcium channel blockers are indicated as this suggests a contribution of coronary spasm. If ischemic events occur during the recovery period, an alternative, especially where myocardial ischemia is associated with hypotension, is to consider emergency coronary angiography followed by coronary angioplasty with or without stenting. This may cause an almost instantaneous symptomatic and hemodynamic improvement. A selection of intravenous drugs for the management of perioperative ischemia is listed in Table 9-7.

Table 9-7. Intravenous drugs used for perioperative ischemia.

Clinical condition	Suitable drug(s)	Mechanism of action	Dose, intravenous
Ischemia, no tachycardia	Nitroglycerin (N) Isosorbide dinitrate (ID)	NO donors	N: 5–200 g/min ID:1.25–5 mg/h*
Ischemia, sinus tachycardia, non-compensatory	Esmolol (E) Atenolol (A) Metoprolol (M)	Beta-blockers. Cardio-selective	E: 50–300 µg/ kg/min A: 5mg 2X M: 5 mg 3 X
Ischemia, SVT	Esmolol (E) Verapamil (V) Diltiazem (D)	Beta-blocker Ca antagonist Ca antagonist	E: as above V:5–10 mg over 2 min; D:0.25 mg/kg over 2 min
Ischemia, poor LV	Nitroglycerin Isosorbide dinitrate	NO donors	N: as above ID: as above*
Ischemia, severe hypertension	Esmolol Nicardipine Verapamil Diltiazem	Beta-blocker Ca antagonist Ca antagonist Ca antagonist	E: as above N: 3–15 mg/h V: as above* D: as above*

* = indication not approved in USA
SVT = supraventricular tachycardia
Poor LV = poor left ventricular function
NO = nitric oxide
Ca = calcium

Management of Patients at High Risk of Ischemia

While routine prophylactic coronary revascularization before vascular surgery or other major operations is impractical, identification of the high risk patients who would benefit from it is important and optimization of medical therapy is crucial. Intensive monitoring during the perioperative period is also of major importance to minimize hemodynamic derangements.

In an important outcome study, Mangano et al (1996) identified high risk patients about to undergo non-cardiac surgery, as those with coronary artery disease (previous myocardial infarct, typical angina, or atypical angina with a positive stress test), or those with at least two of the following: age equal to or greater than 65 years, hypertension, current smoking, serum cholesterol equal to or greater than 240 mg/dL (6.2 mmol/L), or diabetes mellitus. These patients were given atenolol or placebo just before the induction of the anesthesia, immediately after surgery and daily throughout the hospital stay of up to seven days. The first two doses were intravenous (5 mg over 5 minutes, repeated 5 minutes later if tolerated), and the remainder of the doses either by infusion over 12 hours or orally. Mortality was reduced upon discharge, after 6 months, and after 2 years. Event-free survival was prolonged.

There are a number of caveats to this study by Mangano and colleagues. The mean duration of surgery for non-cardiac procedures was approximately 6 hours with a range of 1.5 to 15.6. It is possible that the relatively long duration of surgery was responsible for a relatively high incidence of adverse cardiovascular outcome in the control group. This in turn may have strengthened the relationship between high risk patients, silent ischemia and adverse outcome. *Therefore it is especially high risk patients subject to prolonged operative procedures that should benefit from prophylactic beta-blockade*, which in turn implies the need for more prolonged post-operative monitoring. Thus the advantages of beta-blockade must be balanced against the risk in patients who may have borderline cardiorespiratory problems, not severe enough to contraindicate beta-blockade, but enough to make the postoperative course more hazardous. In the end, it will often be a matter of clinical judgement whether or not to use prophylactic beta-blockade.

MAINTENANCE BETA-BLOCKADE IN THE PERIOPERATIVE PERIOD

The question arises of how to maintain beta-blockade in patients unable to continue to take their usual oral medication. This is particularly important in view of the risk of myocardial ischemia after acute withdrawal of beta-blockade. Highly lipid soluble beta-blockers such as propranolol, and labetalol have a very high first-pass metabolism. Thus, the effective intravenous dose is much lower than the oral dose. Similarly, with less lipid soluble drugs with hepatic clearance such as acebutolol, metoprolol and timolol, a marked reduction of the dose is needed when the intravenous route is used to replace the oral route (Table 9-3). Currently, the agents most used are esmolol, atenolol and metoprolol, all of them cardioselective and the first having a very short half life.

MAINTENANCE OF CIRCULATION AND MYOCARDIAL ISCHEMIA

Hypotension is caused by most inhalational and intravenous anesthetics by a combination of myocardial depression, venodilation and/or vasodilatation. Many reduce sympathetic activity and blunt the baroreflexes. These effects are potentially relevant to the development of ischemia, because hypotension predisposes to impaired myocardial perfusion. The effects on the myocardium itself are usually the result of reductions of the initial inward calcium current and the tail current caused by the release of calcium from the sarcoplasmic reticulum (Terrar and Victory, 1988; Puttick and Terrar, 1992). The respective roles of reduced contractility, venodilation, and vasodilation differ between agents. Halothane and enflurane exert their effects mostly because they depress cardiac contractility. By contrast isoflurane, desflurane and sevoflurane cause both myocardial depression and vasodilation (Bernard et al, 1990; Merin et al, 1994, Ebert et al, 1995). Thiopentone depresses contractility, while propofol causes veno- and vasodilation, though high concentrations also depress contractility (Puttick et al, 1992). Opioids exert little effect on contractility and vascular resistance. The addition of nitrous oxide usually causes a modest degree of myocardial depression (Pagel et al, 1990).

The overall effect of anesthetic agents on *cardiac output* reflects the balance between cardiac depression (if present), venous and arteriolar vasodilation. With agents that cause marked arteriolar dilation such as isoflurane, desflurane and sevoflurane, cardiac output is relatively well maintained, whereas it is reduced in a dose-dependent fashion by agents that do not cause arteriolar dilation such as halothane and enflurane. The mode of ventilation modifies the effects of all anesthetic agents. When patients are artificially ventilated, the effect of raised intra-thoracic pressure may contribute to a reduction of cardiac output. Conversely, when patients are breathing spontaneously during anesthesia and surgery, carbon dioxide tension increases and this causes an hyperdynamic response of the circulation, mediated by increased sympathetic activity. Such responses of the circulation are also modified by the changes in sympathetic activity caused by anesthetic and surgical maneuvers, or by concomitant medications.

Coronary blood flow is reduced in a dose-dependent manner by those many anesthetic agents which decrease blood pressure and contractility (Puttick et al, 1992; Doyle et al, 1989). This reduction in coronary flow is the result of local regulation, matching oxygen supply and oxygen demand. However, several anesthetic agents cause coronary vasodilatation, especially isoflurane, desflurane and sevoflurane (Cutfield et al, 1988; Pagel et al, 1991; Hirano et al, 1995). With these agents, the reduction of arterial pressure exceeds the reduction of coronary blood flow. While in the normal heart coronary vasodilation causes generalized luxury perfusion, in the presence of coronary artery disease, coronary vasodilation may cause redistribution of coronary flow away from the compromised myocardium. (See later in this chapter).

Sympathetic activation with an increased myocardial oxygen demand is caused by some old anesthetic agents such as cyclopropane and ether. The intravenous agent ketamine also causes sympathomimetic effects. Nitrous oxide causes a modest increase in sympathetic activity. Most, if not all modern inhalational and intravenous anesthetics decrease sympathetic activity. However, desflurane increases sympathetic activation especially when its concentration is rapidly increased from 1.0 to 1.5 MAC (Ebert et al, 1993; Weiskopf et al, 1994). This effect also occurs with isoflurane, but only when its concentration is abruptly increased to 5%. As sympathetic activation brought about by desflurane occurs well within the range of concentrations used in clinical practice, caution should be exercised when this agent is used in patients suffering from coronary artery disease, the increase in heart rate being a particular risk.

EFFECTS OF ANESTHETIC AGENTS ON THE COMPROMISED HEART

A large proportion of episodes of myocardial ischemia during the perioperative period occur in association with hemodynamic changes such as hypotension, hypertension, tachycardia and left ventricular dilation. Some of these changes are a direct consequence of the effects of anesthesia on the heart and the circulation. However, the specific effects of anesthetic agents and their associated effects on cardiac mechanics remain difficult to assess as they may differ according to the type of ischemic dysfunction.

Experimental Ischemia and Anesthetic Agents

Following acute coronary occlusion, a large number of studies have shown that inhalational anesthetics and opioid analgesics decrease the extent of ischemia (assessed as summated ST elevation) and lessen the size of infarction (Bland and Lowenstein, 1976). It is generally argued that protection results from reduced myocardial oxygen demand as heart rate and systolic arterial pressure are lower. When a coronary artery is critically narrowed, flow through the stenosis is exquisitely dependent upon the coronary perfusion pressure and the duration of diastole. As inhalational anesthetic agents decrease arterial pressure and some may increase heart rate, exaggerated depression of function in the myocardium supplied by a narrowed coronary artery could be expected (Lowenstein et al, 1981; Priebe and Foëx 1987). Indeed, many experimental studies of the effects of inhalational anesthetics and some intravenous anesthetics, including propofol, have shown such a selectively exaggerated depression of function of the compromised myocardium. This effect is dose-dependent and becomes significant in the presence of high concentrations of inhalational anesthetics or intravenous agents. Even nitrous oxide, whose effects on the circulation are relatively modest, exerts an adverse effect on compromised myocardial segments as evidenced by reduced systolic shortening and appearance of paradoxical wall motion termed post-systolic shortening (Philbin et al 1985; Leone et al, 1988).

Coronary Steal Syndrome

Anesthesia-induced coronary steal syndrome results when arteriolar dilators redistribute coronary blood flow away from the compromised myocardium. Steal is typically induced by exercise, dobutamine and/or the vasodilator dipyridamole. One study showed a high incidence of myocardial ischemia (ST segment depression, lactate production) in patients with documented coronary artery disease anesthetized with isoflurane (Reiz, 1983). As isoflurane causes dose-dependent coronary vasodilation, the authors concluded that the isoflurane-induced myocardial ischemia resulted from coronary steal (Reiz et al, 1983). In a number of experimental models of multiple stenoses or chronic coronary occlusion with development of collateral circulation, there is redistribution of blood flow from endocardium to epicardium and from compromised to normal myocardium (Priebe, 1988; Buffington et al, 1987). This redistribution is associated with regional dysfunction and ST-segment changes suggestive of ischemia.

Whether "steal" is specific to isoflurane has been debated, as other anesthetic agents such as desflurane and sevoflurane also cause coronary vasodilation. With desflurane, a steal phenomenon has been observed and has been attributed to the overall effect of this agent on the circulation as redistribution of coronary blood flow could be partly reversed by returning heart rate and blood pressure to control levels (Hartman et al, 1991). Thus, the effect of desflurane relates significantly to hypotension and tachycardia. Sevoflurane causes less vasodilation than isoflurane and does not appear to cause coronary flow redistribution and steal. By contrast with isoflurane and desflurane, sevoflurane does not increase heart rate in patients and volunteers (Ebert et al, 1995). This may minimize the risk of myocardial ischemia.

The very wide use of *isoflurane* does not appear to be associated with an inordinate incidence of myocardial ischemia or coronary events in clinical practice. Some studies have shown a slight increase in the incidence of myocardial ischemia, yet other studies have shown adverse cardiovascular events to be essentially the same irrespective of the anesthetic agent used (Tuman et al, 1989). This apparent absence of excess adverse cardiovascular events may have several explanations. Firstly, anesthetists titrate the depth of anesthesia as a function of the intensity of the surgical stimulus; it is unlikely that they will allow severe hypotension in patients with known coronary heart disease. Secondly, isoflurane being a vasodilator, a modest amount of afterload reduction may benefit the compromised myocardium. Thirdly, a steal phenomenon implies the presence of collateral vessels. The ideal condition of coronary steal to develop is the presence of an occlusion, a stenosis of a neighboring vessel, and the presence of demonstrable collateral vessels, a situation termed "steal prone" anatomy. This occurs in approximately 25% of patients with coronary heart disease (Buffington et al, 1988). Finally, there is an almost universal confounding factor. When patients recover from anesthesia, they will develop hypercapnia, at least temporarily, unless they are artificially ventilated. Hypercapnia causes coronary vasodilation (Foëx and Ryder, 1979) and, therefore, is a potential steal-inducing agency. This may be another reason why studies have failed to demonstrate a clear increase in risk when isoflurane was compared with opioids.

Studies of cardiac outcome have failed to demonstrate isoflurane-induced adverse events (Tuman et al, 1989; Stuehmeier et al, 1992). The reason for this apparent discrepancy is that isoflurane is often used in relatively low concentrations in association with an opioid. Often the concentration of isoflurane is increased to treat hypertension. When isoflurane is used to this end, it is very unlikely to cause ischemia. By contrast, all the experimental studies have shown that the steal phenomenon occurs with isoflurane in relatively high concentrations in association with significant hypotension. Therefore, when isoflurane is administered to patients with coronary artery disease, its concentration should be low enough to avoid hypotension.

As inhalational anesthetics improve recovery from stunning (next section), the adverse effects of coronary steal may be minimized. This may explain why anesthesia-induced coronary steal is not a major clinical problem.

Recovery from Ischemia and Myocardial Stunning

A number of recent studies have addressed the question of the effects of inhalational anesthetics on the stunned myocardium, ie myocardium that has been temporarily ischemic, has recovered its coronary blood flow but remains functionally impaired. A number of mechanisms have been postulated to explain myocardial stunning. These include calcium overload and free radicals. Several studies have contrasted the incomplete and slower recovery from ischemia in conscious animals and in those anesthetized with opioids, and the faster and more complete recovery in animals anesthetized with inhalational anesthetics such as halothane, enflurane and isoflurane (Freedman et al, 1985; Warltier et al, 1988). As inhalational anesthetics alter calcium fluxes in cardiac cells, it is tempting to conclude that they may facilitate functional recovery of the stunned myocardium. This is in keeping with many observations of the beneficial effects of calcium channel antagonists. Pretreatment with calcium channel antagonists such as verapamil and diltiazem allow a rapid and complete recovery of contractile function after a 15 minute episode of coronary occlusion (Pryzklenk and Kloner, 1988; Taylor et al, 1990). Nifedipine also improves recovery of the stunned myocardium (Pryzklenk et al, 1989). Benefits are also observed when the calcium channel blocker is given after the ischemic insult, either at the time of reperfusion or 30 minutes later. As administration of calcium channel antagonists after the ischemic insult cannot minimize the metabolic effects of ischemia, it is likely that recovery is improved because of an increase in coronary blood flow, a reduction of afterload, or a direct effect on the stunned myocyte.

Whether other properties of halogenated anesthetics play a role in this protective effect is unknown. K_{ATP} channel openers are known to improve the functional recovery from ischemia. As isoflurane activates the K_{ATP} channel in vascular smooth muscle (Cason et al, 1994), it may be that such an effect also occurs in the myocardium. This property of isoflurane and maybe of other anesthetic agents could explain their effect on the stunned myocardium.

CONCLUSIONS: ANESTHETIC AGENTS AND THE COMPROMISED HEART

The effects of anesthetic agents on the compromised heart differ widely as a function of the prevailing conditions. They protect against the consequences of acute coronary occlusion, reducing infarct size; they cause selectively exaggerated depression of critically compromised myocardial segments; they may induce coronary steal (isoflurane, desflurane, sevoflurane); and finally they facilitate recovery of the stunned myocardium. The complexity of the effects explains, inter alia, why it is so difficult to identify an agent that is superior to all the others.

SUMMARY

1. *Coronary heart disease remains one of the leading causes of death*, and is a major threat to patients presenting for anesthesia and surgery. Over the past decade improvements in drug therapy have been complemented by developments in angioplasty, coronary artery stenting and coronary bypass surgery.

2. *Management principles.* Patients can be stratified into three risk groups, low, intermediate and high, on the basis of clinical evaluation. In the surgical setting, it is well established that medication of coronary heart disease should be maintained throughout the perioperative period. In many patients, however, further investigations may be required, in order to determine their coronary reserve and the quality of their left ventricular function and perfusion. Coronary angiography, angioplasty and stenting or coronary bypass surgery may be necessary before major non-cardiac surgery in patients with severe coronary artery lesions. This is due to the fact that major surgery is similar to a prolonged exercise test lasting up to 2–3 days. Therefore, in all patients treatment should be optimized.

3. *Perioperative ischemia.* Control of heart rate and blood pressure throughout the perioperative period, avoidance of hypoxemia, are essential in order to avoid perioperative myocardial ischemia and myocardial infarction. The question of the administration of cardioprotective drugs during the perioperative period is evolving fast and beta-blockers enjoy regained popularity in this setting.

REFERENCES

ACC/AHA Guidelines for perioperative cardiovascular evaluation for noncardiac surgery. *Circulation* 1996; 93: 1280–1317.

Alderman MH, Cohen H, Roqué R and Madhavan S. Effect of long-acting and short-acting calcium antagonists on cardiovascular outcomes in hypertensive patients. *Lancet* 1997; 349: 594–598.

Bernard J-M, Wouters PF, Doursout MF, et al. Effects of sevoflurane and isoflurane on cardiac and coronary dynamics in chronically instrumented dogs. *Anesthesiology* 1990; 72: 659–662.

Bland JHL and Lowenstein E. Halothane-induced decrease in experimental myocardial ischemia in the non-failing canine heart. *Anesthesiology* 1976; 45: 289–293.

Boesgaard S, Iversen HK, Wroblewski H et al. Altered peripheral vasodilator profile of nitroglycerin during long-term infusion of N-acetylcysteine. *J Am Coll Cardiol* 1994; 23: 163–169.

Borzak S and Gheorghiade M. Early intravenous beta-blocker combined with thrombolytic therapy for acute myocardial infarction: the Thrombolysis in Myocardial Infarction (TIMI-2) Trial. *Prog Cardiovasc Dis* 1993; 36: 261–266.

Braunwald E and Kloner RA. The stunned myocardium: prolonged, postischemic ventricular dysfunction. *Circulation* 1982; 66: 1146–1149.

Brown BG, Bolson EL and Dodge HT. Dynamic mechanisms in human coronary stenosis. *Circulation* 1984; 70: 917–922.

Buffington C. Impaired systolic thickening associated with halothane in the presence of a coronary stenosis is mediated by changes in hemodynamics. *Anesthesiology* 1986; 66: 632–640.

Buffington C, Davis K, Gillispie S and Pettinger M. The prevalence of steal-prone coronary anatomy in patients with coronary artery disease: an analysis of the coronary artery surgery study registry. *Anesthesiology* 1988; 69: 721–727.

Buffington C, Ronson J, Levine A, et al. Isoflurane induces coronary steal in a canine model of chronic coronary occlusion. *Anesthesiology* 1987; 66: 280–292.

Carliner NH, Fisher ML, Plotnick GD, et al. The preoperative electrocardiogram as an indicator of risk in major noncardiac surgery. *Can J Cardiol* 1986; 2: 134–137.

Cason BA, Shubayev I and Hickey RF. Blockade of adenosine triphosphate-sensitive potassium channels eliminates isoflurane-induced coronary artery vasodilation. *Anesthesiology* 1994; 81: 1245–1255.

Coetzee A, Holland D, Foëx P, et al. The effect of hypocapnoea on coronary blood flow and myocardial function in the dog. *Anesth Analg* 1984; 63: 991–997.

Coriat P, Fauchet M, Bousseau D et al. Left ventricular dysfunction after non cardiac surgical procedures in patients with ischemic heart disease. *Acta Anaesthesiol Scand* 1985; 29: 804–810.

Cutfield GR, Francis CM, Foëx P, et al. Isoflurane and large coronary artery hemodynamics: an experimental study. *Br J Anaesth* 1988; 60: 784–790.

Cutler BS, Wheeler HB, Paraskos JA and Cardullo PA. Applicability and interpretation of electrocardiographic stress testing in patients with peripheral vascular disease. *Am J Surg* 1981; 141: 501–506.

Dirksen A and Kjoller E. Cardiac predictors of death after non-cardiac surgery evaluated by intention to treat. *British Medical Journal* 1988; 297: 1011–1013.

Dodds TM, Torkelson AT, Fillinger MP and Tosteson A. Prophylactic beta-blockade reduces perioperative myocardial ischemia in high-risk patients undergoing noncardiac surgery. *Anesth Analg* 1994; 78: S92.

Doyle RL, Foëx P, Ryder WA and Jones LA. Effects of halothane on left ventricular relaxation and early coronary blood flow in the dog. *Anesthesiology* 1989; 70: 660–666.

Ebert TJ, Harkin CP and Muzi M. Cardiovascular responses to sevoflurane: a review. *Anesth Analg* 1995; 81: S11–22

Ebert TJ and Muzi M. Sympathetic hyperactivity during desflurane anesthesia in healthy volunteers. A comparison with isoflurane. *Anesthesiology* 1993; 79: 444–453.

European Coronary Surgery Study Group. Long-term results of prospective randomised study of coronary artery bypass surgery in stable angina pectoris. *Lancet* 1982; 2: 1173–1180.

European Study of Prevention of Infarct with Molsidomine (ESPRIM) Group. The ESPRIM trial: short-term treatment of acute myocardial infarction with molsidomine. *Lancet* 1994; 344: 91–97.

Foëx P and Ryder WA. Effect of CO_2 on the systemic and coronary circulations and on coronary sinus blood gas tensions. *Bull Europ Physiopath Resp* 1979, 15: 625–638.

Foster ED, Davis KB, Carpenter JA, et al. Risk of noncardiac operation in patients with defined coronary disease: The Coronary Artery Surgery Study (CASS) registry experience. *Ann Thorac Surg* 1986; 41: 42–50.

Freedman B, Hamm D, Everson C, et al. Enflurane enhances postischemic functional recovery in the related rat heart. *Anesthesiology* 1985; 62: 29–33.

Fung H-L and Bauer JA. Mechanisms of nitrate tolerance. *Cardiovasc Drugs Ther* 1994; 8: 489–499.

Gao ZP, Downey HF, Fan WL and Mallet RT. Does interstitial adenosine mediate acute hibernation of guinea pig myocardium? *Cardiovasc Res* 1995; 29: 796–804.

Gersh BJ. Noninvasive imaging in acute coronary disease. A clinical perspective. *Circulation* 1991a; 84: 1–140 — 1–147.

Gersh BJ, Rihal CS, Rooke TW and Ballard DJ. Evaluation and management of patients with both peripheral vascular and coronary artery disease. *J Am Coll Cardiol* 1991b; 18: 203–214.

GISSI-3 (Gruppo Italiano per lo Studio della Sopravivenza nel'Infarto Miocardico). GISSI-3: effects of lininopril and transdermal glyceryl trinitrate singly and together on 6-week mortality and ventricular function after acute myocradial infarction. *Lancet* 1994; 343: 1115–1122.

Gobel EJ, Hautvast RW, van Gilst WH, et al. Randomised, double-blind trial of intravenous diltiazem versus glyceryl trinitrate for unstable angina pectoris. *Lancet* 1995; 346: 1653–1657.

Goehner P, Hollenberg M, Leung J, et al. Hemodynamic control suppresses myocardial ischemia during isoflurane or sufentanil anesthesia for CABG. *Anesthesiology* 1988; 69: A32.

Hartman JC, Pagel PS, Kampine JP , et al. Influence of desflurane on distribution of coronary blood flow in a chronically instrumented model of multivessel coronary obstruction. *Anesth Analg* 1991; 72: 289–299.

Hertzer NR. Basic data concerning associated coronary disease in peripheral vascular patients. *Ann Vasc Surg* 1987; 201: 616–620.

Hertzer NR, Beven EG, Young JR, at el. Coronary artery disease in peripheral vascular patients. A classification of 1,000 coronary angiograms and results of surgical management. *Ann Surg* 1984: 199: 223–233.

Hertzer NR, Young JR, Beven EG et al. Late results of coronary bypass in patients with peripheral vascular disease. II. Five-year survival according to sex, hypertension, and diabetes. *Cleve Clin J Med* 1987; 54: 15–23.

Hirano M, Fujigaki T, Shibata O and Sumikawa K. A comparison of coronary hemodynamics during isoflurane and sevoflurane anesthesia in dogs. *Anesth Analg* 1995; 80: 651–656.

Holland Interuniversity Nifedipine/Metoprolol Trial (HINT) Research Group. *Br Heart J* 1986; 56: 400–413.

Huber KC, Evans MA, Bresnahan JF, Gibbons RJ, Holmes DR. Outcome of non-cardiac surgery in patients with severe coronary disease treated with preoperative angioplasty. *Circulation* 1990; 82 (Suppl III): III 511.

ISIS-1 (First International Study of Infarct Survival) Collaborative group. Randomised trial of intravenous atenolol among 16027 cases of suspected acute myocardial infarction: ISIS-1. *Lancet* 1986; 2: 57–65.

ISIS-4 (Fourth International Study of Infarct Survival). A randomised factorial trial assessing early oral captopril, oral mononitrate, and intravenous magnesium sulphate in 58 050 patients with suspected acute myocardial infarction. *Lancet* 1995; 345: 669–685.

Lazor L, Russell JC, DaSilva J and Radford M. Use of the multiple uptake gated acquisition scan for the preoperative assessment of cardiac risk. *Surg Gynecol Obstet* 1988; 167: 234–238.

Leone BJ, Philbin DM, Lehot J-J, et al. Gradual or abrupt nitrous oxide administration in a canine model of critical coronary stenosis induces regional myocardial dysfunction that is worsened by halothane. *Anesth Analg* 1988, 67: 814–822.

Lowenstein E, Foëx P, Francis CM et al. Regional ischemic dysfunction in myocradium supplied by a narrowed coronary artery with increasing concentration in the dog. *Anesthesiology* 1981; 55: 349–359.

Mangano DT, Browner WS, Hollenberg M and Tateo IM. Long-term cardiac prognosis following noncardiac surgery. *JAMA* 1992; 268: 233–239.

Mangano D. Anesthetics, coronary artery disease, and outcome: unresolved controversies. *Anesthesiology* 1989; 70: 175–179.

Mangano DT, Layug EL, Wallace A and Tateo I, for the Multicenter Study of Perioperative Ischemia Research Group. Effect of atenolol on mortality and cardiovascular morbidity after noncardiac surgery. *N Engl J Med* 1996; 335: 1713–1720.

Mangano DT. Effects of acadesine on myocardial infarction, stroke and death following surgery. A meta-analysis of the 5 international randomized trials. The Multicenter Study of Perioperative Ischemia (MSPI) Research Group. *JAMA,* 1997; 277: 325–332.

Mehra A, Ostrzega E, Shotan A et al. Overcoming early nitrate tolerance with escalating doses of isosorbide dinitrate in chronic heart failure. *J Am Coll Cardiol* 1993; 21: 252A.

Menasche P, Jamieson WR, Flameng W and Davies MK. Acadesine: a new drug that may improve myocardial protection in coronary artery bypass grafting. Results of the first international multicenter study. Multinational Acadesine Study Group. *J Thorac Cardiovasc Surg* 1995; 110: 1096–1106.

Messin R, Boxho G, De Smedt J and Buntinx IM. Acute and chronic effect of molsidomine extended release on exercise capacity in patients with stable angina, a double-blind cross-over clinical trial versus placebo. *J Cardiovasc Pharm* 1995; 25: 558–563.

Merin RG, Bernard J, Doursout MF, et al. Comparison of the effects of isoflurane and desflurane on cardiovascular dynamics and regional blood flow in the chronically instrumented dog. *Anesthesiology* 1991; 74: 568–574.

Multicenter Study of Perioperative Ischemia (McSPI) Research Group. Effects of acadesine on the incidence of myocardial infarction and adverse cardiac outcomes after coronary artery bypass graft surgery. *Anesthesiology* 1995; 83: 658–673.

Packer M, O'Connor CM, Ghali JK, et al. Effect of amlodipine on morbidity and mortality in severe chronic heart failure. Prospective Randomized Amlodipine Survival Evaluation (PRAISE) Study Group. *N Engl J Med* 1996; 335: 1107–1114.

Pagel PS, Kampine JP, Schmeling WT and Warltier DC. Effects of nitrous oxide on myocardial contractility as evaluated by the pre-load recruitable stroke work relationship in chronically instrumented dogs. *Anesthesiology* 1990; 73: 1148–1157.

Pagel PS, Kampine JP, Schmeling WT and Warltier DC. Comparison of the systemic and coronary hemodynamic actions of desflurane, isoflurane, halothane, and enflurane in the chronically instrumented dog. *Anesthesiology* 1991; 74: 539–551.

Palda VA and Detsky AS. Perioperative assessment and management of risk from coronary artery disease. *Ann Intern Med* 1997; 127: 313–328.

Parker JD and Parker JO. Drug therapy: nitrate therapy for stable angina pectoris. *New Engl J Med* 1998; 338: 520–531

Pasternack PF, Imparato AM and Bear G. The value of radionuclide angiography as a predictor of perioperative myocardial infarction in patients undergoing abdominal aortic aneurysm resection. *J Vasc Surg* 1984; 1: 320–325.

Pfeffer MA, Braunwald E, Moye LA et al. Effect of captopril on mortality and morbidity in patients with left ventricular dysfunction after myocardial infarction. Results of the Survival and Ventricular Enlargement Trial (SAVE). *N Engl J Med* 1992; 327: 669–677.

Philbin DM, Foëx P, Drummond G, et al. Postsystolic shortening of canine left ventricle supplied by a stenotic coronary artery when nitrous oxide is added in the presence of narcotics. *Anesthesiology* 1985, 62: 166–174.

Priebe H-J. Isoflurane causes more severe regional myocardial dysfunction than halothane in dogs with a critical coronary artery stenosis. *Anesthesiology* 1988; 69: 72–83.

Priebe H-J and Foëx P. Isoflurane causes regional myocardial dysfunction in dogs with critical coronary artery stenosis. *Anesthesiology* 1987; 69: 72–83.

Prys-Roberts C, Foëx P, Biro GP and Roberts JG. Studies of anaesthesia in relation with hypertension. V. Adrenergic beta-receptor blockade. *Br J Anaesth* 1973; 45: 671–680.

Przyklenk K, Ghafari GB, Eitzman DT et al. Nifedipine administered postreperfusion ablates systolic contractile dysfunction of postischemic "stunned" myocardium. *J Am Coll Cardiol* 1989; 13: 1176–1183.

Przyklenk K and Kloner RA. Effect of verapamil on postischemnic "stunned" myocardium: importance of the timing of treatment. *J Am Coll Cardiol* 1998; 11: 614–623.

Puttick RM, Diedericks J, Sear JW, et al. Effect of graded infusion rates of propofol on regional and global left ventricular function in the dog. *Br J Anaesth* 1992; 69: 375–381.

Puttick RM and Terrar DA. Effects of propofol and enflurane on action potentials, membrane currents and contraction of guinea-pig isolated ventricular myocytes. *Br J Pharmacol* 1992; 107: 559–565.

Raby KE, Barry J, Creager MA, et al. Detection and significance of intraoperative and postoperative myocardial ischemia in peripheral vascular surgery. *JAMA* 1992; 268: 222–227.

Raby KE, Goldman L, Creager MA et al. Correlation between preoperative ischemia and major cardiac events after peripheral vascular surgery. *N Engl J Med* 1989; 321: 1296–1300.

Rahimtoola SH. The hibernating myocardium. *Am Heart J* 1989; 117: 211–221.

Rao TLK, Jacobs KH, El-Et AA. Reinfarction following anesthesia in patients with myocardial infarction. *Anesthesiology* 1983; 59: 499–505.

Reiz S, Balfors S, Sorensen MB, et al. Isoflurane, a powerful coronary vasodilator in patients with coronary artery disease. *Anesthesiology* 1983; 59: 91–97.

Richer C, Pratz J, Mulder P, et al. Cardiovascular and biological effects of K^+ channel openers, a class of drugs with vasorelaxant and cardioprotective properties. *Life Sci* 1990; 47: 1693–1705.

Roger VL, Ballard DJ, Hallett JW Jr, et al. Influence of coronary artery disease on morbidity and mortality after abdominal aortic aneurysmectomy: a population-based study, 1971–1987. *J Am Coll Cardiol* 1989; 14: 1245–1252.

Schipke JD. Myocardial hibernation. *Basic Res Cardiol* 1995; 90: 26–28.

Schipke JD, Korbmacher B, Dorszewski A, et al. Hemodynamic and energetic properties of stunned myocardium in rabbit hearts. *Heart* 1996; 75: 55–61.

Shah KB, Kleinman BS, Sami H, et al. Reevaluation of perioperative myocardial infarction in patients with prior myocardial infarction undergoing noncardiac operations. *Anesth Anal* 1990; 71: 231–235.

Slogoff S, Keats AS, Does perioperative myocardial ischemia lead to postoperative myocardial infarction? *Anesthesiology* 1985; 62: 107–114.

Smith JS, Cahalan MK, Benefiel DJ et al. Intraoperative detection of myocardial ischemia in high risk patients: electrocardiography versus two dimensional echocardiography. *Circulation* 1985; 72: 1015–1021.

Steen PA, Tinker JH and Tarhan S. Myocardial reinfarction after anesthesia and surgery. *JAMA* 1978; 239: 2566–2570.

Stone JG, Foëx P, Sear J, et al. Myocardial ischemia in untreated hypertensive patients: effect of a single small oral dose of a beta-blocker. *Anesthesiology* 1986; 68: 495–500.

Stühmeier KD, Mainzer B, Sandmann W and Tarnow J. Isoflurane does not increase the incidence of intraoperative myocardial ischemia compared with halothane during vascular surgery. *Br J Anaesth* 1992; 69: 602–606.

Takayama M, Norris RM, Brown MA et al. Post-systolic shortening of acutely ischemic canine myocardium predicts early and late recovery of function following coronary artery reperfusion. *Circulation* 1988; 78: 994–1007.

Talke P, Li J, Jain U, Leung J, et al. Effects of perioperative dexmedetomidine infusion in patients undergoing vascular surgery. The Study of Perioperative Ischemia Research Group. *Anesthesiology* 1995; 82: 620–633.

Taylor AL, Golino P, Eckels R et al. Differential enhancement of postischemic segmental systolic thickening by diltiazem. *J Am Coll Cardiol* 1990; 15: 737–747.

Terrar DA and Victory JG. Isoflurane depresses membrane currents associated with contraction in myocytes isolated from guinea-pig ventricle. *Anesthesiology* 1988; 69: 742–749.

Thadani U, Maranda CR, Amsterdam E et al. Lack of pharmacologic tolerance and rebound angina pectoris during twice daily therapy with isosorbide-5-mononitrate. *Ann Intern Med* 1994; 120: 353–359.

Thaulow E, Guth BD, Heusch G et al. Characteristics of regional myocardial stunning after exercise in dogs with chronic coronary stenosis. *Am J Physiol* 1989; 257: H113–H119.

Tuman K, MaCarthy R, Spiess B, et al. Does choice of anesthetic agent significantly affect outcome after coronary artery surgery. *Anesthesiology* 1989; 70: 189–198.

Vatner SF. Correlation between acute reductions in myocardial blood flow and function in conscious dog. *Circ Res* 1980; 47: 201–207.

Wallace A, Layung E, Tateo I, et al, McSPI Research Group. Prophylactic atenolol reduces postoperative myocardial ischemia. *Anesthesiology* 1998; 88: 7–17.

Warltier D, Al-Wathiqui M, Kampine J and Schmeling W. Recovery of contractile function of stunned myocardium in chronically instrumented dogs is enhanced by halothane and isoflurane. *Anesthesiology* 1988; 69: 552–565.

Warltier DC, Auchampach JA and Gross GJ. Relationship of severity of myocardial stunning to ATP dependent potassium channel modulation. *J Cardiovasc Surg* 1993; 8 (Suppl): 279–283.

Wells PH and Kaplan JA. Optimal management of patients with ischemic heart disease for non cardiac surgery by complementary anesthesiologist and cardiologist interaction. *Am Heart J;* 1981: 102: 1029–1037.

Weiskopf RB, Moore MA, Eger II EI et al. Rapid increase in desflurane concentration is associated with greater transient cardiovascular stimulation than with rapid increase in isoflurane concentration in humans. *Anesthesiology* 1994; 80: 1035–1045.

Yusuf S, Ramsdale D, Peto R, et al. Early intravenous atenolol treatment in suspected acute myocardial infarction. Preliminary report of a randomised trial. *Lancet* 1980; 2: 273–276.

CHAPTER 10

Heart Failure and its Therapy in the Perioperative Period

Gaisford G. Harrison and Lionel H. Opie

Congestive heart failure (CHF) is the predictor most strongly correlated to post-operative cardiac morbidity (PCM), even stronger than previous myocardial infarction (MI). PCM in turn is the leading cause of death following anesthesia and surgery (Mangano et al, 1990; Clarke and Stanley, 1990). Although peri-operative left ventricular failure occurs very rarely in the presence of a normal heart (Skarvan, 1994), the presence of CHF in patients presenting for anesthesia and surgery has been shown to increase the "relative risk" of post-operative mortality 2–10 fold (Cripps and Gareth-Jones, 1989; ACC/AHA Task Force, 1996). Conversely, this risk is very considerably reduced when CHF has been optimally treated pre-operatively (Goldman et al, 1978). This fact predicates the policy that CHF should always be therapeutically controlled to the optimum extent in the pre-anesthetic period, subject only to the constraints and urgency of the condition for which surgical intervention is required.

This chapter will emphasize the drug treatment of chronic CHF which may be defined *as a state in which contractile function of the heart is impaired despite an adequate venous filling pressure*, with congestion of the lungs and other organs and a compensatory neurohumoral response.

Management of *acute cardiac* failure, in which systolic ventricular function and tissue oxygen delivery are impaired over a short period, allowing for little or no development of the compensatory mechanisms which characterize chronic CHF, is dealt with briefly here and at greater length in chapters 11 and 12.

PATHOPHYSIOLOGY OF CONGESTIVE HEART FAILURE

The most common syndrome of CHF is that which follows *failure of the left ventricle* (LV) as a pump, with a consequent fall in stroke volume (SV). This in turn invokes a series of compensatory mechanisms, many of which become ultimately self defeating and the effects of which feature as the major components of the syndrome as well as the principal targets of therapeutic drug intervention (Packer et al, 1996). It is a better understanding of this sequence and in particular the profoundly important role played in it by the renal-angiotensin system (RAS) and activation of the sympathetic nervous system that has led to considerable change in the therapeutic approach to CHF of recent years (Packer et al, 1996).

The initial event in the decline of LV systolic function is a decrease in intrinsic myocardial contractility. This may follow conditions such as severe systemic hypertension (HT) or valvular pathologies which impose volume or pressure overload on the ventricle. Other predisposing conditions such as ischemic heart disease (IHD) or cardiomyopathies result in direct loss of or damage to cardiac muscle. LV function may also be limited by pericardial disease. The consequent reduction in cardiac output (CO) is accompanied by an increase in LV filling pressure or preload and concomitant ventricular dilatation. The increased preload invokes a compensatory increase in the myocardial force of contraction through the Frank-Starling mechanism, but at the expense, in time, of progressive pulmonary congestion and consequent dyspnea. Should this process later progress to a stage when left atrial (LA) or pulmonary capillary wedge pressure (PCWP) exceeds the optimum range of the Frank-Starling curve (15–20 mm Hg), ventricular contractility falls sharply and pulmonary edema will ensue.

The decline in systolic function of the LV activates a gamut of neuroendocrine mechanisms which include sympathetic adrenergic response, stimulation of renin release, angiotensin and aldosterone production (Fig 10-1), secretion of arginine vasopressin and the release from the heart of atrial and brain natriuretic peptide (ANP and BNP). Taken together, these changes, with the exception of ANP and BNP, cause fluid and Na^+ retention, increasing blood volume together with an increase in systemic vascular resistance (SVR). All these effects combine together to increase both pre- and afterload. Increases in the latter engender the vicious cycle:

reduced SV → increased SVR → increased resistance to ejection → further reduction in SV

The fall in the SV is accompanied by early sympathetically-induced sinus tachycardia. This helps maintain the CO at rest but not during exercise, a circumstance which causes dyspnea on exertion, the most reliable symptom of cardiac failure. Systolic wall stress — a function of ventricular pressure, geometry and myocardial mass — becomes increased (in terms of the Laplace Law). According to Laplace:

$$\text{Wall stress} = \frac{\text{Pressure} \times \text{radius}}{2 \times \text{wall thickness}}$$

following the increase in ventricular dimensions secondary to LV dilation and remodeling. In response to the prolonged volume and pressure overload and contributing to a

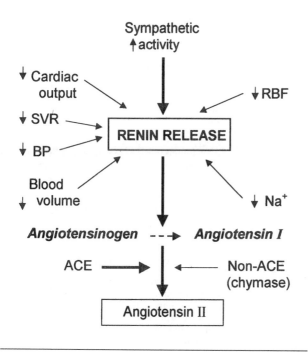

Fig 10-1. Renin release and angiotensin production. *Renin is released by low levels of blood pressure (BP), or a decreased blood volume, or by increased sympathetic beta-adrenergic activity, in response to a decreased systemic vascular resistance (SVR). RBF = renal blood flow; ACE = angiotensin converting enzyme; Non-ACE = conversion by pathways other than ACE, e.g. chymase, cathepsin G. In the human heart, non-ACE paths may account for only 20% of the conversion (Zisman, 1995). (Diagram copyright © GG Harrison, 1997).*

further decline in systolic function and myocardial distensibility are reactive decrease in myocardial ATPase activity (Mercadier et al, 1987), the down-regulation of myocardial β-adrenoceptors (Hausdorff et al, 1990; Collucci et al, 1989), and increased cardiac fibrosis (Weber et al, 1995).

In terms of drug therapy it is also important to distinguish between *systolic (or ejection) heart failure*, in which the primary deficiency is one of myocardial contraction, and *diastolic (or filling) failure*. In the latter, myocardial relaxation is impaired with a resultant decrease in ventricular compliance, and/or decreased filling time (Skarvan 1994; Brutsaert et al, 1993). Only systolic failure is associated with a reduced ejection fraction. Failure of both types is of relevance in the peri-operative period in which large compartmental fluid shifts are commonplace.

Other syndromes of CHF may present in the *absence of LV failure*. These include the pulmonary congestion that follows mitral stenosis and that secondary to *primary failure of the right ventricle (RV)* which may follow pulmonary hypertension secondary to chronic obstructive airways disease (COAD) or repeated pulmonary thromboembolism. In terms of the functional severity of CHF as it presents, the New York Heart Association (NYHA) clinical classification is widely used (Braunwald, 1992) (Table 10-1).

In contrast to CHF, *acute cardiac failure* is characterized by acute impairment of myocardial contractility that is not

Table 10-1. Classification of heart failure (HF) by severity of symptoms

NYHA class	Patient description
I	*Mild Heart Failure.* Patients with cardiac disease but ordinary physical activity does not cause undue fatigue, palpitation, dyspnea, or anginal pain.
II	*Moderate Heart Failure.* Patients with cardiac disease resulting in slight limitation of physical activity. They are comfortable at rest. Ordinary physical activity results in fatigue, palpitation, dyspnea, or anginal pain.
III	*Severe Heart Failure.* Patients with cardiac disease resulting in marked limitation of physical activity. They are comfortable at rest. Less than ordinary physical activity causes fatigue, palpitation, dyspnea, or anginal pain
IV	*Most Severe Heart Failure.* Patient with cardiac disease resulting in inability to carry on any physical activity without discomfort. Symptoms of cardiac insufficiency or of the anginal syndrome may be present even at rest. If any physical activity is undertaken, discomfort increases.

From American Heart Association: New York Heart Association (NYHA) functional classification (Braunwald, 1992).

offset by LV dilation, remodeling and hypertrophy nor the other responses to the neurohumoral compensatory mechanisms that accompany CHF (Weber et al, 1987). Although such failure is very uncommon in the immediate perioperative phase in patients with hearts hitherto normal, patients previously in stable, treated and controlled CHF may develop exacerbation of their failure. The result is clinical instability for reasons such as ill-judged withdrawal of medication, infection, anemia, hemorrhage or fluid loss followed by under or over transfusion or replacement, electrolyte imbalance or hypoxemia. In either event, in addition to treating the cause, the clinical management must focus primarily on the improvement of myocardial contractility and a reduction in afterload, in order to reduce LV filling pressure and attenuate pulmonary venous and capillary pressures.

PRINCIPLES OF DRUG TREATMENT OF CHF

While the close functional interrelationship between the various pathophysiological mechanisms of CHF results in an overlap in the benefits derived from each of the classes of drugs applied to its treatment, these are most conveniently considered in relation to the particular treatment objectives they primarily achieve. Classed in this manner, they will be presented as follows:—

(1) Natriuresis and reduction of preload by diuretics.

(2) Inhibition of the neurohumoral response:—

    (i)   Inhibition of the renin-angiotensin system by

Angiotensin Converting Enzyme (ACE) inhibitors
or by Angiotensin II receptor (AT 1) antagonists.

(ii)   Modification of the sympathetic response with β
or mixed β and α-receptor blockers.

(3)   Reduction of pre- and afterload by vasodilators such as
nitrates and hydralazine.

(4)   Enhancement of myocardial contractility with digoxin,
sympathomimetic amines and phosphodiesterase (PDE)
III inhibitors. The latter also vasodilate (inodilators).

To these must be added prophylaxis for the possible
postoperative sequelae — venous thrombo-embolism and
bacterial endocarditis — for which CHF is a high risk factor.
These are not covered in this text.

Commonly drugs from two, three or sometimes even
all of the above groups are used in combination, the complexity of treatment depending on the severity of symptoms
which, in turn, reflect the severity of the circulatory failure.
Before, or integrated with, the commencement of such treatment the precise cause of the cardiac failure must be investigated and specific treatment — medical or surgical —
applied or planned.

Natriuresis and Reduction in Preload
by Diuretics

Diuretics feature as the standard first line therapy in the
treatment of CHF. Reducing the preload by limiting Na^+
and water retention, diuretics beneficially influence pulmonary and peripheral congestion with a high benefit-to-

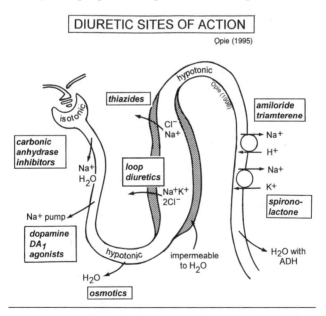

Fig. 10-2. The six sites of action of diuretic agents. *ADH = Anti-
diuretic hormone. A common maximal combination, using the principle of
sequential nephron blockade, is a loop diuretic plus a thiazide plus a K^+-
sparing agent. (Fig. copyright © LH Opie, 1998)*

risk ratio during acute use. For clinical use, diuretics may be classed into three broad groups — thiazide derivatives, loop diuretics and K^+ sparing diuretics — each of which acts at a sequentially different site in the nephron. To act, all but the K^+ sparers must be transported to the luminal aspect of the tubule. This mode of action allows improved diuresis to be achieved by sequential nephron blockade through combined use of drugs from different groups (Fig 10-2).

Thiazide derivatives

The thiazide diuretics are the standard first line therapy for CHF when edema is modest. In more severe cases their use may be safely combined with that of the loop diuretics (Opie et al, 1995). The thiazides act at a proximal site in the distal renal tubules, a site of action just distal to that of the loop diuretics. Here they inhibit the resorption of both Na^+ and Cl^-. Thiazides may also increase the active excretion of K^+ and Mg^{++}, at the same time diminishing that of Ca^{++}. These agents are rapidly absorbed from the gastrointestinal tract producing a diuresis within 1–2 hours of administration. Only oral formulations of these drugs are available.

In the case of the group prototype, *hydrochlorthiazide*, the diuresis lasts for 6–12 hours, a duration of action that is longer than that of the loop diuretics. In that the maximal response to this group of drugs is achieved at low dosage, they are characterized as "low ceiling" diuretics (See Loop Diuretics). A drawback to the use of these drugs in patients suffering the more severe grades of CHF is their decreased effectiveness in the face of renal failure (serum creatinine >2.0 mg/dl or 180 μmol/l, glomerular filtration rate <15–20 ml/min), in contrast to the more effective action of the loop diuretics in similar circumstances. Currently used thiazide diuretics and the thiazide-like agents, together with their dosage and duration of action are listed in Table 10–2. Though the choice of agent seems to be of little moment in

Table 10-2: Low ceiling diuretics for congestive heart failure therapy

Diuretic (generic)	Oral dose, once daily	Duration of diuresis (hours)
Thiazides		
Hydrochlorthiazide	25–100 mg	6–12
	Up to 200 mg	
Hydroflumethazide	25–200 mg	2–24
Bendrofluazide	10 mg	6–12
Benzthiazide	50–200 mg	2–18
Chlorothiazide	250–1000 mg	6–12
Cyclothiazide	1–2 mg	6–24
Trichlormethazide	1–4 mg	24 (approx.)
Cyclopenthiazide	0.125–0.25 mg	6–12
Other		
Chlorthalidone	12.5–50 mg	48–72
Metolazone	5–20 mg	18–25
Indapamide	2.5–5 mg	16–36
Xipamide	20–40 mg	6–12

The onset of diuresis is usually within 1–2 hours.

the treatment of hypertension, in the management of CHF use of the shorter acting diuretics is more appropriate for the greater inherent flexibility this allows. Based largely on a similar pattern of induced electrolyte loss, the *side effects* and *drug interactions* of the thiazide diuretics of clinical anesthetic relevance mirror those of the loop diuretics.

Loop diuretics

Loop diuretics, exemplified by furosemide and its congeners *bumetanide, torsemide,* and *ethacrynic acid,* act on the ascending limb of the loop of Henle inhibiting the $Na^+/K^+/2Cl^-$ cotransporter mechanism. This leads to intraluminal loss of Na^+ and K^+ with a consequent decrease in water resorption and the possible side effects of hyponatremia, hypokalemia and hypochloremia. Na^+/H^+ exchange in the distal tubule, in response to the increased intraluminal Na^+ concentration, adds alkalosis as a further side effect. Increasing doses exert an increasing and prompt diuretic effect before a "ceiling" is reached, so that this group is characterized as "high ceiling" diuretics. In the case of *furosemide* itself, venodilation contributes further to preload reduction. These drugs, which are effective following both oral and intravenous administration, are the diuretics of choice in the management of severe CHF and pulmonary edema, as they induce a more acute Na^+ loss than others and are effective even in renal failure. Furosemide induced venodilation is an added advantage. Dosage and kinetics of the loop diuretics are set out in Table 10–3.

Table 10-3. High ceiling loop diuretics for congestive heart failure therapy

Drug (generic)	Dose	Diuresis		
		Onset (intra-venous)	peak	duration
Furose-mide (Lasix)	20–80 mg × 3 up to 250–300 mg (intrave-nously or oral)	10–20 min	90 min	4–5 hrs
Bumeta-nide (Bumex, Burinex)	0.5–2.0 mg once or twice daily, can re-peat at 4–5 hour intervals to maximum of 10 mg daily	within 10 min	75–95 min	4–5 hrs
Torsemide (Demadex, Torem)	10–20 mg once daily (IV or oral), increasing as needed; usual maxi-mum 40 mg daily, occasion-ally more	10 min	60 min	6–8 hrs
Ethacrynic acid (Ecedrin)	50 mg IV 25–200 mg orally	10–20 min	90 min	4–5 hrs

Side effects and interactions of thiazide and loop diuretics

Electrolyte depletion. In patients on chronic medication with these diuretics presenting for anesthesia and surgery, electrolyte loss features as the side effect of greatest clinical import. Depletion of K^+ and Mg^{++} in particular are potentially arrhythmogenic in the clinical anesthetic environment, in addition to the arrhythmogenic properties of the anesthetic agents themselves e.g. halothane (Forrest et al, 1990). Furthermore, a labile pH status secondary to over- and/or underventilation may bring changes in plasma K^+ levels. Circumstances inherent in the surgical procedures involved, such as blood and fluid loss and their replacement together with intercompartmental shifts, also contribute to this labile electrolyte environment. These factors have an added cogency in patients at high risk for arrhythmias e.g. sufferers from ischemic heart disease and in the presence of cotherapy with digoxin or QT interval lengthening drugs. The merits/demerits of the discontinuance of digoxin medication pre-operatively in these circumstances are discussed in the section on digoxin (to follow). In patients who have been subjected to severe diuresis before anesthesia and surgery, hypovolemia (paradoxically) may also be anticipated. Monitored by measurement of central venous pressure, this defect should be corrected, when possible, before induction of anesthesia.

Dysfunction of the neuromuscular junction. This also may follow electrolyte depletion and lead to a prolongation of the action of nondepolarizing muscle relaxants. Such effects are usually associated only with high dosage of these diuretics. Chronic medication at lower dosage, in particular with a shorter acting loop diuretic, is far less prone to cause hypokalemia, especially if there has been restriction of dietary Na^+ intake and a high K^+ diet. Addition of K^+ and Mg^{++} supplements — formerly much practiced — has not been shown to be reliably effective (Opie et al, 1995; Dorup et al, 1988; Bashir et al, 1993). Better results in regard to K^+ and Mg^{++} homeostasis are achieved by the combined use of K^+ sparing diuretics or ACE inhibitors with a lower diuretic dosage. It must be noted that ACE inhibitors and K^+ sparing diuretics should not be administered simultaneously (except when hypokalemia is documented) because of the risk of hyperkalemia.

Diabetogenesis. Hypokalemia is possibly responsible secondarily for another, though rarer, side effect of these diuretics, namely hyperglycemia with insulin resistance and raised plasma insulin levels (Santoro et al, 1992). These effects occur predominantly in patients familiarly disposed to diabetes mellitus and treated by high diuretic doses. However the precipitation of frank diabetes is rare. When severe, this effect may lead to a nonketotic hyperosmolar state.

Other side effects. Other side effects of less immediate anesthetic relevance include skin rash, hyperuricemia, atherogenic changes in blood lipid profile and, in the case of furosemide, a high-dose related ototoxicity (Opie et al, 1995). Rarely the thiazide derivatives may invoke sulfonamide immune type reactions such as intrahepatic jaundice, pancreatitis and blood dyscrasias.

Drug interactions. Development of hypokalemia may be hastened by steroid or ACTH therapy. Loss of diuretic response may follow administration of indomethacin and other NSAIDs as well as probenecid — though the mechanisms involved differ. *Captopril*, of all the ACE inhibitors, decreases renal excretion of furosemide thereby reducing the diuretic potency of the latter (McLay et al, 1993, Toussaint et al, 1989).

K^+ sparing or retaining diuretics

Three drugs which act on sequential sites in the distal tubule — *amiloride, triamterene* and *spironolactone* — comprise this group of diuretics. Acting on proximal sites in the distal tubules, the first two inhibit the Na^+/H^+ exchange mechanism, while *spironolactone* inhibits aldosterone mediated Na^+/K^+ exchange at a sequential site. All, particularly *amiloride* and *triamterene*, are relatively weak diuretics but achieve their action by natriuresis without major loss of K^+ or of Mg^{++} (Devane and Ryan, 1981; 1983). This property renders them very suitable for use in combination with the thiazide and loop diuretics. Hyperkalemia is a potential hazard with pre-existing renal disease or nephrotoxic agents, diabetes or during cotherapy with ACE inhibitors (antialdosterone effect). Should hyperkalemia occur, it may be controlled by drug withdrawal and, if severe, glucose plus insulin infusions and cation exchange resins may be needed. Dosage and kinetics of this group of diuretics are listed in Table 10-4.

Table 10-4. Potassium and magnesium sparing diuretics

Diuretic drug	Dose	Diuresis	
		Onset	**Duration**
Spironolactone (Aldactone)	Oral 25–200 mg 2–3 × per day; IV 200 mg	2–3 days for maximum effect	3–5 days
Amiloride (Midamor)	Oral 2.5–20 mg Once daily	120 min	6–24 hours
Triamterene (Dytac, Dyrenium)	Oral 25–300 mg Once daily	2–4 hours	8–12 hours

Diuretic combinations

To achieve effective non-hypokalemic diuresis, a number of diuretic combinations have been formulated (Table 10-5).

INHIBITION OF NEUROHUMORAL RESPONSE

The separate, though inter-related components of the neurohumoral response to CHF (Fig 10-1) are manifestations of renin-angiotensin activation and of autonomic sym-

Table 10-5. Proprietary diuretic combinations for congestive heart failure therapy

| Components of combination | Dosage | | Proprietary name |
	Strengths	Oral (tabs/day)	
Hydrochlorthiazide plus Triamterene	25 mg 50 mg	Up to 4	Dyazide
Hydrochlorthiazide plus Triamterene	50 mg 75 mg	1/4–1	Maxide
Hydrochlorthiazide plus Triamterene	25 mg 37.5 mg	1/2–1	Maxide — 25
Hydrochlorthiazide plus Amiloride	50 mg 5 mg	Up to 2	Moduretic
Hydrochlorthiazide plus Spironalactone	25 mg 25 mg	1–4	Aldactazide
Furosemide plus Amiloride	40 mg 25 mg	1–2	Frumil (Not in USA)
Cyclopenthiazide plus Potassium Chloride	0.25 mg 600 mg	1/2–1	Navridex-K (Not in USA)

pathetic stimulation. Basic and clinical research in both these areas, of recent years, has advanced pharmacological control of these systems with great therapeutic benefit in the management of CHF. To our ability to reduce the effects of renin-angiotensin activation by inhibition of angiotensin-converting-enzyme (ACE) has now been added that of angiotensin II receptor blockade. With regard to the sympathetic component, trials have now suggested extraordinary benefit to follow addition of bisoprolol (β-blocker) or carvedilol (mixed β and α-blocker) to conventional CHF therapy.

INHIBITION OF THE RENIN-ANGIOTENSIN SYSTEM (RAS)

ACE inhibition

ACE inhibition therapy of CHF — alone or in combination with diuretics, digoxin or conventional vasodilator agents — is highly effective and well established. The pharmacodynamic effects of ACE inhibitors include a substantial reduction in systemic and pulmonary vascular resistances with consequent reduction (of the order of 40%) in LV and RV filling pressures. Reduction in heart size follows, accompanied by an increase in ventricular stroke volume and cardiac output. It has been suggested that some of this improvement may be in response to direct cardiac actions of the ACE inhibitors (Unger and Gohlke, 1990). These beneficial changes in hemodynamics which are not associated with reflex tachycardia, are maintained in the long term during prolonged treatment (Kellow, 1994). Exercise capacity can be improved by as much as 20% with amelioration of NYHA class. Several well controlled studies [CONSENSUS, 1987; SOLVD, 1991; V-HeFT II, 1991; SOLVD 2, 1992; SAVE, 1992; AIRE 1993] validate the therapeutic efficacy of ACE inhibitors in the therapy and prevention of CHF. "Hard" end points, such as mortality and hospitalization, are reduced and disease progression is slowed or even prevented. Improvement may vary from a delaying of deterioration from mildly symptomatic LV dysfunction without overt CHF, to reduction of mortality in overt grades of failure. Only in a minority of patients do ACE inhibitors fail to benefit and possibly do harm by way of hypotension. The standard combination therapy for mild to moderate CHF comprises co-treatment with diuretics and ACE inhibitors with the addition of digoxin (triple therapy) being reserved for the severer grades of failure. Patients suffering more severe degrees of failure may benefit from a further reduction in SVR achieved by the addition of a conventional vasodilator drug to the treatment regime (quadruple therapy), both *nitrates* and/or *hydralazine* being used. For pharmacokinetic parameters and dosage schedules for ACE-inhibitors in CHF, see Table 10-6.

With regard to the choice of ACE inhibitor, it seems that there is little advantage for any one agent compared with the others. *Captopril* has the widest range of approved indications and, not being a pro-drug, has a rapid onset of action so that it is often chosen as the test drug. *Enalapril*, the standard pro-drug, has been comprehensively tested for all stages of CHF. Used alone or in combination with diuretics and digoxin, in patients in all grades of CHF, it has been documented as being responsible not only for substantial reductions in mortality from CHF at 1 year but also a 37% preventative reduction in the development of CHF in

Table 10-6. ACE inhibitors for congestive heart failure therapy

ACE inhibitor	Elimination $t_{1/2}$ (hours)	Initial dose	Maintenance dose (daily)
CLASS I* Captopril	4–6	6.25 mg	Up to 50 mg × 3
CLASS II ** Enalapril (prototype)	11	2.5 mg	Up to 10 mg × 2
Benazapril	10–11	2.0 mg	5–20 mg × 1
Perindopril	6–17	2.0 mg	2–8 mg × 1
Quinapril	1.8	5.0 mg	5–20 mg × 2
Ramipril	13–17	1.25 mg	2.5–5.0 mg × 2
Trandolapril[a]	10	1 mg	up to 4 mg × 1
CLASS III*** Lisinopril	>7	2.5 mg	5–20 × 1

*   Class I = Drug and metabolites active
**   Class II = Prodrug - Diacid metabolite, only, active
***   Class III = Water soluble, not metabolized, renal excretion in unchanged form
$t_{1/2}$ = Plasma half life; a = post-AMI, LV ejection fraction equal to or below 35%, see Kober al al, *New Engl J Med* 1995; 333: 1670)

patients suffering from asymptomatic LV dysfunction [CONSENSUS 1987; SOLVD, 1991; V-HeFT II, 1991; SOLVD 2, 1992]. Differences from *captopril* that *enalapril* manifests are:-1) being a pro-drug with the requirement of hepatic hydrolysis to its active form, enalaprilat, it has a slower onset of action, 2) a longer half life, and 3) a lower risk of immune based side effects owing to the absence of the SH-group in its structure. *Ramipril*, another pro-drug, has been shown to be associated with significant reduction (27%) in mortality of early post-infarct patients with CHF clinically diagnosed (AIRE, 1993).

Side effects of ACE inhibitors. Hypotension is the most important side effect of ACE inhibition especially from the clinical anesthetic viewpoint. It is a major consideration also when ACE inhibition is to be introduced into the therapeutic regime for CHF patients who have been vigorously diuresed. Patients with serum Na^+ levels less than 130 mM/L should be considered at high risk for this complication. Any such hypotension may precipitate or aggravate renal failure secondary to poor renal perfusion. This is particularly dangerous in patients who suffer from renal artery stenosis.

ACE inhibition reduces urinary K^+ loss secondary to its aldosterone blocking activity and may consequently precipitate hyperkalemia when administered to patients already on treatment with K^+ sparing diuretics. The latter should be discontinued 24–48 hours before ACE inhibitor treatment is initiated. In order to obviate the above risks a test dose followed by BP monitoring for 2 hours is advisable. In the case of *captopril*, 6.25 mg should be administered before dosage is increased to 12.5 mg three times a day, and then to 50 mg three times daily, if tolerated.

While not dangerous, a dry irritating cough features as the most common and troublesome side effect of ACE medication. This and the angioedema noted below, are thought to be manifestations of the proinflammatory action of bradykinin (Hall, 1993; Ferner, 1994), the local production of which is increased by ACE inhibitors. Treatment for this may be difficult, though inhalation of *sodium cromoglycate* may help. A most uncommon (1:1,000) but highly dangerous side effect of ACE inhibitor administration is angioedema. This demands the prompt administration of epinephrine intravenously or subcutaneously.

All ACE inhibitors are embryopathic and so absolutely contraindicated during pregnancy. The 2nd and 3rd trimesters constitute the period of highest risk (Opie, 1996).

ACE inhibitor interaction with clinical anesthesia. In the well hydrated, Na^+ replete patient neither the renin-angiotensin system nor ACE are directly affected by anesthesia. However, these systems are intimately involved in the maintenance of circulatory homeostasis in response to fluid and electrolyte changes induced by surgery and the conditions for which it is required. It is not surprising therefore that several workers have reported the occurrence of hypotension and bradycardia during the anesthesia of patients on ACE inhibitors. Although these conditions may be easily controlled by the infusion of crystalloids, moderate doses of adrenergic agonists and atropine (Mets, 1998; Kellow, 1994), the blunting of baroreceptor homeostatic responses can make difficult the anesthetic management of operations which involve significant blood loss. Thus it may be wise to discontinue ACE inhibitors before such operations (Mirenda and Grissom, 1991), contrary to current anesthetic philosophy of continuing with established medication during the perioperative period. Cardiac performance and electrolyte balance are not adversely affected by the short term withdrawal of ACE inhibition used for CHF therapy, and its discontinuance does not result in rebound hypertension such as follows clonidine withdrawal (Mets, 1998). On the other hand ACE inhibitor medication has been found to be renoprotective during the aortic cross clamping phase of aortic resection continued (Joob et al, 1986; Kataja et al, 1989). Also unclear is the advisability or otherwise of withdrawal of ACE inhibitor medication before spinal or epidural anesthesia when indicated in patients with CHF.

Angiotensin II receptor antagonists

Losartan is the first of a new class of orally active specific AT_1 selective angiotensin II receptor antagonists. By blocking angiotensin II at receptor level it eliminates also the effects of angiotensin produced via the non-ACE inhibitor pathway (Fig 10-1) although these may not be so important in the human heart (Zisman et al, 1995). Favorable results from early short term clinical trials suggest that losartan and other AT_1 blockers will be useful for all the current indications for ACE inhibitors, including CHF (Gottlieb et al, 1993). However, apart from a relatively small positive trial in heart failure in the elderly (Pitt et al, 1997), long term outcome studies are largely unavailable at present. Lacking any effect on bradykinin production, it does not have the ACE inhibitor side effects of cough or angioedema and is better tolerated. Likewise the lack of formation of bradykinin may mean that the proposed benefits of this peptide such as vasodilation, increased formation of nitric oxide, and enhanced fibrinolysis, may be missing. As yet no specific study of its interactions with clinical anesthesia has been published. However, it is unlikely that these and their management will differ from those of ACE inhibitors as already discussed.

Modification of sympathetic response

The benefit of *ACE inhibitors* in CHF can be explained not only by the inhibition of the renin-angiotensin system, but also by their anti-adrenergic effects as shown by a 30% fall in muscle sympathetic nerve traffic (Grassi et al, 1997).

Although α-*adrenoceptor antagonists* have a confirmed place in the treatment of hypertension and reduction in afterload is a logical therapeutic maneuver in the management of CHF, no studies show this class of agent to be of any material benefit in the chronic treatment of CHF (V-HeFT II, 1991).

In contrast, β-*adrenoceptor blockers* have an increasing role in CHF therapy. In congestive cardiomyopathy, low dose β-blockade with *metoprolol*, cautiously added to conventional therapy, may improve the symptoms and prevent clinical deterioration of patients in whom there is persistent tachycardia. Other β-blockers that have been effectively used are the vasodilatory agents *carvedilol* and *bucindolol* (Bristow, 1997). In general, there is a consistent trend for the non-selective β-blockers to prolong survival more than the selective agents, such as metoprolol and bisoprolol (Packer 1996a). Nonetheless, a clear mortality reduction with *bisoprolol* resulted in the recent CIBIS 2 trial being stopped prematurely.

Carvedilol. This drug is now registered for use in the USA, to reduce progression of disease in class II and III patients otherwise fully treated for heart failure. In a multi-center trial (Packer et al, 1996b) in which carvedilol was cautiously added in escalating dosage to standard triple therapy by a diuretic, an ACE inhibitor and digitalis yielded a 65% decrease in mortality and 27% reduction in hospitalizations during a mean follow-up period of 7 months. Certain aspects of this trial, however, are subject to criticism (Pfeffer and Stevenson, 1996), so that further trials are still needed to validate mortality reduction by carvedilol in particular.

Pre-operative β-blockade. In relation to anesthesia and surgery, recent studies suggest that pre-operative administration of β-blockers, e.g. to high risk IHD patients, reduces the incidence of peri-operative myocardial ischemia and may reduce the risk of post-operative myocardial infarction and possibly death. Among the β-blockers used are *metoprolol* (ACC/AHA Task Force Report, 1996), and *atenolol* (Mangano et al, 1996). Accordingly, patients presenting with IHD and recent angina, symptomatic arrhythmias and/or hypertension (especially untreated hypertension) should be considered for β-blocker premedication.

REDUCTION IN PRE- AND AFTERLOAD BY VASODILATORS

The nitrate vasodilators and phosphodiesterase inhibitors are used chiefly in the management of acute heart failure, acting variably by reducing the preload and the afterload so that the position of the failing heart on the Frank-Starling curve is improved, and the cardiac output rises (Fig 10-3).

Nitrates

While the nitrates are primarily used for their coronary vasodilatory and consequently antianginal properties, their venodilatory effects are also of great use in reducing the preload of the failing heart (Thadani and Opie, 1995; Williams and Lake, 1994) (Fig 6-1, page 142). Acting primarily on the venous capacitance vessels, nitrates have a particular value in the treatment of severe CHF accompanied by markedly raised PCWP, pulmonary congestion and pulmonary edema. In patients with pulmonary congestion,

HEMODYNAMICS OF VASODILATORS IN CHF

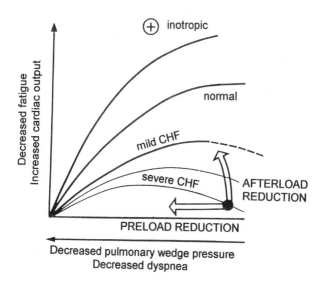

Fig 10-3. Theoretical Frank-Starling curves in CHF. *Note effects of preload reduction on dyspnea and pulmonary wedge pressure, and afterload reduction on cardiac output and muscle fatigue. Nitrates reduce the preload, hydralazine the afterload, and angiotensin-converting enzyme inhibitors and sodium nitroprusside reduce both preload and afterload. Inotropic agents, such as digoxin, put the heart onto a high Frank-Starling curve.*

nitrates administered at night can improve sleep decisively. Both short and long acting nitrates are effective (Table 10-7). In severe CHF nitrates may be used as the sole preload reducing agent or in combination with ACE inhibition or hydralazine for afterload reduction.

In *acute pulmonary edema*, nitroglycerin administered intravenously is most effective, this method of administration allowing for rapid upward or downward adjustment of dosage. This drug is also rapidly effective when administered sublingually. An infusion of nitroglycerin (Fig 11-5, page 333) or repeated doses of 0.8–2.4 mg every 5–10 minutes can relieve coarse crackles and dyspnea within 15–20 minutes, inducing a fall in LV filling pressure together with a rise in cardiac output. In patients suffering severe pulmonary edema with arterial oxygen saturation less than 90%, the addition of low dose furosemide to nitrate therapy has been shown to control the edema effectively and safely (Cotter et al, 1998). However, in mild CHF already being satisfactorily treated by diuretics and ACE inhibitors, the addition of nitrates to the therapy is of little added benefit (Thandani and Opie, 1995). At higher doses nitrates cause significant arteriolar vasodilation, so reducing afterload as well as preload (Gerson et al, 1982). Reduction in left ventricular filling pressure follows, with a reduction in wall stress and MVO_2 together with an improvement in myocardial oxygen supply/demand ratio. The extent to which pre- and afterload reduction separately affect cardiac perfor-

Table 10-7 Nitrate compounds for congestive heart failure therapy

Compound	Route	Dosage	Onset time	Action duration	Comments
Nitroglycerin, Glyceryl Trinitrate (licensed in USA for control of CHF in AMI)	Intravenous	5–200µg/min	1 min	While infused	Titrate against monitored BP, may need increasing dose
	Sublingual	0.3–0.6 mg, can repeat up to 5 times after 5 min	2 min	$t\frac{1}{2}$ = 7 min	Use for acute pulmonary edema
	Transdermal patch	0.2–0.8 mg over 12 hrs on, then 12 hrs off	1–2 hrs	8–12 hrs	Results in CHF variable
Isosorbide dinitrate (licensed for LV failure in UK, not USA)	Intravenous (not in USA)	1.25–5.0 mg/hr	1 min	Elimination $t\frac{1}{2}$ = 18–139 min	Care with PVC tubing, may need increasing dose
	Sublingual	2.5–10 mg	3–4 min	1 hr or more	Use for acute pulmonary edema
	Chewable	5–10 mg	$2\frac{1}{2}$–3 min	2–2½ hr	As above
Isosorbide mononitrate (licensed as adjunct in CHF in UK, not USA)	Oral	20–30 mg, 2–3 times daily; up to 120 mg in divided doses	30–60 min	5 hrs	Interval dosing can lessen nitrate tolerance

Note: tolerance can develop with all longer acting preparations; escalating doses or concurrent hydralazine or interval therapy may be required.

mance depends ultimately on pre-existing LV function (Haber et al, 1993).

Intra-operative nitroglycerin. Apart from its relevance to CHF therapy, the coronary vasodilatory effects of nitroglycerin may also find a particular application in rendering anesthesia and surgery safer for patients suffering IHD. The ability of nitroglycerin to reverse myocardial ischemia intra-operatively has long been of use in anesthetic techniques for cardiac surgery (Tinker and Roberts, 1989). This and recent studies now prompt the recommendation that the use of nitroglycerin infusion (1.0 mg/min) be considered for a similar purpose in high risk IHD patients undergoing non-cardiac surgery (ACC/AHA Task Force Report, 1996). However, it must be recognized that consequent severe hypotension, especially in the presence of hypovolemia, may render this therapy self-defeating. The α agonist, phenylepherine, may be of use in controlling this situation.

Nitrate tolerance. Sustained high dosage of nitrate preparations leads, through poorly understood mechanisms, to tolerance and failing of efficacy. The mechanism is not known but may include impaired conversion of the nitrate moiety to the active form, nitric oxide, in the vascular wall. Another proposal is that the abrupt vasodilation leads to renin-angiotensin stimulation. This major drawback can be managed in the perioperative period by escalating dosage schedules (Mehra et al, 1995) or during chronic therapy by the concomitant use of oral hydralazine (Gogia et al, 1995).

Side effects of nitrates. The most serious complication of nitrate therapy is *hypotension* with possible syncope. This requires recumbency and reassessment of dosage as well as consideration of the wisdom of continuance of such therapy. In non-anesthetized patients, headache is the most troublesome complication of nitrate therapy, leading often to lack of patient compliance during chronic therapy. Three other side effects have particular relevance in clinical anesthetic practice. The first of these is *methemoglobinemia* which may follow prolonged high dosage of nitrate preparations (Kaplan et al, 1985). Not only does this condition reduce the oxygen carrying capacity of the blood but also causes a leftward shift in its dissociation curve, so reducing tissue oxygen delivery at appropriate oxygen tensions (Benumof, 1990). In addition it provides a source of error in pulse oximetry causing it to underestimate true SaO_2 values above 85% while overreading at values below this level (Eisenkraft, 1988; Sykes et al, 1991). Methemoglobinemia can be effectively treated with the intravenous administration of *methylene blue* (1–2 mg/Kg over 5 minutes) (Orkin, 1983). Secondly, *heparin resistance* may follow high dose intravenous nitrate therapy (Williams and Lake, 1994). Thirdly, *hypoxemia* that may follow from ventilation/perfusion mismatch secondary to nitrate inhibition of hypoxic pulmonary vasoconstriction (Berthelson et al, 1986). Despite the above side effects, provided they are kept in mind and monitored, discontinuance of oral nitrate therapy before anesthesia is not necessary.

Sodium nitroprusside

Intravenous sodium nitroprusside (SNP) has an arteriolar/venous vasodilation ratio of close to 1.0 in contrast to the 0.53 of nitroglycerin (Miller et al, 1976). It is a direct nitrate donor, that can only be given intravenously. It is particularly useful for increasing left ventricular stroke volume in severe refractory heart failure caused by mitral or aortic incompetence, heart failure after cardiac surgery, acute exacerbation of CHF and that complicating acute myocardial infarction. Though systemic hypotension results from its administration and must be carefully monitored, the considerable increase in stroke volume that follows the reduction in systemic vascular resistance usually leads to a greater hemodynamic benefit despite a moderate degree of hypotension.

Pharmacokinetics and dosage. The hemodynamic response to intravenous nitroprusside, mediated through vascular endothelially generated nitric oxide, is extremely rapid — an effect which stops equally rapidly on its discontinuation. This property allows for flexible clinical control. Non-enzymatic biotransformation of the drug in the erythrocytes (98%) and plasma (2%) results in the formation of the cyanide ion, cyanocobalamine and cyanmethemoglobin. The potentially toxic cyanide ion is subsequently converted to renally excreted thiocyanate through the action of hepatic rhodanase (Harrison and Bates, 1993). The rate limiting factor in this process appears to be the availability of sulfydryl groups, which is increased by the administration of Na^+ thiosulphate thereby enhancing considerably the production of thiocyanate, so reducing blood cyanide levels (Krapez et al, 1981). In general terms, clinically effective doses of the drug do not produce toxic levels of cyanide. However, in the presence of hepatic or renal failure or following prolonged or high dosage, cyanide toxicity can occur (Robin and McCauley, 1992). This may be avoided by monitoring blood lactate, which mirrors the increase in arterial base deficit, and thiocyanate levels (toxic level 100 mg/ml).

Administration of SNP. For intravenous administration sodium nitroprusside (SNP) should be diluted in a 5% dextrose solution to produce a 0.01% solution and must be shielded from light (a brown paper bag over the container is adequate). Infusion is commenced at 10 μg/min. and increased by this amount every ten minutes up to a dosage of 40–75 μg/min. This dose may be exceeded up to a maximum of 300 μg/min. The infusion rate is judged by careful titration against the mean arterial blood pressure which must be continuously monitored to avoid excessive hypotension. Discontinuance should be gradual to avoid the rebound hypertension which follows secondarily to renin-angiotensin stimulation (Zall et al, 1990), unless the patient is also on an ACE inhibitor. SNP is contraindicated — as are all vasodilators — in the presence of obstructive valvular or cardiomyopathic lesions.

Side effects of SNP: Fatigue, nausea and vomiting may arise especially when treatment is prolonged beyond 48 hours. Pulmonary vasodilation may cause hypoxia due to induced ventilation/perfusion mismatch (Berthelsen et al, 1986).

Hydralazine (Apresoline)

The predominant effect of hydralazine is reduction of systemic vascular resistance coupled with an indirect positive inotropic effect on the heart. Cardiac output is increased with little or no decrease in the pulmonary capillary wedge pressure or right atrial pressure. Although less used in current practice, hydralazine remains an option in the treatment of CHF associated with regurgitation (mitral and aortic), increasing forward stroke volume while decreasing regurgitation. Its chronic oral use in heart failure is limited to combination with chronic oral nitrate therapy. An interesting proposal is that the hydralazine may limit the development of nitrate tolerance when both are used in the treatment of chronic heart failure (Gogia et al, 1995). It should be noted, however, this combination is inferior to treatment with ACE inhibitors in decreasing mortality from severe CHF (V-HeFT II Study, 1991). Regarding *pharmacokinetics,* hydralazine binds to and acts on arteriolar walls, with the precise mode of vasodilation not yet understood. Subject to hepatic acetylation and renal excretion, its metabolites may also be pharmacodynamically active. Hydralazine is rapidly absorbed from the gut reaching peak concentration in one to two hours with a metabolic half life of two to eight hours and a hypotensive effect which extends beyond this. Oral dosage of 50–75 mg 6 hourly is usually adequate but this may be increased to 100 mg 4 times per day in treating patients with severe mitral regurgitation.

Phosphodiesterase-III inhibitors

Inhibition of cyclic AMP breakdown augments myocardial contractility, at the same time reducing afterload through vasodilation — an ideal short-term therapy option in the treatment of severe, intractable or acute heart failure. These conditions are induced by a class of phosphodiesterase (PDE) III inhibitors — the inodilators — of which *amrinone* and *milrinone* are the prototypes. Though increased levels of myocyte cyclic AMP may predispose to arrhythmias, the above effects — inotropic vasodilation — are accompanied by relatively little change in heart rate and/or BP (Marcus et al, 1995). *Amrinone* is excreted largely unchanged in the urine and feces, the remainder being metabolized. Treatment reactions with this group of drugs is indicated for short-term management of severe CHF resistant to conventional therapy. It is contraindicated in AMI (arrhythmia risk) and in outflow tract obstruction or severe aortic stenosis. Serious side effects of these drugs — rare during short term intravenous use — include ventricular arrhythmias, hypotension, thrombocytopenia, hepatotoxicity and hypersensitivity. (For dosage and administration see Table 10-9). These agents are considered in more detail in chapters 3 and 12.

Atrial natriuretic factor (Peptide) (ANF)

ANF is secreted by the cardiac atria in response to volume distention and by the ventricles in LV failure. It induces the powerful cyclic GMP mediated vasodilation of renal vasculature with diuresis. Endopeptidase inhibitors which decrease ANF degradation can improve hemodynamics and renal function in CHF. However, this therapy is likely to be of limited benefit as levels of naturally occurring ANF are already high in CHF and downgrading of ANF receptors occurs. Clinical use of ANF has not yet been established.

CHF WITH PREDOMINANT DIASTOLIC DYSFUNCTION

Of patients presenting with heart failure, as many as 40% have diastolic dysfunction with preserved systolic function and a normal, even raised ejection fraction (Gersh and Opie, 1995). This condition may accompany the left ventricular hypertrophy of hypertension or aortic stenosis, especially in the early compensated phase. Not only does digitalis not benefit the patient but is strongly contraindicated (Bolognesi et al, 1992). Hypothetically, cytosolic Ca^{++} overload is to blame. Strangely, there have been no large scale prospective trials to validate the various therapeutic strategies for this condition. In general terms, drugs which produce a reduction in afterload — and so lessen hypertrophy — are beneficial provided hypotension is avoided. One trial (Gonzalez-Fernandez et al, 1992) reports good results from the use of *ACE inhibition.* It can be conjectured that, by reducing cytosolic Ca^{++} levels, *calcium channel antagonists* would be of benefit. Indeed the outcome of one trial with *verapamil* bears this out (Setaro et al, 1990). When there are symptoms of pulmonary congestion *diuretics* are of help but care must be taken to avoid heavy or over diuresis as this will reduce LV filling pressure, which in these circumstances is critical for LV performance. Logic also supports the use of β-adrenoceptor agonists e.g. *dobutamine*, which enhance Ca^{++} uptake by the sarcoplasmic reticulum, thereby accelerating myocardial relaxation (Zeppelini et al, 1993). Conversely, although β-adrenoceptor blockers may impede LV relaxation, those with vasodilatory action e.g. *carvedilol*, theoretically can help. It needs to be restated that when the contraction phase is normal (normal ejection fraction), then there is no place for the use of positive inotropes such as digitalis in the management of diastolic dysfunction.

ENHANCEMENT OF MYOCARDIAL CONTRACTILITY WITH INOTROPES

Digitalis (Digoxin)

Introduced into therapeutics over 200 years ago, digitalis (as digoxin) remains the only widely used inotrope for the chronic medication of CHF. Its many properties, such as the combination of positive inotropy with vagally induced bradycardia — in contrast to the tachycardia induced by other inotropes — together with AV nodal inhibition and a sympatholytic effect, are uniquely useful in the treatment of CHF. Digoxin is the only such inotrope available in oral formulation. Reservation in regard to the long term efficacy of digoxin has been prompted by the failure of a recent trial to demonstrate any long term survival benefit to follow digoxin therapy of CHF. At the same time, no detrimental effect on survival was validated either (Digitalis Investigation Group, 1997).

A major drawback to use of digoxin is a narrow therapeutic/toxicity ratio which is readily influenced by factors, associated with CHF itself, such as renal failure and response to diuretics or the electrolyte and pH changes which may accompany surgical disease, surgery and anesthesia (Table 10-8).

Table 10-8. Factors enhancing sensitivity to digoxin toxicity

Physiological effects	Enhanced autonomic activity
Systemic disorders	Renal failure Pulmonary diseases Myxedema
Electrolyte disorders	Hypokalemia Hypomagnesemia Hypercalcemia
Cardiac disorders	Acute myocardial infarction Acute myocarditis (rheumatic, viral)
Concomitant drug therapy	Diuretics (electrolyte deficiencies) Anesthetic drugs and techniques Drugs affecting SA and AV nodes: CCAs, β blockers, amiodarone

CCAs = Calcium channel antagonists

Mode of action and pharmacodynamics of digoxin

Inotropic effects. The positive inotropic effects of the digitalis glycosides follow from the increase in cytosolic Ca^{++} ion concentration they induce which, in turn, enhances myocardial contractile force. The underlying mechanism is indirect. It involves the binding of the glycoside to and consequent inhibition of the myocardial sarcolemmal Na^+/K^+ ATPase with inhibition of the Na^+ pump (Fig. 10-4). Decreased outward transport of Na^+ increases the intracellular Na^+ content. This prompts a sarcolemmal Na^+/Ca^{++} interchange mechanism which then increases the cytosolic Ca^{++} ion concentration. Stored by the sarcoplasmic reticulum, this Ca^{++} increases the amount of Ca^{++} released by excitation—contraction—coupling, so enhancing myocardial contractile force (Marcus et al, 1995). Ironically it is this "beneficial" increase in intracellular Ca^{++} which underlies the drug's most troublesome toxic effects.

Positive inotropy counteracts the depressed contractility of the failing left ventricle, shifting its function curve (Frank-Starling) upward (Fig. 10-3). Ejection fraction, stroke volume and cardiac output are all increased with a resultant fall in left ventricular filling pressure. Beneficially, this effect is more pronounced the greater the severity of the failure (Gheorghiade et al, 1987). The improved contractility causes a reduction in left ventricular dimensions which through the Laplace effect reduces wall stress and so MVO_2.

Neurohumoral effects. Improvement in cardiac output reduces or even inhibits, the failure-induced neurohumoral compensatory mechanisms, decreasing plasma noradrenaline, renin and aldosterone levels (Fig. 10-4). Renal vascular resistance, as also systemic vascular resistance, are decreased, so that diuresis may be initiated. Preceding and independent of the above reactions, digoxin displays a sympatholytic effect which is mediated through an increase in baroreceptor sensitivity (Ferguson, 1993). At the same time parasympathetic activation invokes SA nodal slowing and AV nodal inhibition, slowing the heart rate.

While a direct effect of digoxin on blood vessels, raising their cytosolic Ca^{++} concentration, leads to mild vasoconstriction with possible increase in systemic vascular resistance, the autonomic effects usually dominate with a net decrease in peripheral resistance.

Electrophysiology of digoxin. Digitalis glycosides cause a prolongation of the refractory period and reduce conduction velocity through the AV node. These properties together with its autonomic effects make digitalis particularly useful for the control of ventricular response rate to atrial fibrillation or flutter. However, the safety margin is narrow. At toxic levels, with intracellular Ca^{++} overload, digitalis causes a marked reduction in the Action Potential

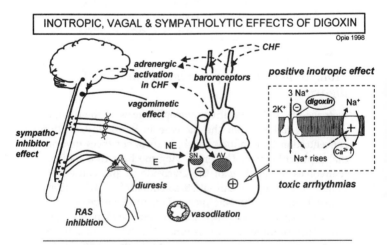

Fig 10-4. Digoxin has both neural and myocardial cellular effects. *The inotropic effect of digoxin is due to inhibition of the sodium pump in myocardial cells. Slowing of the heart rate and inhibition of the atrioventricular node by vagal stimulation and the decreased sympathetic and neurohumoral nerve discharge are important therapeutic benefits. Toxic arrhythmias are less well understood, but may be caused by calcium-dependent afterpotentials. (Fig. copyright © LH Opie, 1998)*

Duration (APD). Digoxin also decreases the resting membrane potential and upstroke velocity of the action potential and may induce oscillatory afterpotentials or delayed after-depolarizations (Kojima and Sperelakis, 1986). All contribute to a dangerous increase in arrhythmogenicity from which a wide spectrum of tachy- and bradyarrhythmias may result.

Kinetics and dosage schedules of digoxin. 75% of the orally administered drug is rapidly absorbed, the rest being inactivated by bacterial action in the lower gut. Circulating in unbound form, digoxin binds to tissue receptors in cardiac and skeletal muscle. An appropriate therapeutic effect is achieved at plasma levels of 1–2 ng/ml (Marcus et al, 1995). With 70% of the circulating drug being renally excreted — glomerular filtration plus tubular excretion — the adequacy of renal function is the most important of the many factors which affect the plasma level. Nonrenal clearance accounts for excretion of the remainder. The drug's half life — relatively long at 36 hours — is a factor which must be considered in the context of its narrow therapeutic/toxicity ratio.

Depending on the urgency to achieve maximum therapeutic effect demanded by the clinical circumstances, several dosage schedules have been recommended, the principal difference between which is the size of the loading dose. This aside, the basic maintenance dose in a 70 kg adult with adequate renal function — the principal factor governing dosage — is 0.25 mg/day. Whichever dosing schedule is adopted, cognizance must be given to the many factors which influence the plasma levels of digitalis achieved, either higher or lower than intended.

Alternative loading dosages are:—

i)   0.5 mg twice daily for two days followed by 0.25 mg/daily.

ii)   0.5 mg thrice daily for one day followed by 0.25 mg daily.

iii) 0.5 mg intravenously followed by 0.25 mg orally, 1 or 2 doses to a total loading dose of 0.75–1.0 mg, thereafter 0.25 mg/daily.

Ultimately each patient's dose must be individually adjusted, by monitoring the plasma level of the drug. The usual therapeutic level ranges from 1–2 ng/ml. Digitalis toxicity should be considered in any patient who develops an arrhythmia or presents with new gastrointestinal, ocular or central nervous complaints.

Indications for digoxin. For long traditionally regarded as an essential component of CHF therapy, current opinion is still ambivalent. Some clinicians feel that chronic medication should be instituted only for clearly defined indications, such as heart failure with atrial fibrillation. Otherwise, the benefits derived will be limited and acquired at the risk of toxicity. In the case of paroxysmal atrial fibrillation or chronic atrial fibrillation without CHF, *digoxin* is not as effective as specific antiarrhythmics such as flecainide, sotalol, propafenone, amiodarone or verapamil. In the case of mild to moderate CHF (NYHA 1–2), in sinus rhythm a combination of diuretic and ACE inhibitor is now regarded as the most appropriate therapy. Only when the grade of failure is more severe (NYHA 3–4) does addition of digoxin confer real benefit in lessening effort intolerance and reducing morbidity but not mortality. In *acute or intractable failure* initial intravenous use of the more potent and therapeutically flexible sympathomimetic inotropes such as *dobutamine* or the phosphodiesterase inhibitors, such as *amrinone* or *milrinone*, should precede the addition of digoxin.

Contraindications to digoxin. Contraindications, both absolute and relative, are based on inotropy and arrhythmogenesis — both related to cytosolic Ca^{++} increase — and its autonomically mediated inhibitory dromotropic effects on SA and AV nodal activity. The first group includes CHF with predominantly diastolic dysfunction, hypertrophic obstructive cardiomyopathy and low output states due to valvular stenosis or chronic pericarditis as well as the high output states associated with chronic cor pulmonale and thyrotoxicosis. The arrhythmogenic category includes the Wolff-Parkinson-White syndrome, early acute myocardial infarction or myocarditis and atrial fibrillation not due to CHF.

Contraindications based on the autonomic actions include any degree of disease or drug induced depression of AV nodal conduction or SA nodal activity. The former includes sinus bradycardia and sick sinus syndrome; the latter, actions of such drugs as verapamil, diltiazem, amiodarone, reserpine, methyldopa and clonidine.

Digoxin during the perioperative period. The management of the patient on digitalis medication presenting for anesthesia and surgery places the clinician on the horns of a dilemma. It is accepted that CHF must be controlled before a patient is submitted to anesthesia. Yet at the same time, the narrow therapeutic/toxicity ratio of digitalis considered in the context of the anesthetic, surgical and surgical diseases environment which may sensitize the patient to digitalis toxicity, make it difficult to achieve simultaneously optimal digoxin tissue levels and yet avoid toxicity. Indeed, peri-operative digoxin is associated with an increased incidence of postoperative ventricular tachycardia (Mangano et al, 1990). On the other hand, two recent studies report that withdrawal of digoxin from treatment regimes of patients in CHF with sinus rhythm, caused a progressive worsening in functional capacity, a decrease in ejection fraction and an increase in heart rate (PROVED, 1993; RADIANCE, 1993).

How can this dilemma be resolved? Various trials (Captopril Multicentre Study, 1983; V-HeFT II, 1991; SOLVD, 1991) have now demonstrated that in patients in mild to moderate CHF (NYHA 1–2) in sinus rhythm, maximum therapeutic benefit is achieved by medication with diuretics and ACE inhibitors alone or in combination. Digoxin medication confers no additional benefit. The "prophylactic" pre-anesthetic digitalization of patients in sinus rhythm considered to be in mild or so called "incipient" cardiac failure, advocated by some authors in the past, can no longer to be recommended.

On the other hand when atrial fibrillation or flutter is present, continuation of established digoxin therapy to maintain the heart rate within the normal range is still acceptable. If, however, the patient presents for urgent surgery in atrial fibrillation with a rapid ventricular response rate, this should not be treated in the first instance with intravenous digoxin. Rather, the ventricular response rate should be cautiously slowed by intravenous titration of cardio-selective β-adrenoceptor blockers, e.g. esmolol, or the calcium antagonists verapamil or diltiazem under ECG control (Prys-Roberts and Foëx, 1989). In patients in the more severe grades of failure on established therapy with digitalis, it is important to monitor digitalis plasma levels, to prevent possible digoxin toxicity and to maintain K^+ and Mg^{++} at physiological levels. If the anesthetic technique involves spontaneous respiration, care must be taken to avoid underventilation with consequent respiratory acidosis, especially when halothane is administered. Contrariwise, when IPPV techniques are utilized, volumes of ventilation, appropriately monitored by capnography, must be regulated to maintain normocapnia. Respiratory alkalosis with resultant hypokalemia must be stringently avoided. With regard to the choice of anesthetic agents, those with arrhythmogenic and/or myocardial depressant action should be omitted or, if considered necessary, used with monitored caution (Forrest et al, 1990; ACC/AHA Task Force Report, 1996).

Digoxin mediated arrhythmias. Atrial, junctional and ventricular ectopy are especially amenable to treatment with *phenytoin* (100 mg intravenously over 5 minutes, up to 1000 mg). Lidocaine is also effective. Treatment with either drug may be accompanied by the infusion of $MgSO_4$. Phenytoin may be effective also for the relief of the high degree of AV block, though temporary transvenous pacing is preferable. Atropine administration may be sufficient for less severe bradycardia. Patients suffering very severe life threatening toxicity should be treated with digoxin specific Fab antibody fragments. Fab binds digoxin and enhances its renal excretion (Atlee, 1997).

ACUTE OR INTRACTABLE HEART FAILURE

For those patients who present for surgery and anesthesia in deteriorating severe or intractable CHF, decompensated by surgical disease, anesthesia and/or effects of surgery, the management is essentially the same as for *acute cardiac failure*. In these circumstances improvement of ventricular contractility demands the use of acute sympathomimetic inotropes and vasodilator drugs or drugs which combine these actions, the *inodilators*. These agents are administered by continuous intravenous infusion under surveillance by continuous multichannel hemodynamic monitoring. This should include the use of a pulmonary artery flotation catheter, so enabling real time assessment of all parameters of cardiac performance. The aim of treatment should be an increase in the cardiac index to 2.0–2.2 liters per minute per meter square. This should provide whole body oxygen delivery of the order of 500 ml per minute, with a pulmonary capillary wedge pressure of 18–22 mm Hg. This level of wedge pressure should provide adequate LV filling and stroke volume, yet alleviate pulmonary congestion (Weber et al, 1987; Russell et al, 1970). Inotrope induced improvement in ventricular contractility may be enhanced by afterload reduction induced by vasodilator agents. Maintenance of coronary perfusion is paramount and must not be compromised. Systolic BP should be maintained at above 90 mm Hg. Should a patient present with a systolic pressure of below 90 mm Hg, it may be essential initially to raise this by an increase in systemic vascular resistance induced by cotherapy with an α-*adrenoceptor agonist* agent. These agents must be administered cautiously as severe or rapid increase in afterload will produce severe LV strain, further LV ischemia and possibly VT or VF. Reduction in preload and pulmonary congestion may be achieved by the acute induction of diuresis and the use of venodilators.

Sympathomimetic inotropes. These improve the circulation in acute cardiac failure through three mechanisms, each of which is subject to a drawback:—

(1) β_1 ino- and chronotropic effect. In some circumstances these effects may precipitate arrhythmias and tachycardia which can worsen myocardial ischemia.

(2) β_2 mediated arterial vasodilation and inotropic effect. β_2 effects may cause hypokolemia which will enhance the risk of arrhythmias.

(3) α_1 induced vasoconstriction counteracting hypotension — the increased afterload may prove detrimental.

The specific circumstances in which various inotropes may be of benefit in acute failure depends on each agent's pattern of receptor stimulation and the careful management of dosage. The latter is predicated by the monitored response. The acute inotropes, their individual pattern of receptor stimulation and dosage schedules, are listed in Table 10-9.

Co-therapy with inotropes. In the treatment of severe heart failure there is logic in combining the use of agents which achieve their inotropic action through differing mechanisms. β-adrenoceptor agonists like *dobutamine* may be rapidly rendered ineffective by increasing down regulation of the β receptors. Some patients may indeed present in severe failure with pre-existing β receptor desensitization which reduces their response to the acute β agonists. In both these circumstances the increased cytosolic cyclic AMP resulting from *PDE inhibition* will augment the failing myocardial contractility.

In the long term, all positive inotropes the effects of which are mediated through the adenyl cyclase-cyclic AMP mechanisms, and this includes all the sympathomimetic inotropes and PDE inhibitors, may adversely influence mortality. This may be for the reasons that the hemodynamic benefit from these agents is bought at the catabolic cost of an increased myocardial energy and oxygen requirement (Hasenfuss, 1992; Hiesmayr et al, 1995). Alternatively, or

Table 10-9. Sympathomimetic inotropes for acute cardiac failure therapy

Drugs and mediating receptors	Dobutamine β1, β2, α	Dopamine Dopaminergic High dose α	Norepinephrine β1, α	Epinephrine β1, β2, α	Isoproterenol β1 > β2	Amrinone PDE inhibitor	Milrinone PDE inhibitor	Phenylephrine α - agonist
Dose infusion µg/kg/min	2–15	2–5 renal effect 5–10 inotropic 10–20 SVR↑	0.01–0.03 max. 0.1	0.01–0.03 max. 0.1–0.3	0.01–0.1	Bolus 750 Drip 2–10	Bolus 50–75 (10 min) Drip 0.375–0.75	0.2–0.3
Elim t½ minutes	2.4	2.0	3.0	2.0	2.0	240*	150*	20
Inotropic effect	↑↑	↑↑	↑	↑↑	↑↑↑	↑	↑	–
Arteriolar Vasodilation	↑	↑↑	–	↑	↑	↑↑	↑↑	→
Vasoconstriction	↑	HD↑	↑↑	HD↑	–	–	–	↑↑↑
Chronotropic effect	↑	↑–	↑	↑↑	↑↑↑	–	–	–
Blood pressure effect	↑	HD↑	↑	–↑	↑	→	→	↑↑↑
Diuretic effect (direct)	–	↑↑	↑	–	–	–	–	→
Arrhythmia risk	↑↑	HD↑	↑	↑↑↑	↑↑↑	↑↑	↑	–

↑= increase; - = no change; ↓ = decrease. HD = high dose. Elim t½ = elimination half life, SVR = systemic vascular resistance.
*Note duration of action of milrinone 3-5 HR, versus amrinone 30–120 min (Fahmy, 1987).

additionally, the increase of myocardial cyclic AMP may be arrhythmogenic. Because of this, the period of inotropic support with such agents should be as short as is absolutely necessary. Their use should constitute a bridging operation only to re-establishment of the conventional chronic therapy for CHF. Alternatively, the energy substrate supply of the myocardium may be improved anabolically by the short term continuous intravenous infusion of insulin, K^+ and glucose (Haider et al, 1984a, b).

Novel Therapies

Calcium sensitizers

These agents, not yet approved for clinical use, act by sensitizing the contractile proteins to the prevailing level of cytosolic calcium. As a group, they also often have phosphodiesterase activity that contributes to their action, and, possibly, to their side-effects. Early results have been disappointing from the point of view of long-term outcome, which has been either slightly worse or the same as placebo when added to otherwise maximal therapy for CHF.

Endothelin receptor antagonists

Circulating levels of the powerful vasoconstrictor, endothelin, are increased in heart failure, the source of the endothelin being, at least in part, the failing ventricles. Endothelin, by promoting myocardial calcium overload, has a direct toxic effect, induces hypertrophy, and is a positive inotrope which may be a disadvantage in the failing heart. An endothelin receptor antagonist lessens mortality in experimental heart failure, and improves hemodynamics in humans (Kiowski et al, 1995). There is a large trial underway in patients with CHF, testing the hypothesis that endothelin receptor blockade may reduce mortality.

Cytokine inhibitors

Cytokines are locally acting polypeptides that increase the severity of cellular injury. Examples are the inflammatory cytokines, such as the interleukins, derived from macrophages and leukocytes. Such cells produce cytokines especially in ventricles damaged by infective cardiomyopathies. One current hypothesis is that failing myocytes can produce cytokines such as tumor necrosis factor alpha (TNFα) and interleukin-6 which then exaggerates the degree of cell damage. Of interest, the calcium antagonist *amlodipine* may exert at least part of its benefit in dilated cardiomyopathy by inhibition of cytokine production (Mohler et al, 1997).

Management Policy for Patients in CHF Requiring Surgery

In deciding the management of the high risk patient in CHF presenting for essential surgery, we would suggest the following to be the most appropriate policy:—

1) Patients with no or minimal functional deficit — proceed to surgery with appropriate hemodynamic monitoring.

2) Patients with moderate correctable functional deficit — delay surgery until the patient's physical condition has been optimised by appropriate treatment, thereafter proceed to surgery with appropriate monitoring.

3) Patients in advanced uncorrectable or intractable functional deficit — defer surgery when possible; if not, choose an alternate minimal palliative surgical procedure. Hemodynamic monitoring should include the use of a Swan-Ganz catheter together with appropriate computer data processing enabling real time assessment of all parameters of cardiac performance.

A major contribution to the safe conduct of anesthesia and the manipulation of drug therapy in these patients has come from the considerable recent advances in sophisticated "real time" monitoring of all parameters of cardiovascular function. However, characterization of what constitutes "appropriate" monitoring in particular circumstances is still the topic of wide debate. The outcome cost/benefit status of the various modalities of monitoring such as the use of Swan-Ganz catheterization, computerized ST segment monitoring and transesophageal echocardiography (TEE) have yet to be established.

In the context of CHF during the perioperative period, the actual choice of anesthetic technique and agent, surprisingly, appears to be of little relevance in terms of outcome (Mangano et al, 1990; Forrest, 1990). Such choice broadly concerns the use of regional versus general anesthesia, and inhalational versus narcotic techniques. The answer, as with so many outcome aspects in clinical anesthesia, depends on the quality and expertise of the management of the technique rather than on the technique itself. Thereafter outcome appears to be more affected by the nature of the cardiac pathology and the site and duration of the surgery (Cohen, 1988)

INTRAVENOUS INOTROPES FOR HEART FAILURE: FDA WARNING

The Cardiovascular Panel of the Food and Drug Administration (FDA) has now warned that these drugs are for use only on hospitalized patients with acute decompensated heart failure. There is no evidence of safety when they are used for more than 24 to 48 hours. Prolonged use of these drugs, whether continuously or intermittently, may be associated with the same risks as chronic oral administration, that is increased hospitalization and death (see Thadani and Roden, *Circulation* 1998; 97: 2295).

SUMMARY

For the patient who presents for surgery in CHF or on therapy for CHF, it is essential that the anesthesiologist ensures that the failure is controlled, treatment optimal and the patient's physical status is stable before anesthesia and surgery are embarked on. In terms of its pathophysiology, the objectives of the peri-operative management of CHF are:

1. *Diuretics* for natriuresis and reduction of pre-load.

2. *Inhibition of the neurohumoral response* by suppression of activity of the renin-angiotensin system and modification of the autonomic sympathetic response. The former is accomplished with the use of ACE inhibitors, with the blockade of angiotensin receptors currently being explored. With regard to autonomic modification, current trials of the adrenoceptor blockers carvedilol, bisoprolol and metoprolol have produced promising beneficial results. ACE inhibitors also act by reduction of sympathetic outflow.

3. *Reduction of pre- and after-load by vasodilators.* For reduction of pre-load, pulmonary congestion and edema, the nitrates are of particular use. When reduction in after-load more than that which follows from administration of ACE inhibitors is required, the use of hydralazine is beneficial.

4. *Enhancement of myocardial contractility by inotropes.* These include digitalis, the sympathomimetic amines and phosphodiesterase-III inhibitors. Combined with diuretic and ACE inhibitor medication, digitalis is still the standard inotrope for the chronic management of CHF of the severer grades. The sympathomimetic amines and PDE inhibitors (inodilators) find application only in the short-term management of acute or intractable cardiac failure.

5. *Important changes* from older conventional treatment patterns of CHF are the early intervention with ACE inhibitors, and the addition of mixed beta- and alpha-adrenoceptor blockade with drugs like carvedilol or beta-blockade with metoprolol or bisoprolol.

REFERENCES

ACC/AHA Task Force Report. Guidelines for peri-operative cardiovascular evaluation for non-cardiac surgery. *Circulation* 1996; 93: 1278–1317.

AIRE Study. The Acute Infarction Ramipril Efficacy (AIRE) Study Investigators. The effect of ramipril on mortality and morbidity of survivors of acute myocardial infarction with clinical evidence of heart failure. *Lancet* 1993; 342: 821–828.

Atlee JL. Perioperative cardiac dysrhythmias. *Anesthesiology* 1997; 86: 1397–1424.

Bashir Y, Sneddon JF, Staunton HA, et al. Effects of long term oral magnesium chloride replacement in congestive cardiac failure secondary to coronary artery disease. *Am J Cardiol* 1993; 72:1156–1162.

Benumof JL. Respiratory physiology and function during anesthesia. In: *Anesthesia.* 3rd Ed. Miller RD Editor. Churchill Livingstone. New York. Edinburgh. London. 1990, 505–550.

Berthelsen P, Havholdt OS, Husun, B et al. PEEP reverses nitrogly-cerine induced hypoxaemia following coronary artery bypass surgery. *Acta Anaesthesiol Scand* 1986; 30: 243–246.

Bolognesi R, Cucchini F, Lavernaro A et al. Effects of strophanthi-din administration on left ventricular relaxation and filling phase in coronary artery disease. *Am J Cardiol* 1992; 69: 169–172.

Braunwald E. *Heart Disease*. 4th Ed. WB Saunders Company, Phila-delphia, 1992, 452.

Bristow R. Mechanism of action of beta-blocking agents in heart failure. *Am J Cardiol* 1997; 80(11A): 26L–40L.

Brutsaert DL, Sys SU and Gilbert TC. Diastolic failure: Pathophy-siology and therapeutic implications. *J Am Coll Cardiol* 1993; 22: 318–325.

Captopril Multicenter Research Group. A placebo-controlled trial of captopril in refractory chronic congestive heart failure. *J Am Coll Cardiol* 1983; 2: 755–763.

Clark NJ and Stanley TH. Anesthesia for vascular surgery. In: *Anesthesia*. Third Ed. Ed. Miller RD. Churchill Livingstone. New York. 1990, 1693–1736.

Cohen MM. Does anesthesia contribute to operative mortality? *JAMA* 1988; 260: 2859–2863.

Colucci WF, Ribiero JP, Rocco MB, et al. Impaired chronotropic response to exercise in patients with congestive heart failure: Role of postsynaptic beta adrenergic desensitization. *Circulation* 1989; 80: 314–323.

CONSENSUS. Co-operative North Scandinavian Enalapril Survival Study. Effects of enalapril on mortality in severe heart failure: *N Engl J Med* 1987; 316:1429–1435.

Cotter G, Metzkor E, Kaluski E. et al. Randomised trial of high-dose isosorbide dinitrate plus low-dose furosemide versus high-dose furosemide plus low-dose isosorbide dinitrate in severe pulmonary edema. *Lancet*, 1998; 351: 389–93.

Cripps TP and Gareth-Jones J. Preoperative assessment of the patient with pre-existing disease of the circulatory system for non-cardiac surgery. In: *General Anesthesia*. 5th ed. Eds. Nunn JF, Utting JE, Brown BR. Butterworth, London 1989, 366–382.

Devane J and Ryan MP. The effects of amiloride and triamterene on urinary magnesium excretion in conscious saline-loaded rats. *Br J Pharmacol* 1981; 72: 285–289.

Devane J and Ryan MP. Evidence for a magnesium sparing action by amiloride during renal clearance studies in rats. *Br J Pharmacol* 1983; 79: 891–896.

Digitalis Investigation Group. The effect of digoxin on mortality and morbidity in patients with heart failure. *New Engl J Med*, 336: 525–533, 1997.

Dorup I, Skajaa K, Clausen T and Kjeldsen K. Reduced concentra-tion of K^+, Mg^{++} and Na^+-K^+ pumps in human skeletal muscle dur-ing treatment with diuretics. *Br Med J* 1988; 296: 455–458.

Eisenkraft JB. Pulse oximeter desaturation due to methemoglo-binemia. *Anesthesiology* 1988; 68: 279–282.

Fahmy NR. Cardiovascular drugs, in: *Practical Anesthetic Pharmacol-ogy* 2nd ed. Eds Rafik RA, Grogonon AW, Domer FR. Appleton-Century-Crofts Norwalk, CT. 1987, 195–236

Ferguson DW. Sympathetic mechanisms in heart failure — patho-physiological and pharmacological implications. *Circulation* 1993; 87(supplement 4): 97–103.

Ferner RE. Adverse effects of angiotensin converting enzyme inhibitors. *Adv Drug React Bull* 1994; 141: 528–531.

Forrest JB, Cahalan MK, Rehder K, et al. Multicentre study of general anesthesia. II Results. *Anesthesiology* 1990; 72: 262–268.

Gersh BJ and Opie LH. Which drug for which condition? In: *Drugs for the Heart.* 4th edition. Ed. Opie LH. WB Saunders Co. Philadelphia. 1995, 308–342.

Gerson JI, Allen FB, Seltzer, et al. Arterial and venous dilatation by nitroprusside and nitroglycerine — is there a difference? *Anes Analg* 1982; 61: 256–260.

Gheorghiade M, St. Clair J, St. Clair C. and Bella GA. Hemodynamic effects of intravenous digoxin in patients in severe heart failure initially treated with diuretics and vasodilatation. *J Am Coll Cardiol* 1987; 9: 849–857.

Gilbert EM, Ohlsen SI, Renlund DG and Bristow MR. Beta-adrenergic receptor regulation and left ventricular function in idiopathic dilated cardiomyopathy. *Am J Cardiol* 1993; 71: 223C–229C.

Gogia H, Mehra A and Parikh S. Prevention of tolerance to hemodynamic effects of nitrates with concomitant use of hydralazine in patients with chronic heart failure. *J Am Coll Cardiol* 1995; 26: 575–580.

Goldman LG, Caldera DL, Southwick FS, et al. Cardiac risk factors and complications of non-cardiac surgery. *Medicine* 1978; 57:357–370.

Gonzales-Fernandez RA, Altieri PI, Diaz LM, et al. Effects of enalapril on heart failure in hypertensive patients with diastolic dysfunction. *Am J Hypertens* 1992; 5:480–483.

Gottlieb SS, Dickstein K, Fleck E, et al. Hemodynamic and neurohumoral effects of angiotensin II receptor antagonist losartan in patients with congestive heart failure. *Circulation* 1993; 88:1602–1609.

Grassi G, Cattaneo BM, Seraville G, et al. Effects of chronic ACE inhibition on sympathetic nerve traffic and baroreflex control of the circulation in heart failure. *Circulation* 1997; 96: 1173–1179.

Haber HL, Simek CL, Bergen JD, et al. Bolus intravenous nitroglycerine predominantly reduces afterload in patients with excessive arterial elastance. *J Am Coll Cardiol* 1993; 22:251–257.

Haider W, Eckersberg F and Wolner E. Preventative insulin administration for myocardial protection during cardiac surgery. *Anesthesiology* 1984a; 60:422–429.

Haider W, Benzer H, Schultz W and Wolner E. Improvement of cardiac preservation by pre-operative high insulin supply. *J Thorac Cardiovasc Surg* 1984b; 88:294–300.

Hall JM. Braydkinin receptors: pharmacological properties and biological roles. *Pharmacol Ther,* 1993; 56: 131–190.

Harrison DG and Bates JN. The nitro vasodilators: New ideas about old drugs. *Circulation* 1993; 87:1461–1467.

Hasenfuss G. Neue Kardiotonika/Inodilatoren: Energetische Aspekta. *Zeits Kardiol* 1992; 81:(supp 4) 57–63.

Hausdorff WP, Caron MG and Lefkowitz RJ. Turning off the signal: Desensitization of beta adrenergic receptor function. *FASEB* 1990; 4:881–889.

Hiesmayr M, Haider WJ, Grubhofer G, et al. Effects of dobutamine versus insulin on cardiac performance, myocardial oxygen demand, and total body metabolism after coronary artery bypass grafting. *J Cardiothor Vasc Anes,* 1995; 9: 653–658.

Joob AW, Human PK, Kaiser DL, and Kron IL. The effect of renin-angiotensin system blockade on visceral blood flow during and after thoracic aortic cross clamping. *J Thorac Cardiovasc Surg* 1986; 91:411–418.

Kaplan KJ, Taber M, Teagarden JR, et al. Association of methemoglobinemia and intravenous nitroglycerine administration. *Am J Cardiol* 1985; 55:181–183.

Kataja JH, Kaukenin S, Namaki OV, et al: Hemodynamic and hormonal changes in patients treated with captopril for surgery of abdominal aorta. *J Cardiothor Anes* 1989; 3:425–432.

Kellow NH. The renin-angiotension system and angiotensin converting enzyme (ACE) inhibitors. *Anaesthesia* 1994; 49:613–622.

Kiowski W, Sutsch P, Hunziker P, et al. Evidence for endothelin-1-mediated vasoconstriction in severe chronic heart failure. *Lancet* 1995; 346: 732–736.

Kojima N and Sperelakis N. Effects of calcium channel blockers on ouabain-induced oscillatory afterpotentials in organ cultured young embryonic chick heart. *Eur J Pharmacol* 1986; 182:65–73.

Krapez JR, Vesey CJ, Adams L and Coe EL. Effects of cyanide antidotes used with sodium nitroprusside infusion: sodium thiosulphate and hydroxycobalamine given prophylactically to dogs. *Br J Anaesth* 1981; 53: 793–804.

Mangano DT. Peri-operative cardiac morbidity. *Anesthesiology* 1990; 72: 153–184.

Mangano DT, Browner WF, Hollenburg M, et al. Association of perioperative myocardial ischemia with morbidity and mortality in men undergoing noncardiac surgery. *N Engl J Med* 1990; 323:1781–1788.

Mangano DT, Layug EL, Wallace A, Multicentre Study of Perioperative Ischemia Research Group. Prevention of myocardial ischaemia after noncardiac surgery. Effect of atenolol on mortality and cardiovascular morbidity after noncardiac surgery. *New Engl J Med* 1996; 335: 1713–1720.

Marcus FI, Opie LH, Sonnenblik EH and Chatterjee K. Digitalis and other inotropes. In: *Drugs for the Heart.* 4th ed. Ed: Opie LH. WB Saunders Company. 1995, 145–173.

McLay JS, McMurray JJ, Bridges AB, et al. Acute effects of furosemide in patients with chronic heart failure. *Am Heart J* 1993; 126: 879–886.

Mehra A, Shotan A, Ostrzega T, et al. Escalating nitrate dose overcomes early attenuation of hemodynamic effect caused by nitrate tolerance in patients with heart failure. *Am Heart J* 1995; 130: 692–697.

Mercadier JJ, de la Bastie D, Menasche D, et al. Alpha -myosin heavy chain isoform and atrial size in patients with various types of mitral valve dysfunction: A quantitative study. *J Am Coll Cardiol* 1987; 9: 1024–1030.

Mets BM. The renin-angiotensin system and ACE inhibitors in the perioperative period, in Balliere's *Clinical Anaesthesiology.* Vol II. No 4. In press, 1998.

Miller RR, Vismara LA, Williams DO, et al. Pharmacological mechanisms for left ventricular unloading in clinical congestive cardiac failure: Differentiated effects of nitroprusside, phentolamine and nitroglycerine on cardiac function and peripheral circulation. *Circ Res* 1976; 39: 127–133.

Mirenda JV and Grissom TE. Implications of renin angiotensin system and angiotensin converting enzyme inhibitors. *Anes Analg,* 1991; 72: 667–683.

Mohler ER III, Sorensen LC, Ghali JK, et al. Role of cytokines in the mechanism of action of amlodipine: the PRAISE heart failure trial. *J Am Coll Cardiol* 1997; 30: 35–41.

Opie LH. ACE inhibition in pregnancy — how to avoid the sting in the tail. *S Afr Med J,* 1996; 86: 326–327.

Opie LH, Kaplan NN and Poole-Wilson PA. Diuretics. In: *Drugs for the Heart.* 4th ed. Ed. Opie LH. WB Saunders Co. Philadelphia, 1995, 83–103.

Orkin FK. Acquired methemoglobinaemia and sulf-hemoglobine-mia. In: *Complications in Anesthesiology.* Eds. Orkin FK & Cooperman LH. JB Lippincott Co, Philadelphia, 1983, 495–504.

Packer M. Beta-blockade in the management of chronic heart failure. Another step in the conceptual evolution of a neurohormonal model of the disease. *Eur Heart J:* 1996a:7(suppl B): 21–23.

Packer M, Bristow M R, Cohn J N, et al (for US Carvedilol Heart Failure Study Group). The effect of carvedilol on morbidity and mortality in patients with chronic heart failure. *N Engl J Med* 1996b: 334;1349–1355.

Pfeffer M A and Stevenson L W. β-adrenergic blockade and survival in heart failure. *N Engl J Med* 1996; 334: 1396–1397.

Pitt B, Segal R, Martinez FA et al, Randomised trail of losartan versus captopril in patients over 65 with heart failure (Evaluation of losartan in the Elderly Study, ELITE). *Lancet,* 1997; 349: 747–752.

PROVED Study. Uretsky BF, Young JB, Shahidi E et al. Randomized study assessing the effects of digoxin withdrawal in patients with mild to moderate chronic congestive heart failure. Results of the Prospective Randomized Study of Ventricular Failure and the Efficacy of Digoxin (PROVED) trial. *J Am Coll Cardiol,* 1993; 22: 955–962.

Prys-Roberts C and Foëx P. Anaesthesia for patients with dysfunction of the circulatory system. Chapter in: *General Anaesthesia.* 5th edition. Eds. Nunn JF, Utting JE & Brown BR. Butterworth, London, 1989, 704–713.

RADIANCE Study. Packer M, Gheorghiade M, Young JB, et al. Withdrawal of digoxin from patients with chronic heart failure treated with angiotensin converting enzyme inhibitors. Randomized assessment of the effect of Digoxin on Inhibitors of the Angiotensin-Converting Enzyme (RADIANCE) Study. *N Engl J Med* 1993, 329:1–7.

Robin ED and McCauley R. Nitroprusside related cyanide poisoning — time (long past due) for urgent effective intervention. *Chest,* 1992; 102:1842-1845.

Russell RO, Rackley CE, Pombo JS, et al. Effects of increasing left ventricular filling pressure in patients with acute myocardial infarction. *J Clin Invest,* 1970; 49: 1539–1550.

Santoro D, Natally A, Palumbo C, et al. Effects of chronic angiotensin converting enzyme inhibition on glucose tolerance and insulin sensitivity in essential hypertension. *Hypertension,* 1992; 20:181–191.

SAVE Study. Pfeffer MA, Braunwald E, Moye LA, et al Effect of captopril on mortality and morbidity in patients with left ventricular dysfunction after myocardial infarction. Results of the Survival and Ventricular Enlargement (SAVE) Trial. *N Engl J Med,* 1992; 327: 669–677.

Setaro JF, Zarret VL, Schulman DS, et al. Usefulness of verapamil for congestive heart failure associated with abnormal left ventricular diastolic filling and normal left ventricular systolic performance. *Am J Cardiol,* 1990; 66:981–986.

Skarvan K. Perioperative left ventricular failure: The rationale for the use of vasoactive drugs. Chapter in: *Vasoactive drugs.* Ed. Skarvan K. Ballière's Clinical Anaesthesiology. Vol. 8 No. 1. Ballière Tindall, London. 1994, 215–242.

SOLVD Investigators. Effect of enalapril on survival in patients with reduced left ventricular ejection fractions and congestive cardiac failure. Studies of Left Ventricular Dysfunction (SOLVD). *N Engl J Med,* 1991; 325: 293–302.

SOLVD Investigators II. The effect of enalapril on mortality and development of heart failure in asymptomatic patients with reduced left ventricular fractions. Studies of Left Ventricular Dysfunction (SOLVD). *N Engl J Med,* 1992; 327: 685–691.

Sykes MK, Vickers MD and Hull CJ. *Principles of measurement and monitoring in anesthesia and intensive care.* 3rd ed. Blackwell Scientific Publications, London 1991, 262–270.

Thadani U and Opie LH. Nitrates. In: *Drugs for the Heart.* 4th edition. Ed. Opie LH. W B Saunders Co. Philadelphia, 1995, 31–49.

Timmermans PB, Wong PC, Chiu AT, et al. Angiotensin II receptors and angiotensin II receptor antagonists. *Pharmacol Rev* 1993; 45: 205–251.

Tinker JH and Roberts S. Anaesthesia for Cardiac Surgery. In: *General Anaesthesia* 5th Ed. Eds. Nunn JF, Utting JE and Brown BR. Butterworths, London, 1989, 894–910.

Toussaint C, Masselink A , Gentges A, et al. Interference of different ACE inhibitors with the diuretic action of furosemide and hydrochlorthiazide. *Klinische Wochenschrift* 1989; 67: 1138–1146.

Unger T and Gohlke P. Tissue renin angiotensin system in the heart and vasculature: Possible involvement in the cardiovascular actions of converting enzyme inhibitors. *Am J Cardiol,* 1990; 65: 3I–10I.

V-HeFT II Study. Cohn JN, Johnson G, Ziesche S, et al. A comparison of enalapril with hydralazine — isosorbide dinitrate in the treatment of chronic congestive cardiac failure. Vasodilator Heart Failure Trial (V-HeFT) study. *N Engl J Med,* 1991; 325: 303–310.

Weber KT, Janicki JS, Campbell C and Replogle R. Pathophysiology of acute and chronic cardiac failure. *Am J Cardiol,* 1987; 60: 3c–9c.

Weber K T, Sun Y, Katwa L C and Cleutjens J P. Connecting tissue: a metabolic entity. *J Mol Cell Cardiol,* 1995; 27: 107–120.

Williams EF and Lake CL. Nitrates. In: Vasoactive drugs. Ed. Skarvan K. Ballière's *Clinical Anaesthesiology.* Vol. 8 No. 1. Ballière Tyndall, London, 1994, 87–108.

Zall S, Eden E. Winso I, et al. Controlled hypotension with adenosine or nitroprusside during cerebral aneurysm surgery : effects on hemodynamics, excretory function and renin release. *Anesthesia Analg* 1990; 71: 631–636.

Zeppelini R, Polognesi R, Iavernaro A, et al. Effect of dobutamine on left ventricular relaxation and filling phase in patients with ischemic heart disease and preserved systolic function. *Cardiovasc Drugs Therap* 1993; 7: 325–331.

Zisman LS, Abraham WT, Meixell GE, et al. Angiotensin II formation in the intact human heart. *J Clin Invest* 1995; 95: 1490–1498.

CHAPTER 11

Cardiopulmonary Resuscitation and Critical Care Management

Thomas J. Monaco, Jr. and James Ramsay

Cardiopulmonary resuscitation and advanced cardiac life support are essential abilities required of the clinical anesthesiologist. Equally important is the ability to provide care for the unstable patient who may progress to cardiac arrest and to manage the patient who has been successfully resuscitated from cardiac arrest. A sound knowledge of the pathophysiology of cardiovascular collapse, the mechanisms of resuscitation, and the pharmacology of agents used to restore normal circulation is essential in treating the patient with cardiac arrest.

Cardiopulmonary Arrest

Etiology

Cardiopulmonary arrest may occur in any clinical setting. While the etiology of cardiovascular collapse is most commonly related to ischemic cardiac disease, primary cardiac arrhythmias, cardiac valvular disease, or trauma, a number of other causes or contributing events are possible (Table 11-1). Especially in hospitalized patients, an acute pulmonary event such as tension pneumothorax should always be considered in the setting of cardiopulmonary arrest. In general terms, one can classify a cardiac arrest as either arrhythmic in nature or due to myocardial failure. An arrhythmic arrest is characterized by an immediate loss of consciousness and loss of pulse without a preceding collapse of the circulation. An arrest due to cardiac failure is best characterized by a gradual collapse of the circulation before loss of the pulse (Hinkle and Thaler, 1982).

Effects of Tissue Ischemia

Whether immediate or gradual, cessation of cardiac output leads to tissue ischemia and the beginnings of cellular

TABLE 11-1 Conditions associated with cardiovascular collapse and sudden death in adults

1. **Ischemic heart disease**

   a) Coronary atherosclerosis
   b) Coronary artery spasm (Prinzmetal's angina)
   c) Nonatherosclerotic coronary disease (Kawasaki disease)

2. **Valvular heart disease**

3. **Cardiac arrhythmias**

   a) *Primary Rhythm Disturbance*
      1. sinoatrial node disease
      2. accessory tract disease
      3. atrioventricular block

   b) *Conduction System Disease*
      1. amyloid
      2. sarcoid
      3. myotonia dystrophica

   c) *Electrolyte Disturbances*
      1. hypo/hyperkalemia
      2. hypomagnesemia

   d) *Drug Toxicity/Overdose*
      1. digoxin
      2. quinidine
      3. tricyclic antidepressants

4. **Cardiomyopathy**

   a) Ischemic
   b) Infectious
   c) Idiopathic

5. **Infective endocarditis**

6. **Cardiac tumor**

7. **Tamponade**

8. **Ruptured aortic aneurysm/aortic dissection**

9. **Acute pulmonary disease**

   a) Tension Pneumothorax
   b) Pulmonary Thromboembolism

death within minutes. For tissues with a high oxygen extraction which are dependent on aerobic metabolism, several minutes of complete ischemia can mean irreversible organ dysfunction or failure. The low perfusion state leading to or following cardiac arrest results in profound derangements in cellular metabolism. For instance, in cerebral tissue, complete cessation of blood flow leads to an exhaustion of available oxygen within fifteen seconds and a conversion to anaerobic glycolysis. Anaerobic metabolism proceeds until stores of glucose and glycogen are exhausted. This results in a mixed hypercarbic and metabolic (lactic) acidosis at the tissue level. Within five minutes, substrate for the production of high energy phosphate compounds is depleted and energy requiring processes of the cell cease (Siesjo, 1981). With loss of the energy-dependent membrane Na/K ATPase, transmembrane gradients of sodium and potassium decline, uncontrolled entry of calcium into cells occurs, and an ischemic cascade leading to cellular death ensues (Cheung, 1986). Thus, it is imperative that resuscitative attempts be instituted rapidly and effectively following cardiac arrest if end-organ function is to be preserved.

RESUSCITATION PHYSIOLOGY

Re-establishing an effective spontaneous circulation with delivery of oxygen to vital organs is the ultimate goal in resuscitating the cardiac arrest patient. The goal of basic life support (artificial ventilation and chest compressions) is to provide an adequate flow of oxygenated blood to the heart and brain until more definitive therapy is instituted.

Mechanisms for Blood Flow

The predominant mechanism of blood flow during cardiopulmonary resuscitation is controversial. One mechanism is the physical compression of the heart between the sternum and vertebral column (Kouwenhaven et al, 1960). In theory, compression of the chest ejects blood into the great arteries from the ventricles. Relaxation between compressions allows the heart to refill passively. This theory requires that the tricuspid, mitral, pulmonic, and aortic valves remain competent — preventing retrograde flow. This is contradicted by the observation with transesophageal echocardiography that cardiac valvular incompetence occurs with chest compressions in humans. Another, and likely more important, mechanism for blood flow during CPR involves the manipulation of intrathoracic pressure. By compressing the chest cavity during CPB, "forward" or systemic blood flow is favored because of valves in the venous system which prevent the transmission of the increased intrathoracic pressure. Thus, blood flow is explained by the establishment of a peripheral arterial to venous pressure gradient with the heart functioning as a passive conduit during blood flow (Chandra, 1993). A number of investigators have suggested that this is the predominant mechanism for blood flow during CPR in humans (Swenson et al, 1988; Chandra, 1993; Paradis et al, 1989).

Actual blood flow during conventional chest compressions without use of vasopressors is far below that required to meet the metabolic needs of the brain and heart. This has been convincingly demonstrated in animal models and is likely true in man. In fact, coronary and cerebral blood flows may be only 10% of normal (Ditchey et al, 1982) and renal and hepatic blood flow less than 5% of normal (Koehler et al, 1983) during CPR.

The use of alpha adrenergic agonists during CPR greatly augments blood flow to the heart and brain. Coronary blood flow during CPR is proportional to the gradient between aortic diastolic pressure and right atrial pressure (Luce et al, 1983). By increasing arterial vascular tone, alpha agonists increase diastolic pressure, coronary perfusion pressure, and thus coronary blood flow (Fig 11-1). Alpha agonists increase cerebral blood flow by increasing carotid artery pressure during CPR in a manner analogous to aortic pressure and the heart. Alpha adrenergic agonist therapy during cardiac arrest also redistributes blood flow from the peripheral circulation to the central circulation. With effective chest compressions and use of alpha agonists, cerebral and coronary blood flow may approach 30–60% of normal flow and cardiac output may approach 25–35% of normal during CPR (Voorhees et al, 1980).

Electrical Therapy

Frequently, an essential component of cardiac resuscitation is the use of electrical current to terminate malignant ventricular or supraventricular arrhythmias. Ventricular fibrillation is the most common initial rhythm in sudden cardiac arrest. Electrical defibrillation is the passage of electrical current across the heart to depolarize the entire myocardium. This allows natural pacemaker tissue to resume normal activity (Cummins, 1994). The fibrillating heart rapidly consumes available myocardial high energy phosphate compounds. Severe depletion of these energy stores lessens the likelihood that the myocardium will reestablish a spontaneous rhythm (Kern et al, 1990). Thus, when indicated, prompt defibrillation substantially improves the chances for successful resuscitation. Synchronized cardioversion is the application of electrical current to treat hemodynamically significant supraventricular or ventricular tachyarrhythmias. It differs from defibrillation in that the delivery of the shock is synchronized to the refractory period of the cardiac cycle to minimize the chance of inducing ventricular fibrillation.

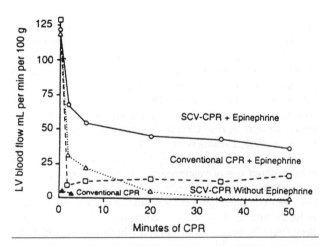

*Fig 11-1. **Left ventricular blood flow** in dogs during CPR with and without epinephrine. SCV indicates simultaneous compression ventilation technique of CPR. (Reproduced with permission Textbook of Advanced Cardiac Life Support 1994). Copyright American Heart Association.*

PRINCIPLES OF RESUSCITATION

With the passage of time after cardiac arrest, the probability of successful resuscitation of the patient declines sharply (Cummins, 1994) (Fig 11-2). Clinicians or rescuers need to rapidly and efficiently execute the series of interventions known as basic life support and advanced cardiac life support. The successful resuscitation of a patient from cardiac arrest mandates prompt recognition of the arrest, immediate initiation of basic life support (CPR), defibrillation if indicated, then rhythm-directed pharmacological management.

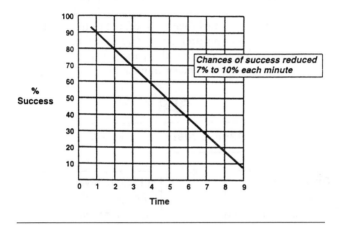

Fig 11-2. Resuscitation success versus time following ventricular fibrillation. (Reproduced with permission Textbook of Advanced Cardiac Life Support 1994). Copyright American Heart Association.

The Resuscitation Team

While an individual can initiate cardiopulmonary resuscitation, successful advanced cardiac life support requires the presence of a team of health professionals who are able to work together to treat the patient. Depending on the scene of the cardiac arrest, this team may be comprised of physicians, physician assistants, nurses, or emergency medical technicians. The team approach affords the simultaneous accomplishment of a number of tasks. For instance, one individual can manage the airway while another performs chest compressions, and yet another obtains intravenous access. Other important tasks include preparing and administering resuscitative drugs, keeping a record of events and times, and limiting access to the scene to only those personnel involved in care of the patient. The successful resuscitation team must have a leader who is able to delegate tasks and make decisions at critical junctures during the resuscitation.

Various groups have constructed algorithms for many of the situations encountered in life threatening cardiac disturbances. The best known in North America are those published by the American Heart Association (AHA, 1992; Cummins, 1994). More recently the International Liason Committee on Resuscitation (ILCOR) published the first of its "advisory statements" (Cummins and Chamberlain,

1997). Knowledge or familiarity with algorithms such as these enables the resuscitation team to function efficiently. Each member of the team can anticipate the next required step and the resuscitation can proceed smoothly. The following discussion is in the context of several of these algorithms.

Basic Cardiopulmonary Resuscitation

Basic life support (Fig 11-3) describes the general approach to the patient with a presumed cardiac emergency. After confirmation of unresponsiveness in a collapsed individual, the first person on the scene of an arrest should call for assistance and initiate basic life support (BLS). In a hospital setting, the monitor/defibrillator is brought directly to the scene. For assessment and optimal resuscitation, the caregivers should then position the patient supine on a firm surface. In the setting of major trauma, the patient's cervical

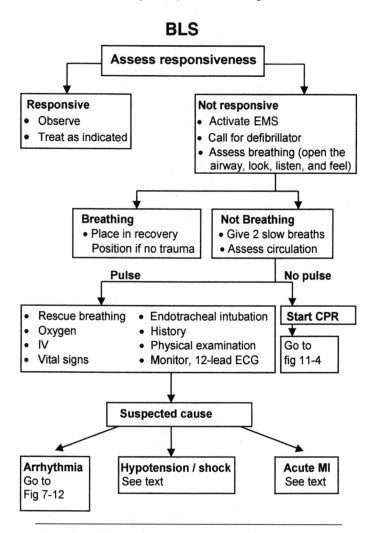

Fig 11-3 Basic life support algorithm (universal algorithm) for adult emergency cardiac care. Reproduced with permission, Journal of the American Medical Association 1992; 268: 2199–2241.
EMS = emergency medical services; MI = myocardial infarction.

spine should be stabilized during movement of the patient to prevent injury to the cervical spinal cord. This stabilization is accomplished by maintaining the head and neck "in line" in a neutral position during movement of the patient and manipulation of the airway (Thal, 1989).

The initial "ABCs" of life support are quickly begun by the caregiver after recognizing the cardiac arrest, where ABC represents Airways, Breathing and Circulation (see the BLS algorithm, Fig 11-3). The initial steps are to open the airway *("A" for airway)*, remove vomitus or foreign bodies, and assess for the presence or absence of spontaneous ventilation. If the patient is not breathing, the caregiver then initiates artificial ventilation *("B" for breathing)* by giving two breaths delivered by mouth, pocket face mask, or ideally, a self-inflating bag. Ventilation with 100% oxygen should commence as soon as oxygen is available. Each breath is delivered with low peak inspiratory pressure (<25 cm H_2O) to prevent overcoming lower esophageal tone and distension of the stomach, and with sufficient time (2–3 sec) for exhalation. The caregiver may need to overcome obstruction to ventilation by altering the head and neck position with a chin-lift or jaw-thrust maneuver or by using an airway adjunct such as an oral or nasopharyngeal airway. Anterior cricoid pressure may be applied to decrease the risk of aspiration of gastric contents. This maneuver produces compression of the esophagus by the posterior cricoid cartilage and helps prevent passive regurgitation of gastric contents or insufflation of the stomach with air during ventilation.

Following an assessment of the airway and initiation of ventilation, the caregiver evaluates the *circulation ("C")* by checking a carotid pulse for 5–10 seconds. If a pulse is present, then the caregiver should continue management of the airway and initiate a diagnostic evaluation to identify and address the primary cause of the patient's clinical deterioration (Fig 11-3). Some of the possibilities may include acute myocardial infarction, pulmonary edema, cardiogenic shock, sepsis or cardiac arrhythmias. Management of some of these clinical scenarios is presented later in this chapter.

If no carotid pulse is detected, a *"precordial thump"* may be administered and cardiac compressions are started at a rate of 80–100 per minute (Fig 11-4). In the adult, each compression should depress the sternum 4–5 cm, and the duration of each compression should be approximately 50% of the time required for an entire compression-relaxation cycle. Ventilation and chest compressions continue until a monitor/defibrillator arrives at the scene of the cardiac arrest, when the Universal Advanced Life Support Algorithm (Fig 11-4) should be followed.

Drug Therapy/Route of Administration

Intravenous access is obtained as soon as possible after CPR is initiated. Medications should be given either intravenously or via an endotracheal tube during advanced cardiac life support. Central administration of drugs produces a relatively rapid delivery of drugs to the myocardium and brain during CPR (Redding and Pearson, 1967).

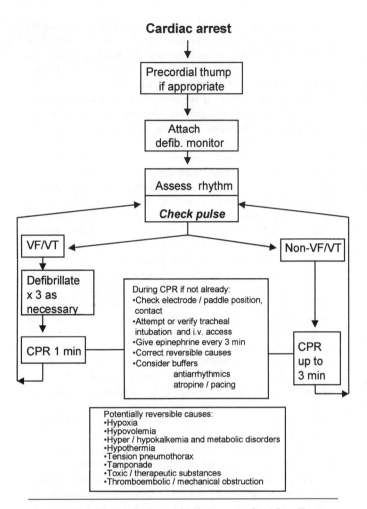

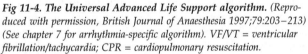

Fig 11-4. The Universal Advanced Life Support algorithm. (Reproduced with permission, British Journal of Anaesthesia 1997;79:203–213) (See chapter 7 for arrhythmia-specific algorithm). VF/VT = ventricular fibrillation/tachycardia; CPR = cardiopulmonary resuscitation.

Because venous return is slow from the peripheral circulation during arrest conditions, drugs administered via a peripheral vein during cardiac arrest should be followed by twenty ml of 0.9% sodium chloride to insure delivery to the central circulation. Elevating the extremity after injection may also hasten delivery of the drug to the heart. If establishment of intravenous access is delayed; atropine, lidocaine, and epinephrine may be delivered via an endotracheal tube during cardiac arrest. The dose of a drug given via an endotracheal tube should be 2.5 times the suggested intravenous dose. Dilution of the drug in at least 10 ml of 0.9% sodium chloride or water and administration via a long catheter extending beyond the tip of the endotracheal tube seems to help increase drug bioavailability (Cummins, 1994).

Fluid Therapy for Resuscitation

Initial fluid therapy during resuscitation from cardiac arrest should be crystalloids in most clinical scenarios. For the arrest caused by hemorrhagic shock, colloid volume expanders or whole blood may be the best fluid for resuscitation based on the clinical judgment of the care team. When using crystalloid solutions for volume expansion or drug delivery during CPR, glucose containing solutions should be avoided except when documented or suspected hypoglycemia exists.

Hyperglycemia has been linked to poor neurologic outcome in the setting of cerebral ischemia in both animal and human studies (Longstreth and Inui, 1984). The proposed mechanism for worsened neurologic outcome is that increased cerebral levels of glucose provide additional substrate for the formation of lactic acid during anaerobic metabolism in ischemic tissue. The resultant worsened tissue acidosis accentuates neuronal injury (Kraig et al, 1987). As the ultimate goal of resuscitation from cardiopulmonary arrest is a neurologically intact patient, avoidance of glucose-containing solutions for resuscitation of the patient appears prudent until future studies confirm or refute the observed relationship between hyperglycemia and poor neurological outcome.

VENTRICULAR FIBRILLATION/ PULSELESS VENTRICULAR TACHYCARDIA

The cardiac rhythm of the patient in full cardiac arrest should be determined as soon as a defibrillator/monitor is available. The majority of patients having sudden cardiac arrest will have ventricular tachycardia (VT) or ventricular fibrillation (VF) as their initial rhythm (Cummins, 1994). The only effective treatment of this arrhythmia is cardiac defibrillation (Figs 11-4; 7-13, page 205). As ventricular fibrillation usually quickly deteriorates to asystole within 5–10 minutes of the arrest, prompt defibrillation is a prime determinant of the successful resuscitation. Usually, asystole represents a state of diffuse, severe cardiac injury from which resuscitation of the patient is unlikely.

Because the identification of ventricular fibrillation (VF) has important therapeutic and prognostic implications, examination of the rhythm should proceed quickly but carefully. Ventricular fibrillation may be quite "fine" in character thus giving the appearance of asystole. More rarely, VF or VT may have a "vector of VF" and thus appear to be asystole (McDonald, 1982). The true rhythm can usually be determined by checking more than one ECG lead. While defibrillation is not an appropriate treatment for asystole, if the clinician has any doubt that the rhythm could be "fine" VF, the patient should be treated as such.

Cardiopulmonary resuscitation is briefly interrupted to allow an examination of the cardiac rhythm. The patient who has either ventricular fibrillation or pulseless ventricular tachycardia should have three successive countershocks in an attempt to defibrillate the heart. The first countershock is delivered at 200 Joules, the second at 200–300 Joules, and the third at 360 Joules. The caregiver pauses between shocks only long enough to examine the cardiac rhythm. If VF or pulseless VT persists or recurs following three shocks, the care team resumes CPR and obtains a definitive airway (intubation) and intravenous access if these tasks have not already been accomplished. Following unsuccessful defibrillation, a series of pharmacologic interventions may be performed to increase the likelihood of converting VF with defibrillation. After each drug is administered during resuscitation from VF, attempts at defibrillation should be repeated.

Epinephrine

As indicated in Fig 11-4, the initial drug given during resuscitation from VF or pulseless VT is epinephrine (at a dose of 1.0 mg). In addition to raising coronary and cerebral perfusion pressures during CPR, epinephrine may make ventricular fibrillation more susceptible to direct current countershock. This is likely an alpha agonist effect of epinephrine (Otto and Yakaitis, 1984). After intravenous administration of the epinephrine, CPR is continued for 30–60 seconds, and then 3 successive shocks are delivered at 360 Joules. The dose of epinephrine is then repeated at 3–5 minute intervals during the continued cardiac arrest.

Epinephrine is the first drug given to patients with VT/VF arrest because it is the only drug which has been clearly shown to make a difference in outcome from VT/VF arrest (Cummins, 1994). Following epinephrine, other medications which may be of benefit include lidocaine, procainamide, bretylium, amiodarone, magnesium sulfate, and sodium bicarbonate. If VF/VT persists after effective ventilation, chest compressions, intravenous epinephrine, and multiple defibrillation attempts, then the caregiver should administer an antifibrillatory agent such as lidocaine, bretylium or amiodarone. Lidocaine and bretylium have, in some studies, reduced the amount of energy necessary to defibrillate the heart (Kerber et al, 1986).

Lidocaine, Bretylium, Procainamide and Amiodarone

Lidocaine is the antiarrhythmic drug of first choice for malignant ventricular arrhythmias. The initial dose of lidocaine is 1.5 mg/kg with a second dose of 1.5 mg/kg given 3–5 minutes after the first for a total loading dose of 3.0 mg/kg. If defibrillation is successful following administration of bolus IV lidocaine, then an infusion of lidocaine is continued at 2–4 mg/min. Bretylium may be used for refractory VF after failure of lidocaine and defibrillation. The initial dose is 5 mg/kg with subsequent doses of 10 mg/kg every 5 minutes to a maximum dose of 30 mg/kg. If spontaneous circulation returns following administration of bretylium and defibrillation, then a continuous infusion of bretylium should be started at 1–2 mg/min. Rarely, a procainamide infusion may be of use in the setting of refractory VF. The recommended dosage is 30 mg/min up to a maximum dose of 17 mg/kg. The maintenance infusion of procainamide is 1–4 mg/min.

Amiodarone. Growing experience with amiodarone in less acute settings (Kowey et al, 1995) has led cardiologists and other clinicians to use this drug increasingly in the setting of resuscitation. Although not reflected in published algorithms, it is probably fair to suggest that, amiodarone, 150–300 mg IV over 15 min is a reasonable second line drug if lidocaine is ineffective. Repeat doses of 150 mg can be given, and/or an intravenous loading dose of 1 mg/min for 6 hr, then 0.5 mg/min thereafter for up to 48 hr.

Magnesium

Another medication that may be considered in the setting of refractory VT/VF is magnesium sulfate. Magnesium has, in some trials, reduced the incidence of VT/VF when given a prophylactic manner to patients who have sustained an acute myocardial infarction (Heesch, 1994). Because of this possible benefit in preventing VT/VF, many clinicians have advocated its use in the management of the VT/VF cardiac arrest (Tobey et al, 1992). This is likely of most benefit in those patients who are hypomagnesemic or in those whose VT has a torsades de pointes pattern. Magnesium sulfate 1–2 grams can be given as an intravenous bolus dose for the treatment of refractory VT in this scenario.

Buffers

Finally, sodium bicarbonate ($NaHCO_3$) or other buffer therapy is indicated in recurrent VT/VF only in certain circumstances. Known hyperkalemia or tricyclic antidepressant overdose are settings in which buffer therapy is appropriate. As intravenous administration of sodium bicarbonate generates large amounts of carbon dioxide, intracellular levels of carbon dioxide rapidly increase owing to the ease with which CO_2 can diffuse across cell membranes. This intracellular accumulation of CO_2, in the setting of diminished perfusion (CPR), may lead to worsened acidosis at the cellular level. The use of buffer agents to correct acidosis in the setting of cardiac arrest is controversial. This controversy is elaborated later in this chapter.

PULSELESS ELECTRICAL ACTIVITY

Although VT/VF is often the initial rhythm in the patient with cardiac arrest, clinicians may encounter pulseless electrical activity or asystole as the presenting rhythm. Pulseless electrical activity (PEA) or electromechanical dissociation (EMD) denotes a scenario wherein organized depolarization of the myocardium occurs in the absence of a palpable pulse or detectable blood pressure. The organized electrical complexes may be fast or slow, narrow or broad. As depicted in Fig 7-14 (page 206), this arrhythmia occurs in a number of specific clinical situations. It is incumbent upon the clinician to consider the possible causes of this arrhythmia as soon as it is recognized because each has a specific treatment or antidote that may prove to be life-saving. For instance, the most common cause of PEA is hypovolemia. This may be absolute hypovolemia such as hemorrhagic shock in which rapid volume replacement is indicated or relative hypovolemia such as occurs in cases of cardiac tamponade or tension pneumothorax in which case prompt pericardiocentesis or needle decompression is indicated.

As in all cases of cardiac arrest, the care team's priorities for the patient in PEA begin with the fundamentals of cardiopulmonary resuscitation. That is, the clinician establishes a patent airway, ventilates with 100% oxygen, and performs effective chest compressions. In addition to addressing the underlying cause for the arrest, the clinician may employ non-specific pharmacologic interventions. For instance, epinephrine 1.0 mg may be administered intravenously every 3–5 minutes to raise central aortic pressure during chest compressions and thus improve coronary and cerebral blood flow. If the patient's cardiac electrical activity is slow, atropine 1.0 mg IV every 3–5 minutes to a maximum dose of 40 μg/kg is acceptable. As in the VT/VF arrest, the use of buffer therapy is controversial. Clearly, for known hyperkalemia or preexisting acidosis sodium bicarbonate is likely a beneficial adjunct in treating PEA.

Asystole

Finally, asystole represents another initial presenting rhythm for the patient in cardiac arrest. In most clinical scenarios, this absence of organized electrical activity portends a very poor prognosis. The diagnosis of asystole should be confirmed in more than one lead to rule out an "isoelectric vector" of VF. If any doubt exists as to whether the rhythm represents fine ventricular fibrillation, it should be treated as VF because of the better chance of intact neurological survival in VF compared to asystole. Once CPR has been initiated the treatment of a bradyasystolic cardiac arrest is nonspecific pharmacologic therapy (epinephrine and atropine), while the care team searches for and attempts to correct underlying conditions responsible for the arrest (Fig 7-14, page 206).

Attempts at electrical defibrillation should not be utilized for asystolic rhythms. As some cases of asystolic arrest may be initiated and sustained by high levels of parasympathetic tone, electrical shocks may impart a higher degree of parasympathetic tone and thus preclude the heart from responding to any further therapeutic interventions. As depicted in Fig 7-14, cardiac pacing is a treatment option for select patients suffering a bradyasystolic arrest. Patients most likely to respond favorably to this intervention are hospitalized patients in whom the arrest is immediately recognized and treated with transcutaneous pacing.

CONTROVERSIES IN RESUSCITATION PHARMACOLOGY

While the algorithms for emergency cardiac care provide the clinician a structured response to the cardiac arrest patient, many of the pharmacologic agents recommended are not without controversy. In fact, controversy regarding selection of agents, dosing, and contraindications to use of some drugs persists despite extensive published basic and clinical science research devoted to this area. Pharmacologic controversies in cardiopulmonary resuscitation include use of adrenergic agonists, anticholinergic agents, antiarrhythmic agents, buffering agents, and calcium and magnesium.

Adrenergic Agonists

As previously indicated, adrenergic therapy is appropriate in the setting of cardiac arrest to improve coronary and cerebral perfusion pressure during chest compressions (Michael et al, 1984), and to make ventricular fibrillation more susceptible to direct countershock (Otto and Yakaitis, 1984). These agents are specifically indicated for cardiac arrest secondary to VF or pulseless VT, pulseless electrical activity, and asystole. Which agents are superior, what dose is optimal, and how they exert their observed effects are all controversial topics.

Alpha-Agonist Effects

Clearly, the most important pharmacologic action of an adrenergic agent used in resuscitation from cardiac arrest is its ability to stimulate alpha receptors. Alpha adrenergic receptor stimulation is responsible for maintaining vascular tone in the cardiac arrest patient. By increasing systemic arteriolar tone and redistributing blood from the peripheral to the central circulation, adrenergic agents elevate coronary and cerebral perfusion. The coronary perfusion pressure during CPR is an excellent predictor to the likelihood of resumption of spontaneous circulation in humans (Paradis, et al, 1990). Potential detrimental effects of agonist stimulation include marked systemic vasoconstriction, decreased cardiac output, and production of a metabolic (lactic) acidosis due to underperfusion of splanchnic and muscular capillary beds (Ornato, 1993).

Beta-Agonist Effects

The usefulness of beta adrenergic receptor stimulation during resuscitation is unclear. Potential detrimental myocardial effects include increases in heart rate and myocardial oxygen consumption. As many patients suffering cardiac arrest have atherosclerotic ischemic heart disease, use of an agent with β_1 agonist effects seems to be counterproductive under conditions of reduced myocardial oxygen supply (CPR). Some investigators have examined choice of adrenergic agonists during arrest conditions and have suggested that β_1 stimulation is either not helpful (Midei et al, 1990) or is harmful (Brown and Werman, 1990).

Epinephrine versus Pure Alpha Agonists

Epinephrine, a mixed alpha and beta adrenergic agonist is the recommended adrenergic agonist for use during cardiopulmonary resuscitation. Although epinephrine increases myocardial oxygen demand by receptor stimulation, it enhances oxygen supply to a greater extent. It more favorably affects the balance of myocardial oxygen supply and demand in animal models of cardiac arrest when compared to pure alpha agonists (Brown and Taylor, 1988). The beta agonist effects of epinephrine may also play a role in increasing cerebral blood flow during CPR. In animals, epinephrine produces a greater increase in regional cerebral blood flow than equipotent doses of phenylephrine (Brown and Werner, 1987) or methoxamine (Brown and Davis, 1987). Comparisons of pure alpha agonists to epinephrine for resuscitation from cardiac arrest in humans have failed to convincingly demonstrate a superiority of pure alpha agonists (Paradis and Koscove, 1990). None has proved more effective in producing neurologically intact outcome when compared to epinephrine.

Dose of Epinephrine

The traditional dose of epinephrine administered intravenously for cardiac arrest is 1.0 mg every 5 minutes during the resuscitation. This dose likely originates from anecdotal reports of intracardiac injections of epinephrine for cardiac arrest in the operating room (Beck and Rand, 1949). A dose-dependent pressor effect relationship for epinephrine has been described in both animals (Brunette and Jameson, 1990) and humans (Gonzalez, 1989) during CPR. In animals, the optimal response to epinephrine during cardiac arrest occurs in the dose range of 0.045–0.20 mg/kg (Cummins, 1994). This is a larger dose than that commonly used clinically for adult humans (0.0075–0.015 mg/kg) during CPR.

Clinical reports have suggested that higher doses of epinephrine may be beneficial in resuscitating humans from cardiac arrest. For instance, higher coronary perfusion pressures were documented using high dose epinephrine therapy in prolonged resuscitations attempts in adults when compared to traditional doses (Gonzalez et al, 1989). Improved survival to hospital discharge using high dose epinephrine (0.2 mg/kg) was reported in pediatric patients who failed to respond to two "standard" doses during resuscitation (Goetting and Paradisi, 1991).

The question of optimal dose of epinephrine in adults in cardiac arrest has been addressed in four multicenter, randomized, blinded, clinical trials (Linder et al, 1991; Stiell et al, 1992; Callahan et al, 1992; Brown and Martin, 1992). These trials failed to demonstrate any significant increase in survival rates to hospital discharge for those patients treated with high dose epinephrine compared to those treated with standard dose epinephrine. This was valid even for all subsets analyzed such as patients with VT/VF arrest, patients with short arrest to institution of therapy interval, and in-hospital compared with out of hospital arrests. Also noted in these studies was a lack of consistent adverse effects attributed to higher doses of epinephrine.

Based on observations made from laboratory and clinical studies, the initial dose of epinephrine given intravenously for adults in cardiac arrest should remain 1.0 mg

(10 ml of a 1:10,000 dilution). Subsequent doses of epinephrine may be increased at the discretion of the care team. Alternative dosing regimens are depicted on the AHA algorithms for emergency cardiac care and include an intermediate (2–5 mg IV), escalating (1, then 3, then 5 mg IV), or high (0.1 mg/kg) dose of epinephrine. As the peak effect following an intravenous bolus injection of epinephrine is achieved in 3–4 minutes during arrest conditions (Paradis et al, 1991), doses of this drug should be administered every 3–5 minutes of continued cardiac arrest to maintain drug effect.

Anticholinergic Agents

Another controversial topic in resuscitation pharmacology is the indication for and dosage of atropine in the cardiac arrest patient. Atropine, an antimuscarinic tertiary amine, produces clinical effects predominately by competitive inhibition of acetylcholine at muscarinic cholinergic receptors located in the heart, salivary glands, and smooth muscle of the gastrointestinal, genitourinary, and respiratory tracts. By virtue of its vagolytic effects on the heart, atropine increases heart rate and enhances conduction through the AV node. Atropine is more appropriate in the setting of cardiac arrest than other anticholinergics such as glycopyrrolate or scopolamine because it is more potent with respect to its ability to increase heart rate (Stoelting, 1991).

The heart's conducting system receives extensive sympathetic and parasympathetic neural input. High vagal tone, by suppressing cardiac automaticity, may play an important role in some forms of cardiac arrest. Anesthesiologists, in the operating theatre, are familiar with the severe bradycardia or bradyasystolic arrest that can occur during procedures invoking marked vagal stimulation (laryngoscopy, extraocular muscle traction, peritoneal traction).

Atropine is most effective in treating progressive symptomatic bradycardia or vagally-mediated hypotension in the patient who still has a pulse. Because ventricular asystole may represent the last stage of a progressive bradycardia, atropine is indicated for those patients who present with asystole to initiate or sustain cardiac electrical activity and to help restore atrioventricular conduction. It also may be helpful in the pharmacologic treatment of PEA. Usually, ventricular asystole in adults is a terminal rhythm indicating a severe myocardial hypoxic-ischemic insult that renders the myocardium unresponsive to any intervention. In studies of adults with asystole, atropine has failed to demonstrate an increased likelihood of restoring spontaneous circulation or improving long-term outcome (Gonzalez, 1993). However, because there is excellent theoretical basis for its use and little evidence to suggest detrimental effects in the setting of cardiac arrest, atropine should be given empirically for cardiac arrest when asystole or PEA is present.

Atropine dosage. When given for symptomatic bradycardia, atropine should be given in 0.5 mg doses intravenously every 5 minutes until a desired effect is reached. Doses less than 0.5 mg should not be administered to the adult patient because of paradoxical slowing of the heart that can occur secondary to weak central or peripheral parasympathomimetic effects of atropine (Kottmeier and Gravenstein, 1968). In those patients with severe bradycardia and myocardial ischemia or infarction, atropine should be used cautiously because of its ability to produce tachycardia, increased myocardial oxygen consumption, and ventricular fibrillation. For ventricular asystole or PEA, atropine should be given in 1.0 mg doses every 3–5 minutes during continued cardiac arrest. A maximal vagolytic dose in humans appears to be 0.04 mg/kg or approximately 3.0 mg in the 70 kg adult (Chamberlain et al, 1967).

Antiarrhythmic Agents in Resuscitation

Choice of antiarrhythmic therapy during resuscitation from cardiac arrest is an area that has been subject to intense laboratory and clinical investigation in the last decade. The premise for the use of antiarrhythmic agents in the setting of cardiac arrest is their demonstrated efficacy in the treatment of malignant ventricular arrhythmias in patients with myocardial ischemia. Although widely used in ventricular fibrillation and pulseless ventricular tachycardia, there is little scientific data to confirm or refute their efficacy in resuscitation from cardiac arrest (Jaffe, 1993).

Lidocaine and bretylium are the most common antiarrhythmic agents utilized for resuscitation from VF/VT. Lidocaine (Class 1B antiarrhythmic agent) is the first line choice in VF/VT refractory to electrical defibrillation and epinephrine. Although it does not have primary antifibrillatory effects (Harrison, 1981), lidocaine elevates the fibrillation threshold and can prevent recurrences of VF/VT after successful defibrillation. Lidocaine also increases the defibrillation threshold (Kerber, 1986). In contrast to lidocaine, bretylium (Class 3 antiarrhythmic agent) likely possesses primary antifibrillatory activity (Bacaner, 1968). Like lidocaine, bretylium raises the fibrillation threshold in cardiac tissue.

Two randomized controlled trials comparing lidocaine and bretylium in resuscitation of humans from ventricular fibrillation have demonstrated that these agents are probably of comparable efficacy (Haynes et al, 1981; Olson et al, 1984). Lidocaine should remain the "first line" agent in resuscitation for now because clinicians are apt to be more familiar with its dosage, pharmacologic effects, and potential adverse effects than for bretylium. Because reduced clearance of lidocaine occurs during the low blood flow state of CPR, a single 1.5 mg/kg dose will produce therapeutic plasma concentrations in adults for the duration of most resuscitations (Barsan et al, 1981).

In the published algorithms for malignant ventricular arrhythmias, bretylium appears as a second-line drug, after lidocaine. It has been suggested that bretylium and lidocaine act synergistically on the VF threshold (Hanyok et al, 1988). This reported synergism may warrant the use of these two medications sequentially in the setting of VT/VF arrest. For instance, after a 1.5 mg/kg IV dose of lidocaine and subsequent unsuccessful defibrillation in the adult patient suffering ventricular fibrillation, it may be beneficial to proceed to a 5 mg/kg dose of bretylium rather that repeating the same dose of lidocaine.

Consideration should be given to the use of *procainamide* in the scenario of recurrent malignant ventricular arrhythmias after the use of lidocaine and bretylium. Procainamide, a Class 1A antiarrhythmic, is an excellent drug for controlling ventricular arrhythmias after successful defibrillation but would rarely be of use in the full cardiac arrest because of the time required to establish an effective serum level. Rapid administration can result in hypotension and widening of the QRS complex, and ventricular function is depressed.

Amiodarone, a drug with multiple antiarrhythmic actions (i.e. Class I, II, III, and IV properties), has been successfully used in managing recurrent VF/VT and in treating supraventricular arrhythmias (Rothenberg, 1994). As already suggested, experience with this drug has convinced many clinicians that it might be the most appropriate second line drug (i.e. after failure of lidocaine). This is because acute administration has fewer adverse effects than bretylium (Kowey et al, 1995), there is very little tendency to proarrhythmia, little or no myocardial depression, and the drug appears to be very effective for prevention of both ventricular and supraventricular arrhythmias. The major unanswered question regarding amiodarone is the ability to achieve therapeutic tissue levels in the acute setting. Due to its high lipid solubility, in the treatment of chronic arrhythmias a long period of amiodarone administration (days) is required to achieve effective tissue levels. In the acute setting intravenous bolus dosing must be accompanied by a longer (i.e. 24–48 hour) intravenous loading to assure effective tissue concentrations. As more scientific evidence accumulates regarding the efficacy of amiodarone for the treatment of acute ventricular rhythm disturbances, amiodarone appears likely to supplant bretylium and procainamide in the algorithms for resuscitation of the patient with recurrent VT/VF.

Buffering Agents

Recommendations for the use of buffer therapy in the treatment of cardiopulmonary arrest have undergone substantial revision in the last decade. Other than treatment of hyperkalemic-associated cardiac arrest, buffer therapy probably adds little to the resuscitation of most patients from cardiac arrest. In fact, there is little scientific evidence to suggest that low blood pH impairs ability to defibrillate the heart, restore the rhythm, or that it confers poorer chance for neurologically intact survival (von Planta et al, 1993). It is important to appreciate the acid-base changes that occur during CPR when deciding whether to use buffer therapy for resuscitation from cardiac arrest.

Acid–Base Changes During CPR

Standard CPR along with use of epinephrine produces only 25% of normal cardiac output. The resultant tissue hypoperfusion leads to reduced oxygen delivery, increased anaerobic metabolism, and a progressive accumulation of tissue CO_2 and lactate. Carbon dioxide rapidly builds up in tissue and venous beds owing to its ongoing generation by tissue and poor elimination secondary to poor peripheral perfusion and decreased pulmonary elimination. Lactic acid will also accumulate and over time produce a metabolic lactic acidosis. Coincident with the hypercarbic venous acidemia is frequently a hypocarbic arterial alkalemia secondary to vigorous hyperventilation. This simultaneous venous acidemia and arterial alkalemia has been termed the "venoarterial paradox" (Grunaler et al, 1986).

As the accumulation of lactic acid is relatively slow, the tissue and venous hypercarbia is of principle importance in the setting of cardiac arrest. As carbon dioxide rapidly accumulates, it easily diffuses across cell membranes. Intracellular hypercarbic acidosis may occur fairly rapidly following cardiac arrest. In cardiac tissue, elevated carbon dioxide increases hydrogen ion content. The hydrogen ions compete with calcium for interaction with troponin and thus inhibit actin-myosin interactions. This interference with crossbridging may partially explain the observed contractile dysfunction of ischemic myocardium (von Planta et al, 1993).

Treatment Principles

Elimination of CO_2 is clearly a priority in resuscitation of the patient from cardiac arrest. This is best accomplished by providing effective ventilation and chest compressions, and restoring a spontaneous circulation as quickly as possible. Administration of a CO_2 generating buffer such as sodium bicarbonate during CPR may cause a tremendous increase in tissue CO_2 as it is poorly removed from tissue secondary to diminished perfusion. This may lead to a markedly worsened intracellular acidosis which can impair efforts to reestablish a spontaneous perfusing cardiac rhythm. When administered without epinephrine therapy, sodium bicarbonate given as an intravenous bolus frequently reduces coronary perfusion pressure thus negating potential benefit derived from the buffering action. Other adverse effects of bicarbonate therapy include hyperosomolality, hypernatremia, and leftward shifts of the oxyhemoglobin dissociation curve.

Treatment Options

In addition to sodium bicarbonate ($NaHCO_3$), other alkalizing options during CPR include inorganic buffers such as sodium carbonate (Na_2CO_3), organic buffers such as Tris-Hydroxy-Amino-Methan (THAM), and mixtures like Carbicarb ($NaHCO_3$ and Na_2CO_3) While these alternatives have a theoretical advantage over sodium bicarbonate because they do not generate CO_2, there is little current published clinical data that support the use of these as primary buffer therapy in the management of cardiac arrest. Furthermore, each alternative buffer has properties that would not be favorable during cardiac arrest. For instance, THAM is a potent vasodilator and may decrease the coronary perfusion pressure when given as a bolus while sodium carbonate solution has a very alkaline pH which may be injurious to tissue.

The strongest indication for bicarbonate therapy during resuscitation from cardiac arrest is known or suspected hyperkalemia. Other scenarios where buffer therapy may be helpful are in the patient with known pre-existing bicarbonate-responsive metabolic acidosis, or in the patient requiring alkalization of the blood (tricyclic antidepressant overdose) or urine (barbiturate overdose). Empiric administration of buffer therapy during prolonged resuscitation efforts or in the setting of hypoxic lactic acidosis likely offers little improvement in the chances of restoring a perfusing rhythm. Perhaps the best use of buffer therapy is after successful restoration of a spontaneous circulation. In this setting, sodium bicarbonate could be expected to help buffer the acid load that would be washed out of underperfused capillary beds. The generated CO_2 would then be eliminated effectively by the lungs because of the restoration of pulmonary perfusion.

When utilized during cardiac arrest, sodium bicarbonate should be given as an intravenous bolus at a dosage of 1 mEq/kg. One half of this initial dose can be repeated every 10 minutes of continued cardiac arrest. Once spontaneous circulation is restored, subsequent buffer therapy should be directed by results of arterial blood gas measurements.

Calcium

The intravenous administration of calcium to the patient suffering cardiac arrest is a concept that has naturally developed out of the understanding of the calcium ion's central role in cardiac muscle contraction. Calcium enters the sarcoplasm of the myocyte in response to electrical stimulation of the cell. This calcium entry into the cytoplasm of the cell comes from extracellular sources and from the sarcoplamic reticulum located inside the cell. Calcium facilitates the interaction between actin and myosin filaments, promotes myofibril shortening, and thus plays an important role in the coupling of myocyte excitation to myocyte contraction.

Exogenous calcium administration increases cardiac inotropy in the setting of ionized hypocalcemia and increases systemic vascular resistance when serum ionized calcium levels are normal (Drop, 1985). Clinical studies examining the effectiveness of calcium administration during PEA or asystole have not shown consistent favorable improvement in outcome. Calcium's inotropic and vasopressor characteristics might be beneficial during cardiac arrest, but there are also potential detrimental effects in administering calcium. For instance, excessive cellular calcium can potentiate reperfusion injury of ischemic myocardium (Katz and Reuter, 1979), and can diminish the inotropic and vasoconstrictive effects of catecholamines (Zaloga et al, 1990). Hypercalcemia can lead to severe arrhythmias, particularly life-threatening bradycardias, and may exacerbate digoxin toxicity.

Thus, calcium should only be given to the cardiac arrest patient with known or suspected ionized hypocalcemia or to those patients who have hyperkalemia or hypermagnesemia. Calcium administration does not lower serum potassium or magnesium levels but rather reverses the adverse cardiac electrophysiologic effects of hyperkalemia or hypermagnesemia. Calcium may also be of value in treating calcium channel blocker overdosage.

Either calcium chloride or calcium gluconate may be administered. *Calcium chloride* is preferable as it has increase bioavailability when compared to calcium gluconate (Broner et al, 1990). An initial dose of 8–10 mg/kg has been recommended by the American Heart Association for the treatment of hyperkalemic cardiac arrest (AHA, 1992). A dose of 4–5 mg/kg may be more appropriate in other settings. The dose of calcium chloride may be repeated every ten minutes of continued cardiac arrest. Calcium should only be administered into central veins as its extravasation into peripheral subcutaneous tissue can produce a severe chemical burn.

Magnesium

Magnesium is an important cofactor of numerous enzyme systems. Hypomagnesemia may lead to reduced sodium-potassium ATPase activity. This enzyme is responsible for establishing and maintaining intracellular to extracellular gradients of sodium and potassium. With alteration of potassium homeostasis, the depolarization and repolarization of cardiac tissue can occur abnormally. Thus, magnesium deficiency can be associated with cardiac arrhythmias because of its indirect effect on potassium homeostasis or because of a direct electrophysiologic effect from the ion (Zaritsky, 1994).

There has been much enthusiasm for the use of magnesium in the resuscitation of the patient with ventricular fibrillation. The use of magnesium during ACLS stems from studies that have documented its efficacy in suppressing supraventricular and ventricular arrhythmias after acute myocardial infarction. An appropriate dose in the treatment of ventricular fibrillation or pulseless ventricular tachycardia is 2 grams of magnesium sulfate given as an intravenous bolus. For treatment of atrial or ventricular ectopy, 1–2 grams of magnesium sulfate may be administered intravenously over 10–15 minutes.

ICU MANAGEMENT

While management of the cardiac arrest patient is extremely important, the clinician has a much better opportunity to favorably influence patient outcome by preventing cardiopulmonary arrest in the unstable patient. Similarly, effective stabilization of the patient after successful resuscitation from cardiac arrest is necessary to limit end-organ damage

SHOCK, HYPOTENSION, PULMONARY EDEMA

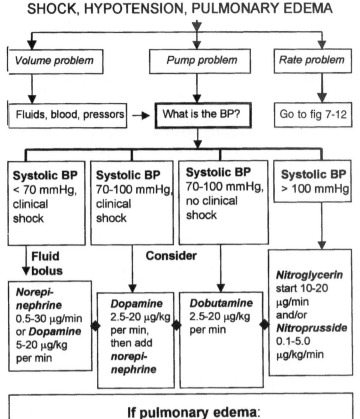

*Fig 11-5. Algorithm for shock, hypotension, pulmonary edema.
Management is based on clinical assessment. Simplified from original
algorithm: for detail see Journal of the American Medical Association,
1992; 268:2199–22410. Reproduced with permission.*

initiated by the low flow state associated with the arrest. In
this section, acute management of conditions commonly
leading to cardiac arrest: "shock", myocardial infarction,
and arrhythmias is presented.

Shock

The common factor in all "shock states" is inadequate tissue oxygenation. This is manifest clinically by confusion or
obtundation, signs of peripheral vasoconstriction (pallor,
coolness), hypotension, tachycardia, and oliguria. Although
a complete description of different classifications of shock is
beyond the scope of this chapter, a simplified approach is
to attempt to ascribe the primary mechanism for the shock
state to absolute or relative hypovolemia, cardiac failure,
vasodilatation, or heart rate and rhythm abnormalities
(Fig 11-5).

Initial Therapy

The clinician must usually initiate therapy based on physical examination findings, noninvasive blood pressure

recordings, and pulse rate. If a patient is hypovolemic or markedly vasodilated (sepsis) and hypotensive, initial therapy is volume resuscitation. Vasopressor support with drugs such as dopamine or norepinephrine may also be appropriate as a temporizing or adjunctive therapy to complement volume resuscitation. The hypotensive patient with presumed cardiogenic shock is most appropriately first treated with a combined and adrenergic agonist such as dopamine or epinephrine. In cardiogenic shock with normal to elevated blood pressure, initial therapy might include an agent capable of reducing afterload (nitroprusside) or one that is both an inotrope and vasodilator (dobutamine, amrinone, milrinone). Therapy should be guided by measurements from a pulmonary artery catheter when possible. Finally, clinical shock produced by cardiac arrhythmia may be reversed by terminating the arrhythmia.

Shock can result from several simultaneous underlying causes and may not fit into a typical hemodynamic pattern. For instance, septic shock can occur in the patient experiencing an exacerbation of congestive heart failure secondary to ischemic cardiomyopathy. In complex clinical scenarios, use of a pulmonary artery should be considered.

Invasive Monitoring

By measuring the pulmonary artery occlusion pressure (PAOP) and cardiac index (CI), a characteristic hemodynamic pattern for each type of shock may be identified. When available, bedside transthoracic or transesophageal echocardiography yields additional diagnostic information. Echo images allow the clinician to "see" ventricular function and volume, and valvular function. Early hypovolemic shock is characterized by a low PAOP and low CI. Cardiac echocardiography would reveal hypovolemia by demonstrating a small ventricular cavity size at end-diastole. Cardiogenic shock presents with high filling pressures (PAOP), associated with a low CI. An echocardiogram in this setting may reveal global or regional myocardial wall motion abnormalities and ventricular dilation. It may reveal valvular pathology that is contributing to the cardiac failure. Finally, the patient with vasogenic or "distributive" shock has a low PAOP and high CI demonstrating a hypercontractile, "empty" heart. These diagnostic tools allow the clinician to administer appropriate treatment, and to monitor its effect.

Volume Resuscitation

While the underlying cause for hypovolemic or distributive shock is being identified, intravascular volume expansion should be performed. In many patients, the end point or guiding parameter can be the blood pressure and heart rate. In patients with cardiac disease or complex problems, intravascular pressure measurement (PAOP) should be performed. Initial fluids should be crystalloid, followed by colloids and red blood cells as required. In cardiogenic shock, fluid administration must be cautious, and should be guided by PAOP measurements.

Inotropic Support (Table 3-1)

Dopamine is an excellent first choice for many shock states because of its combined agonist effects. Starting at a dose of 2.5 µg/kg/min and titrating upward through the "beta agonist range" (5–10 µg/kg/min) then predominately "alpha range" (up to 20 µg/kg/min), the salutary or detrimental hemodynamic effects of primarily beta adrenergic and then alpha adrenergic stimulation from a single drug are observed. If greater than 20 µg/kg/min of dopamine is required to maintain the cardiac output and blood pressure, the clinician should consider the use of a more potent agent such as norepinephrine or epinephrine. Because dopamine acts in part by stimulated release of endogenous norepinephrine from nerve terminals, its use may be associated with diminished drug effect over time (tachyphylaxis). Changing to norepinephrine or epinephrine may be indicated, especially with doses of dopamine exceeding 10 µg/kg/min. Finally, concomitant use of "renal dose" (2 µg/kg/min) dopamine with other inotropes in an attempt to preserve urine output appears to be a reasonable. Whether or not this therapy affects renal blood flow in the presence of potent alpha agents is controversial.

Dobutamine, a synthetic, pure beta agonist, is appropriate therapy for the patient in cardiogenic shock. In the dose range of 5–20 µg/kg/min, dobutamine could be expected to raise the cardiac output while possibly also lowering the blood pressure. As such, dobutamine has often been classified an "inodilator". The non-catecholamine inotropes that work by phosphodiesterase inhibition (amrinone and milrinone), are also inodilators with similar hemodynamic effects. Amrinone is administered as a loading dose of 0.75-1.5 mg/kg over 30-40 minutes, followed by an infusion of 5-20 µg/kg/min. The milrinone loading dose should be 0.05 mg/kg (over 30-40 minutes) followed by an infusion of 0.5-0.75 µg/kg/min. Phosphodiesterase inhibitor therapy can be combined with other adrenergic agents for additive treatment of cardiogenic shock. Also, by using an adrenergic agent with some alpha agonist activity, the principal adverse hemodynamic side effect of use of milrinone and amrinone (lowered blood pressure) can be avoided or minimized.

For the patient whose shock state is principally secondary to peripheral vasodilatation (sepsis, spinal shock), use of a mixed alpha and beta agonist agent may prove helpful in providing vasoconstriction and increased inotropy. Norepinephrine or "alpha range" dopamine (10-20 µg/kg/min) are appropriate choices. Pure alpha agonists such as phenylephrine or methoxamine should rarely be employed in shock states. Their use may be associated with excessive arteriolar vasoconstriction resulting in inadequate organ perfusion or depressed cardiac output.

Monitoring Adequacy of Resuscitation

Monitoring the PAOP and CI give objective evidence of the adequacy of global perfusion. Clinical signs of improved perfusion and oxygenation include cleared sensorium, normalized blood pressure and heart rate, warm extremities with brisk capillary refill, and increased urine output. Unfortunately, global or nonspecific indices of perfusion do not reliably indicate whether specific organs are resuscitated. An example is the elevated CI and mixed venous oxygen saturation seen in sepsis despite the development of lactic acidosis and multiple organ failure. Recently, a gastrointestinal tonometry device has been used to assess the pH of the stomach mucosa (Mythen and Webb, 1995). In critically ill patients, decreases in gastric mucosal pH were associated with a poorer outcome. Currently, tonometry must be considered experimental; however, it presents the possibility of clinical assessment to adequacy of specific organ (GI) perfusion.

ACUTE MYOCARDIAL INFARCTION

Most cases of cardiac arrest are due to myocardial infarction. Once resuscitated, the patient should be transferred to a critical care setting for continuous cardiovascular monitoring and appropriate therapy or intervention. Patients with new onset chest pain (i.e. unstable angina or suspected myocardial infarction) should be managed similarly. Supplemental oxygen therapy delivers more oxygen to the ischemic myocardium and should be given to all patients with known or suspected myocardial ischemia or infarction.

Treatment of myocardial infarction or patients with unstable angina should be guided by a cardiologist and should follow a defined protocol. The American College of Cardiology and American Heart Association have published detailed practice guidelines for acute myocardial infarction (Ryan et al 1996). The initial priority is to relieve ischemia and pain, with first-line therapy being organic nitrates, followed by opioids. Rapid treatment may limit ischemic damage and infarct size. In addition to immediate medical therapy, early aggressive attempts to revascularize the heart are appropriate for some patients. This may be in the form of thrombolytic therapy, percutaneous transluminal angioplasty, or even emergency coronary artery bypass grafting.

Early Revascularization by Thrombolytic Therapy

Early use of thrombolytic agents can limit or prevent myocardial necrosis caused by acute thrombosis in coronary arteries. Both intravenous and intracoronary injection can be effective. Urokinase, streptokinase, anistreplase and tissue plasminogen activator (TPA) are enzymes capable of producing in-vivo thrombolysis. Dosing of these potent thrombolytic agents should be guided by institutional-specific protocols. Contraindications include active hemorrhage, traumatic CPR, recent surgery, head trauma or cerebrovascular accident.

In patients with a large, anterior myocardial infarction or ongoing ischemia, anticoagulation with heparin is indicated. In the former case, intracardiac clot formation (as a result of ventricular wall akinesis) is inhibited and in the latter, intracoronary thrombosis is prevented. Oral aspirin is effective in inhibiting platelet aggregation, and can significantly reduce mortality in acute myocardial infarction if given within 24 hours of the first symptoms (ISIS 2, 1989).

Percutaneous Transluminal Coronary Angioplasty (PTCA)

For the patient with contraindications to thrombolytic therapy, early use of PTCA offers an alternative method of restoring flow to an acutely occluded coronary artery. Other candidates for "early angioplasty" are patients with previous coronary artery bypass grafting with new onset ischemia from graft closure, or the hospitalized patient who develops new onset ischemia. Performed in the cardiac catheterization laboratory, angioplasty entails percutaneously placing a small balloon into an occluded or nearly occluded coronary artery. By intermittently inflating the balloon, the obstruction can frequently be resolved.

Medical Therapy of AMI: Nitrates

Nitroglycerin has a number of beneficial effects in the setting of myocardial ischemia. Via release of nitric oxide, nitroglycerin produces vascular smooth muscle relaxation. This effect predominates in the venous system and the hemodynamic result is decreased venous return, diminished left ventricular volume and wall tension, and thus decreased myocardial oxygen consumption. Nitroglycerin also dilates epicardial coronary arteries, antagonizes coronary vasospasm, and improves collateral blood flow to ischemic myocardium. All of these actions may restore a more favorable balance between myocardial oxygen supply and demand. Nitrates can be given sublingually, intravenously, or topically (Table 10-7, page 292). One approach to using nitrates is to give 0.3 mg of nitroglycerin sublingually every 5 minutes until pain control is achieved. Intravenous nitroglycerin can then be started at 10 μg/min and titrated upward in 10 μg increments every 3–5 minutes until pain control is achieved. Top dose may be 200 μg/min or even higher.

Important potential adverse effects of nitrate therapy during cardiac ischemia must be appreciated. Nitroglycerin is a potent venodilator and weak arterial vasodilator, and causes hypotension in some patients. A reduction in coronary perfusion pressure could reduce myocardial oxygen supply to a greater extent than the reduction in oxygen demand. Hypovolemia exacerbates nitroglycerin induced hypotension, and volume infusion to correct hypovolemia minimizes the adverse hemodynamic effects of nitroglycerin. Other potential detrimental effects of nitroglycerin include inhibition of hypoxic pulmonary vasoconstriction which may cause hypoxemia, and methemoglobinemia. Tachyphylaxis is observed with continuous treatment.

Opioids in AMI

If nitroglycerin does not fully relieve chest pain, opioid drugs should be given. Morphine 2–4 mg IV every 5–10 minutes until pain is diminished or relieved is one effective regimen. In addition to pain relief, morphine produces favorable hemodynamic changes in the patient with ischemia. By release of histamine, morphine causes increased venous capacitance and reduced blood pressure. These changes can reduce the heart's oxygen demand. Because of these expected changes in hemodynamics, morphine should be used cautiously in the hypovolemic or hypotensive patient.

Beta Adrenergic Blockers

Beta blocker therapy is another treatment modality that is usually beneficial for the patient with acute myocardial ischemia or infarction. By reducing heart rate, blood pressure, and myocardial contractility, beta blockers reduce myocardial oxygen consumption and thus can likely limit the size of the myocardial infarction (Antman, 1992). Because of its depressant effect on the heart, β-adrenergic blockade should be carefully initiated in the setting of acute myocardial infarction. Hypotension, bradycardia, and cardiogenic shock are contraindications to use of beta blockers. A brief trial of the ultra short acting beta blocker, esmolol, is one method to assess the effect of beta blockade in the patient with suspected marginal cardiac reserve. If 0.25–0.5 mg/kg of esmolol does not produce adverse hemodynamic changes, then beta blockade can usually safely be continued. As the elimination half life of esmolol is approximately nine minutes, an infusion (50–200 μg/kg/min) must be started following the loading dose for continued drug effect with esmolol. Alternatively, a more practical approach is to administer a longer acting beta blocker. Metoprolol, atenolol, or propranolol are suitable agents. One effective dosing regimen is to administer metoprolol 2.5 mg IV every 2–5 minutes up to a maximum of 15 mg to achieve a heart rate in the 60s. The intravenous dose required to produce this heart rate is then repeated every 6–8 hours.

ACE inhibitors in AMI

When there is overt clinical heart failure in early phase AMI, their use is essential (AIRE study, Ch 10). A new trend is to use ACE inhibitors for all patients at enhanced risk of early death, including diabetics, hypertensives, and those with prior infarcts or higher heart rates or anterior infarcts (Pfeffer, 1998).

Antiarrhythmic Agents in AMI

Although supraventricular or ventricular arrhythmias may arise as complications of acute myocardial infarction, most current scientific evidence discourages the routine use of drugs in a prophylactic manner to prevent these arrhythmias. For instance, *lidocaine*, once touted as an effective prophylactic measure to prevent ventricular tachycardia/

ventricular fibrillation in acute myocardial infarction, has not been shown to change mortality rates in this setting (Jaffe, 1992). Lidocaine should be used when ventricular ectopy results in hypotension, syncope, or angina. It also should be employed when the following ECG patterns of premature ventricular contractions (PVCs) are recognized: 1.) multifocal PVCs 2.) PVCs that occur in couplets or triplets 3.) >6 PVCs per minute and 4.) PVCs that fall on the T wave of the preceding beat (Cummins, 1994). Each of these conditions may be a harbinger of future malignant ventricular arrhythmias. In this situation, lidocaine therapy is initiated with a 1.0–1.5 mg/kg bolus followed by a continuous infusion of 2–4 mg/min. Additional boluses of 0.5–0.75 mg/kg may be given up to a maximum of 3.0 mg/kg if initial dosing does not control the ventricular ectopy.

Magnesium sulfate is another agent that has been considered for routine use in patients with acute myocardial infarction. Initial enthusiasm for use of magnesium in the setting of myocardial infarction came from trials that documented improved survival in those patients treated with magnesium (Woods, 1987). While it was speculated that magnesium provided a benefit via an antiarrhythmic effect, a large study has neither confirmed improved survival nor documented a decreased incidence of arrhythmias (ISIS, 1993). Magnesium deficiency is associated with arrhythmia and sudden cardiac death (Chippenfield, 1973), therefore magnesium sulfate (1–2 grams IV over 15 minutes) should be given to the myocardial infarction patient with documented or even suspected magnesium deficiency. As previously described, magnesium has a well documented role in the treatment of "torsades de pointes" ventricular tachycardia.

Mechanical Adjuncts: Intra-Aortic Balloon Pump (IABP)

In the patient's with ongoing ischemia refractory to pharmacologic therapy, the placement of an IABP should be considered. This device reduces left ventricular afterload and increases diastolic perfusion pressure, often eliminating refractory angina. Once the pain is controlled, elective coronary angiography can be performed to guide further intervention (i.e. thrombolysis, angioplasty, or bypass surgery).

CARDIAC ARRHYTHMIAS

The initial evaluation of the patient with a cardiac rhythm disturbance requires that the clinician make a judgment as to whether or not the patient has signs of hemodynamic compromise. This judgment dictates if there is time for further workup and testing and determines the rapidity with which therapy is instituted. Immediate, definitive treatment is required when the patient has confusion, lapse of consciousness, angina, acute onset of pulmonary edema, significant hypotension, or other evidence of shock.

Tachyarrhythmia

An initial approach for the patient with a tachyarrhythmia is given in Fig 7-12 (page 203). For the patient with hemodynamic compromise, the caregiver should proceed immediately to synchronized cardioversion (Fig 11-6). If time permits, the patient is given an amnestic and an analgesic prior to cardioversion. For the patient with stable hemodynamics, the clinician should initiate pharmacologic interventions based on the type of arrhythmia.

Atrial Fibrillation / Atrial Flutter

The initial goal in treatment of atrial fibrillation or atrial flutter with rapid ventricular response is to control the ventricular rate. This is best accomplished with the use of an intravenous calcium channel blocker (diltiazem or verapamil) or beta blocker (esmolol). Once the ventricular rate is controlled, synchronized cardioversion (Fig 11-6) or pharmacologic methods may be utilized to convert the arrhyth-

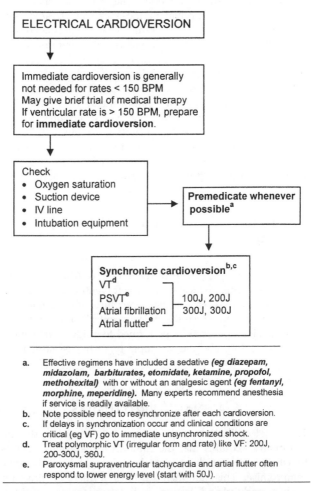

a. Effective regimens have included a sedative *(eg diazepam, midazolam, barbiturates, etomidate, ketamine, propofol, methohexital)* with or without an analgesic agent *(eg fentanyl, morphine, meperidine).* Many experts recommend anesthesia if service is readily available.
b. Note possible need to resynchronize after each cardioversion.
c. If delays in synchronization occur and clinical conditions are critical (eg VF) go to immediate unsynchronized shock.
d. Treat polymorphic VT (irregular form and rate) like VF: 200J, 200-300J, 360J.
e. Paroxysmal supraventricular tachycardia and artial flutter often respond to lower energy level (start with 50J).

Fig 11-6. Electrical Cardioversion Algorithm (for the patient not in cardiac arrest). (Reproduced with permission, Journal of the American Medical Association 1992;268:2199–2241) Use of propofol for sedation did not appear in the published algorithm, and is an alternative to the other drugs listed. BPM = beats per minute.

mia back to sinus rhythm. Quinidine or procainamide are Type IA antiarrhythmics which may be effective in converting these rhythms. Recently *ibutilide*, a short-acting class III drug has become available for the chemical conversion of new onset atrial fibrillation or flutter. This drug appears to be effective in 40–50% of cases, with greater efficacy for flutter than fibrillation (Stambler et al, 1996). There is a risk of proarrhythmia (polymorphic ventricular tachycardia), especially in patients with reduced ventricular function and/or preexisting ventricular arrhythmias.

Digoxin. While useful for the control of ventricular rate in chronic atrial fibrillation, the onset of action of intravenous digoxin may be 30–60 minutes. This makes digoxin of questionable value in urgent rate control for new atrial fibrillation and atrial flutter. The clinician should appreciate the potential for intracardiac thrombus formation in the patient with atrial fibrillation of several days duration. In this circumstance, systemic anticoagulation is warranted to diminish the risk of arterial embolization once sinus rhythm is reestablished.

Paroxysmal Supraventricular Tachycardia (PSVT)

Initial therapy of PSVT may be non-pharmacologic. By performing carotid sinus massage on the patient with PSVT, the clinician can increase vagal output to the AV node and effectively terminate the reentry cycle. Carotid sinus massage and other vagal maneuvers such as facial immersion in cold water, and Valsalva maneuver should only be performed on a patient with continuous monitoring. The risk of performing carotid massage (i.e. syncope, embolic or ischemic stroke, asystole) (Cummins, 1994) must be appreciated by the clinician. The first-line pharmacologic therapy of PSVT is adenosine. The dose of adenosine is 6.0 mg given as a rapid IV bolus. This dose is then doubled in two minutes if there has been no effect. If adenosine fails to convert PSVT, then other appropriate therapy may include verapamil, diltiazem, digoxin, or beta blockers. Use of intravenous β-blocker therapy and intravenous calcium channel blockers within 30 minutes of one another is contraindicated because high grade atrioventricular block, bradycardia, or asystole blockers may result. If at any time the patient becomes hemodynamically unstable, synchronized cardioversion is the therapy of choice.

Ventricular Tachycardia (VT)

The treatment of known or suspected VT depends on the presence or absence of hemodynamic stability. Pulseless VT is treated like ventricular fibrillation with CPR, defibrillation, epinephrine, then antiarrhythmic medications. Ventricular tachycardia in the patient with a pulse but with signs of circulatory compromise (altered mental status, hypotension, angina) is treated with immediate synchronized cardioversion (Fig 11-6). The treatment of choice for VT in the hemodynamically stable patient is a series of antiarrhythmic agents (Fig 7-12, page 203). Lidocaine is utilized first, fol-

lowed by procainamide, bretylium or amiodarone if lidocaine is unsuccessful. As with the other tachyarrhythmias,
elective synchronized cardioversion is indicated in the
stable patient if none of the pharmacologic measures prove
helpful.

Wide Complex Arrhythmias of Unknown Etiology

It may be difficult to tell whether a wide-complex tachyarrhythmia represents ventricular tachycardia or a supraventricular tachycardia with aberrant ventricular conduction.
Although there are a number of subtle electrocardiographic
differences between the two, in an urgent clinical scenario,
it should be assumed that the arrhythmia is ventricular
tachycardia and treatment should be intravenous lidocaine.
If lidocaine is unsuccessful, a trial of adenosine is acceptable, as it may convert the wide complex rhythm if it originates in the atria (Fig 7-11, page 198). As verapamil has
been reported to cause death in the patient with VT (Cummins, 1994), it should never be used to treat a wide-complex tachyarrhythmia.

Bradyarrhythmia

Regardless of the type of bradycardia, if signs or symptoms
of hemodynamic compromise are present, the clinician
should proceed directly to cardiac pacing. Otherwise, first-
line pharmacologic therapy consists of atropine or cathecholamines with beta-1 agonist effects (Fig 7-12).

Those patients who are asymptomatic, yet have bradycardia secondary to Type II second degree atrioventricular
block (AVB) or third degree AVB, should have a temporary
transvenous pacing wire placed. In this type of AVB at the
His-Purkinje level, there is an increased risk of progression
to either complete heart block or cardiac arrest.

Transcutaneous Pacing (TCP)

TCP is an option for treating the symptomatic bradycardia
that, if readily available, can be instituted as quickly as giving medications. In addition to being an effective primary
therapy, TCP can serve as a "back up" while transvenous
pacing is accomplished. Because TCP is often uncomfortable to the awake patient, amnestic/sedatives (benzodiaze-
penes) and analgesics (narcotics) serve as useful adjuncts in
treatment.

Atropine

The anticholinergic agent, atropine, is first-line pharmacologic therapy for symptomatic bradycardia. The adult patient
should be given a dose of 0.5–1.0 mg of IV atropine every
3 minutes of continued severe bradycardia until a maximum dose of 40 µg/kg is reached. As previously discussed,
caution should be exercised in giving the patient with acute
myocardial infarction atropine because of the drug's propensity to greatly increase myocardial oxygen demand if
tachycardia results.

Catecholamine Therapy

Alternatively, an infusion of a catecholamine that possesses beta-1 agonist properties is often an effective treatment of symptomatic bradycardia because of the positive chronotropy that results. Epinephrine (1–2 μg/min) and dopamine (5–20 μg/kg/min) are preferable to the pure beta-agonist agent isoproterenol. The former two cathecholamines tend to better support blood pressure secondary to agonist effects.

SUMMARY

1. *The pathophysiology of cardiac arrest* and its immediate consequences must be understood, as well as the principles of resuscitation. These are essential for the practice of anesthesia. A large body of evidence indicates that early, effective cardiopulmonary resuscitation techniques can improve outcome.

2. *Basic life support* (chest compressions and ventilation) provides critical oxygen to the tissues, while more advanced techniques aid in diagnosis and treatment of specific pathologies.

3. *Algorithms* designed to rapidly deal with specific situations are endorsed by national and international groups. These algorithms standardize the language of resuscitation and incorporate the most recent knowledge regarding routes of administration, specific techniques and drugs.

4. *Epinephrine and lidocaine* are widely known therapies that continue to form the first line of attack in asystole and ventricular arrhythmias (respectively).

5. *Newer techniques* such as transcutaneous pacing for asystole and intravenous amiodarone for refractory arrhythmias appear to provide additional benefit.

6. *Some previously standard therapies* such as sodium bicarbonate for acidosis, are now controversial.

7. *Aftercare.* Once a patient has been resuscitated from a life threatening episode, continued monitoring and therapy, and early intervention in the presence of acute myocardial infarction, are essential in order to prevent further life threatening events.

REFERENCES

AHA (American Heart Association) Emergency Cardiac Care Committee. Guidelines for cardiopulmonary resuscitation and emergency cardiac care. Part III. Adult advanced cardiac life support. *JAMA*, 1992; 268: 2199–2241.

Antman EM, Lau J, Kupelnick B, et al. A comparison of results of meta-analysis of randomized control trials and recommendations of clinical experts: treatments for myocardial infarction. *JAMA*. 1992; 208: 240–248.

Bacaner MB: Treatment of ventricular fibrillation and other acute arrhythmias with bretylium tosylate. *Am J Cardiol* 1968; 21: 530–543.

Barsan WG, Levy RC and Weir H. Lidocaine levels during CPR: Differences after peripheral venous, central venous, and intracardiac injection. *Ann Emerg Med*. 1981; 10: 73–78.

Beck CS and Rand HJ III. Cardiac arrest during anesthesia and surgery. *JAMA*. 1949; 141: 1230–1233.

Broner C, Stidham G, Westen D and Watson D. A prospective, randomized, double-blind comparison of calcium chloride and calcium gluconate therapies for hypocalcemia in critically ill children. *J Pediatr* 117: 986–989, 1990.

Brown CG, Davis EA, Werner HA and Hamlin RL. Methoxamine versus epinephrine on regional cerebral blood flow during cardiopulmonary resuscitation. *Crit Care Med* 1987; 15: 682–686.

Brown CG, Martin DR, Pepe PE, et al. A comparison of standard-dose and high-dose epinephrine in cardiac arrest outside the hospital: the Multicenter High-dose Epinephrine Study Group. *N Engl J Med* 1992: 327: 1051–1055.

Brown CG, Taylor RB, Werman HA, et al. Myocardial oxygen delivery/ consumption during cardiopulmonary resuscitation: A comparison of epinephrine and phenylephrine. *Ann Emerg Med* 1988; 17: 302–308.

Brown CG and Werman HA. Adrenergic agonists during cardiopulmonary resuscitation: Collective review. *Resuscitation* 1990; 19: 1–16.

Brown CG, Werner HA, Davis EA, et al. The effect of high dose phenylephrine versus epinephrine on regional cerebral blood flow during CPR. *Ann Emerg Med* 1987; 16: 743–748.

Brunette DD and Jameson SJ. Comparison of standard versus high dose epinephrine in the resuscitation of cardiac arrest in dogs. *Ann Emerg Med* 1990; 19: 8–11.

Callahan M, Madsen CD, Barton CW, et al. A randomized clinical trial of high-dose epinephrine and norepinephrine vs standard-dose epinephrine in prehospital cardiac arrest. *JAMA* 1992; 268: 2667–2672.

Chamberlain DA, Turner P and Sneddon JM. Effects of atropine on heart rate in healthy man. *Lancet* 1967; 1: 12–15.

Chandra, N C. Mechanisms of Blood Flow During CPR. *Ann Emerg Med* 1993; 22 (pt 2): 281–288.

Cheung J, Bonventre J, Malis C and Leaf A. Calcium and ischemic injury. *N Engl J. Med* 314:1670–1676, 1986.

Chipperfield B. Heart-muscle magnesium, potassium, and zinc concentrations after sudden death from heart disease. *Lancet*. 2(824): 293–6, 1973.

Cummins R.O. (editor). *Textbook of Advanced Cardiac Life Support*. American Heart Association; Dallas, Texas, 1994.

Cummins RO and Chamberlain DA (Co-chairs). Advisory Statements of the International Liason Committee on Resuscitation. *Circulation* 1997; 95:2172–2212.

Cummins RO. From concept to standard-of-care? Review of the clinical experience with automated external defibrillators. *Ann Emerg Med* 1989; 18: 1269–1275.

Ditchey RV, Winkler JV and Rhodes CA. Relative lack of coronary blood flow during closed chest resuscitation in dogs. *Circulation* 1982; 66: 297–302.

Drop L. Ionized calcium, the heart, and hemodynamic function. *Anesth Analg* 64: 432–451, 1985.

Goetting MG and Paradis NA. High dose epinephrine improves outcome from pediatric cardiac arrest. *Ann Emerg Med* 20: 22–26, 1991.

Gonzalez ER; Ornato JP, Garnett AR, et al. Dose-dependent vaso-pressor response to epinephrine during CPR in humans. *Ann Emerg Med*, 1989; 18: 920–926.

Gonzalez GR. Pharmacologic controversies in CPR. *Ann Emerg Med* 1993; 22 (2): 317–323.

Grunaler WG, Weil MH and Rackow EC. Arteriovenous carbon dioxide and pH gradients during cardiac arrest. *Circulation* 1986; 74: 1071–1074.

Hanyok J, Chow MSS, Kluger J, et al. Antifibrillatory effects of high dose bretylium and a lidocaine-bretylium combination during cardiopulmonary resuscitation. *Crit Care Med* 1988; 691–694.

Harrison EE. Lidocaine in prehospital countershock refractory ventricular fibrillation. *Ann Emerg Med* 1981; 10: 420–423.

Haynes RE, Chinn TL, Copass MK, et al. Comparison of bretylium tosylate and lidocaine in management of out-of-hospital ventricular fibrillation: A randomized clinical trial. *Am J. Cardiol* 1981; 48: 353–356.

Heesch R. Magnesium in acute myocardial infarction. *Ann Emerg Med* 1994; 24: 1154–60.

Hinkle LE Jr and Thaler HT. Clinical Classification of Cardiac Deaths. *Circulation* 1982; 65:457–464.

ISIS Collaborative Group. ISIS-2. A randomized trials of intravenous streptokinase, oral aspirin, both or neither among 17187 cases of suspected acute myocardial infarction. *Lancet* 1988; 2: 349–360.

ISIS Collaborative Group. ISIS-4. A randomized factorial trial assessing early oral captopril, oral mononitrate, and intravenous magnesium in 58,050 patients with suspected acute myocardial infarction. *Lancet* 1995; 345: 669–685.

Jaffe AS. Prophylactic lidocaine for suspected acute myocardial infarction? *Heart Dis Stroke*. 1992; 1: 179–183.

Jaffe AS. The use of antiarrhythmics in advanced cardiac life support. *Ann Emerg Med* 1993; 22:2 Part 2; 307–316.

Katz A and Reuter H. Cellular calcium and cardiac cell death. *Am J Cardiol* 44: 188–190, 1979.

Kerber RE, Pardian NG, Jensen SR, et al. Effect of lidocaine and bretylium on energy requirements for transthoracic defibrillation: experimental studies. *J Am Coll Cardiol* 1986; 7: 397–405.

Kern KB, Garewal HS, Sanders AB, et al. Depletion of myocardial adenosine triphosphate during prolonged untreated ventricular fibrillation: effect on defibrillation success. *Resuscitation* 1990; 20: 221–229.

Koehler RC, Chandra N, Guerci AD et al. Augmentation of cerebral perfusion by simultaneous chest compression and lung inflation with abdominal binding following cardiac arrest in dogs. *Circulation* 1983; 67: 266–275.

Kottmeier CA and Gravenstein JS. The parasympathomimetic activity of atropine and atropine methylbromide. *Anesthesiology* 1968; 29: 1125–1133.

Kouwenhaven WR, Jude JR and Knickerbocker GG. Closed Chest Cardiac Massage. *JAMA*. 1960; 173: 1064–1067.

Kowey PR, Levine JH, Herre JM et al. Randomized, double-blind comparison of intravenous amiodarone and bretylium in the treatment of patients with recurrent hemodynamically destabilizing ventricular tachycardia or fibrillation. *Circulation* 1995; 92: 3255–3263.

Kraig RP, Petito CK and Plum F. Hydrogen ions kill brain at concentrations reached in ischemia. *J Cereb Blood Flow Metab* 1987, 7: 379–386.

Lindner KH, Ahnefeld FW and Prengel AW. Comparison of standard and high-dose adrenenaline in the resuscitation of asystole and electromechanical dissociation. *Acta Anesthesiol Scand*. 1991; 35: 253–256.

Longstreth WT and Inui TS. High blood glucose level on hospital admission and poor neurological recovery after cardiac arrest. *Ann Neurol* 1984; 19:59–63.

Luce JM, Ross BK, O'Quin RJ, et al. Regional blood flow during cardiopulmonary resuscitation in dogs using simultaneous and nonsimultaneous compression and ventilation. *Circulation* 1983; 67: 258–265.

McDonald JL. Coarse ventricular fibrillation presenting as asystole or very low amplitude ventricular fibrillation. *Crit Care Med* 1982; 10: 790–791.

Michael JR, Guerci AD, Koehler RC, et al. Mechanisms by which epinephrine augments cerebral and myocardial perfusion during cardiopulmonary resuscitation in dogs. *Circulation* 1984; 69: 822–835.

Midei MG, Sugiura S, Margham WL, et al. Preservation of ventricular function by treatment of ventricular fibrillation with phenylephrine. *Circulation* 1990, 16: 489–494.

Mythen MG and Webb AR. Perioperative plasma volume expansion reduces the incidence of gut mucosal hypoperfusion during cardiac surgery. *Arch Surg* 1995; 130: 423–429.

Olson DW, Thompson BM, Daqrin JC, et al. A randomized comparison study of bretylium tosylate and lidocaine in resuscitation of patients with out-of-hospital ventricular fibrillation in a paramedic system. *Ann Emerg Med* 1984; 13: 807–810.

Ornato, JP. Use of adrenergic agonists during CPR in adults. *Ann Emerg Med* 1993, 22:2, 145–149.

Otto CW and Yakaitis NE. The role of epinephrine in CPR: a reappraisal. *Ann Emerg Med* 1984; 13 (pt 2) 840–843.

Paradis NA and Koscove EM. Epinephrine in cardiac arrest: A critical review. *Ann Emerg Med* 1990; 18: 1288–1301.

Paradis NA, Martin GB, Goetting M, et al. Simultaneous aortic, jugular bulb, and right atrial pressures during cardiopulmonary resuscitation in humans: Insights into mechanisms. *Circulation* 1989, 80: 361–368.

Paradis NA, Martin GB, Rosenberg J, et al. The effect of standard and high dose epinephrine on coronary perfusion pressure during prolonged cardiopulmonary resuscitation. *JAMA* 265: 1139–1144, 1991.

Paradis NA, Martin GB, Rivers EP, et al. Coronary perfusion pressure and the return of spontaneous circulation in human cardiopulmonary resuscitation. *JAMA* 263: 1106–1113, 1990.

Pfeffer MA. ACE Inhibitors in acute myocardial infarction. Patient selection and timing. *Circulation*. 1998; 97: 2192–2194.

Redding JS and Pearson JW. Effective routes of drug administration during cardiac arrest. *Anesth Analg* 1967; 46: 253–258.

Robertson CE. Advanced life support guidelines. *Brit J Anaes* 1997;79:172–177.

Rothenberg R. Use, value, and toxicity of amiodarone. *Heart Dis Stroke.* 1994; 3: 19–23.

Ryan TJ (Chair). ACC/AHA Guidelines for the management of patients with acute myocardial infarction. *JACC* 1996; 28:1328–1428.

Siesjo BK. Cell damage in the brain: A speculative synthesis. *J. Cereb Blood Flow Metab.* 1981; 1:155–185.

Stambler BS and Wood MA, Ellenbogen KA, et al: Efficacy and safety of repeated intravenous doses of ibutilide for rapid conversion of atrial flutter or fibrillation. *Circulation* 1996; 94:1613–1621.

Stiell IG, Hebert PC, Weitzman BN et al. High-dose epinephrine in adult cardiac arrest. *N Engl J Med* 1992; 327: 1047–1050.

Stoelting RK. *Pharmacology and Physiology in Anesthetic Practice* JB Lippincott Co., Philadelphia, 1991. pp 242–251.

Swenson RD, Weaver WD, Nisaken RA et al. Hemodynamics in humans during conventional and experimental methods of cardiopulmonary resuscitation. *Circulation* 1988; 78: 630–639.

Thal, E.R. (editor). *Textbook of Advanced Trauma Life Support.* American College of Surgeons, Chicago, Illinois 1993.

Tobey RC, Birnbaum GA, Allegra JR et al. Successful resuscitation and neurologic recovery from refractory ventricular fibrillation after magnesium sulfate administration. *Ann Emerg Med.* 1992; 21: 92–96.

von Planta M, Bar-Joseph G, Wiklund L, et al. Pathophysiologic and therapeutic implications of acid-base changes During CPR. *Ann Emerg Med.* 1993; 22 (pt 2): 404–410.

Voorhees WD, Jaeger CS, Babbs CR, et al. Regional blood flow during cardiopulmonary resuscitation in dogs. *Crit Care Med* 8; 134–136, 1980.

Woods KL, Fletcher S, Roffe C and Haider Y. Intravenous magnesium sulphate in suspected acute myocardial infarction: results of the second Leicester Intravenous Magnesium Intervention Trial (LIMIT-2). *Lancet* 1992; 339: 1553–1558.

Zaloga GP, Strickland RA, Butterworth JF IV, et al. Calcium attenuates epinephrine's α-adrenergic effects in post-operative heart surgery patients. *Circulation* 81: 196–200, 1990.

Zaritsky, AL. Resuscitation Pharmacology. In Chernow B (ed). *The Pharmacologic Approach to the Critically Ill Patient, Third Edition* Williams and Wilkins, Baltimore, MD 1994, pp. 233–246.

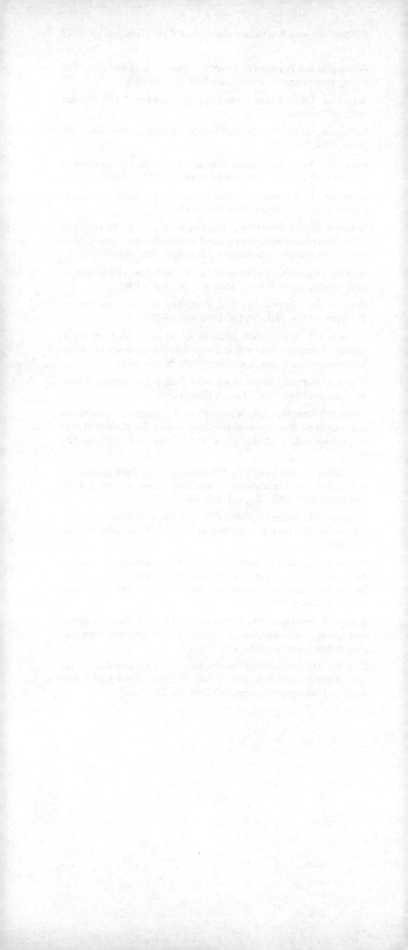

CHAPTER 12

Vasoactive Drugs and Cardiopulmonary Bypass

Lisa Wollman and Dan Philbin

The cardiac anesthesiologist clinically manages the acute care of the critically ill patients through the induction of anesthesia, the course of surgery, and the separation from cardiopulmonary bypass. This requires expertise in administration of vasoactive drugs in the manipulation of hemodynamics as well as the anticipation of the profound side effects of these pharmacological agents. Cardiopulmonary bypass and many of the interventions implicit to cardiac surgery commonly result in clinical myocardial dysfunction; this has been shown to occur in patients with both normal and impaired preoperative ventricular function. The degree of such dysfunction correlates with the length of aortic cross clamping, adequacy of myocardial protection (Swanson and Myerowitz, 1983), hypothermia, completeness of revascularization, inflammatory responses, and reperfusion injury (Swanson and Myerowitz, 1983). The effects of positive pressure ventilation and the rewarming process also contribute to the acute, yet transient, deterioration in myocardial function and hemodynamic instability (Przyklenk and Kloner, 1989).

Many studies, employing an assortment of techniques to assess function, have documented the occurrence of this phenomenon and consistently demonstrate that in the minutes following the separation from cardiopulmonary bypass, ventricular performance initially improves, but predictably and gradually deteriorates over a period of four to eight hours (Przyklenk and Kloner, 1989). The cause of this deterioration is not clear but may involve incomplete rewarming with a further decline in temperature, microemboli of air or particulate matter, mechanics of chest closure, reperfusion injury, or early myocardial edema. Ischemic or hibernating myocardium now reperfused may improve in function, can become arrhythmogenic, or remain hypo- or dyskinetic. Over time, function recovers toward baseline, usually within twenty-four hours. The time course of these events can often be quite protracted in patients with pre-existing dysfunction.

RATIONALE OF INOTROPIC ADMINISTRATION

The pharmacological regimen

Despite numerous studies correlating preoperative factors with outcome in cardiac surgery, few studies have looked at predictors of inotropic drug requirements. Goenen et al found that patients with ejection fractions less than 40% required significantly more inotropic therapy than patients with ejection fractions which were higher (Goenen et al, 1987). Royster et al showed that factors related to the use of inotropes included lower ejection fraction, older age, cardiac enlargement, female sex, higher baseline filling pressures, and longer bypass and cross-clamp times (Royster et al, 1991). Rational use of medications and interventions requires a thorough understanding of the balance of myocardial oxygen supply and demand, and the ability to promptly assess the myocardial inotropic state and changing Starling curve in the post bypass period (Fig 10-3, page 291). Pharmacological therapies, which are commonly administered to support patients through this reperfusion process and to avoid any further ischemic insult will be reviewed in this chapter.

The pharmacological regimen selected during the *recovery phase post-bypass* must take into account the pathophysiology of heart failure. The patient with pre-existing dysfunction undergoing cardiac surgery suffers the ischemic insult of cardioplegic arrest in addition to the pathophysiology of the underlying diseased condition. The failure of the myocardium to return to baseline function after episodes of hypoxic injury and subsequent reperfusion has been called "stunned myocardium" (Braunwald and Kloner, 1982). While the pathophysiology has not been clearly defined, it is a function of intracellular calcium overload, the generation of free radicals, and disturbances in the microcirculation involving white blood cells and platelets (Kloner et al, 1989). It is clear, however, that this "stunned myocardium" does respond to inotropic administration and function will improve. This is not true of actively ischemic and dysfunctional myocardium (Ellis et al, 1984; Bolli et al, 1985). Myocardial blood flow must be redistributed to the ischemic regions prior to the instituting of inotropic therapy for the repletion of the ATP stores and improvement in function.

After bypass, areas of incomplete revascularization are going to be at risk of ischemic injury. Raised intracavitary pressures can compress subendocardial vessels further reducing blood flow; wall tension is increased as well, leading to higher oxygen requirements. Increases in heart rate shorten diastolic filling time which can also put the subendocardium at risk for worsening ischemia. For all of these reasons, it is crucial to maintain adequate coronary perfusion pressure to deliver the oxygen demanded by a recovering ventricle. Inotropic support, although it increases the energy requirements of the myocardium, theoretically improves the net balance of supply and demand by lowering diastolic filling pressures and the raising coronary perfusion pressure. In addition, inotropes have been shown to significantly increase blood flow in new saphenous vein grafts and not adversely affect flow in internal mammary artery grafts in the immediate post bypass period (DiNardo et al, 1991). Inotropes should be titrated as needed for function and in attempt to avoid tachycardia. Tachycardia has been shown to increase reperfusion injury and worsen contractile function whether it is caused by drug effect or pacing (Lederman et al, 1987; Vatner and Baig, 1979).

INOTROPIC AGENTS

The myocardial inotropic state is defined as the intrinsic ability of the myocytes to contract. The intensity of this systolic contractile force is related to the availability of calcium within the cells to bind troponin C which leads to increased cross-bridging of actin and myosin. The opposite occurs in diastole: calcium is sequestered within the cell and there is less crossbridging, which, in turn, results in relaxation (Fig 3-2). Inotropic agents act by either raising the intracellular levels of calcium or by sensitizing the contractile apparatus to this ion. In general, pharmacologic agents which raise the inotropic state of the heart, increase the myocardial oxygen consumption, and therefore, can create or worsen ischemia. In the failing or "stunned" ventricle, however, inotropes are employed to increase contractility. If increased arterial blood pressure is the result, the perfusion pressure and coronary blood flow will likely improve, thereby increasing the oxygen supply to the myocardial cells.

There are currently three principal classes of inotropic agents available in intravenous form for clinical use by the cardiac anesthesiologist. These are catecholamines, sympathomimetics, and phosphodiesterase inhibitors (Table 3-1, page 65).

Endogenous Catecholamines

Catecholamines are a class of agents characterized by the structure of a catechol ring, hydroxyl groups, and a variety of attached side chains. The naturally occurring catecholamines include epinephrine (adrenaline), norepinephrine (noradrenaline) and dopamine. These chemicals, when endogenously released or exogenously administered, increase the inotropic state of the heart by stimulation of both the $beta_1$ and $beta_2$ receptors on myocardial cells. Alpha receptors are also stimulated to a varying degree and while this has been shown to result in an increased inotropic effect in vitro, it has not been shown to be clinically significant. Catecholamines bind to these adrenergic receptors which then activate the stimulatory guanine nucleotide binding protein (G-protein); G-protein stimulation results in activation of the adenylyl cyclase enzyme cascade. Adenylyl cyclase is a catalyst for the creation of cyclic AMP, the second messenger, from ATP, which, in turn, stimulates protein phosphorylation and raises the intracellular calcium level. Proteins are phosphorylated at subcellular sites, the sarcolemma, the sarcoplasmic reticulum, and the troponin-tropomyosin regulatory complex on myofilaments. This chain of events ultimately raises the contractile state of the cardiac muscle fibers (Fig 3-2, page 61). In the clinical doses at which these catecholamines are administered, there are often significant peripheral effects; vasoconstriction or vaso-dilatation can be seen as a result of the balance of the alpha and beta receptors stimulation (Fig 1-9, page 11). As Hoff-man and Lefkowitz (1996) noted, there are several predomi-nant effects of these catecholamines: a) peripheral excitatory action on certain types of smooth muscle such as blood ves-sels to skin, mucous membranes, and glands; b) inhibition of smooth muscle in the GI tract and the bronchial tree; c) excitation of cardiac muscle via increased heart rate and contractility; d) increased glycogenolysis and free fatty acid release; e) modulation of renin, pituitary hormones and insulin; f) decreased appetite and increased alertness or wakefulness by direct central effects (Hoffman and Lefko-witz, 1996). These are all teleologically important survival mechanisms in the ability to fight or flee from a threatening stimulus.

Epinephrine (adrenaline)

Epinephrine is a crucial drug in the cardiac anesthesiolo-gist's armamentarium, with indications for use varying from bronchospasm and anaphylaxis to cardiogenic failure and cardio-pulmonary resuscitation. It is not often used as a first line agent for myocardial dysfunction in the post bypass period in adults. However, it can be a safe and life-saving treatment for patients otherwise unable to wean from bypass. Acute asthmatic episodes can be broken by its administration as it has a dramatic ability to relax bronchial smooth muscle. Drug reactions characterized by hemody-namic instability are effectively treated with epinephrine as it increases the cyclic AMP levels in mast cells which pre-vents further degranulation. These effects are achieved with relatively low dosages (roughly 0.5-2 μg/min.) of epinephr-ine at which the beta receptor stimulation predominates. However in cardiopulmonary resuscitation, relatively high doses (1-5 mg) are currently recommended given either intravenously, via the endotracheal tube, or by intraventri-cular injection. At these higher doses vasoconstriction results from predominant alpha receptor stimulation (Table 3-1, page 65).

Epinephrine is a potent myocardial inotrope. It increases heart rate, stroke volume, and myocardial blood flow. It does have notable arrhythmogenic potential. Any rhythm from sinus tachycardia to ventricular fibrillation may be seen in patients receiving the drug. Cardiac arrhythmias can be seen at extremely low doses of epi-nephrine, especially in the presence of inhalation anes-thetics. It is an extremely potent vasoconstrictor predominantly affecting the small arterioles and precapil-lary vasculature. The vasoconstriction is quite pronounced in the beds supplying the kidneys and skin while vasodila-tation is seen in the skeletal muscles. At low doses epi-nephrine can cause a reduction in blood pressure by producing more beta$_2$-stimulated vasodilatation than alpha-mediated constriction. However, at most clinical doses used after cardiopulmonary bypass, an increased mean arterial blood pressure results. The systolic pressure often is raised to a greater degree than the diastolic pressure, creating a widened pulse pressure (Hoffman and Lefkowitz, 1996).

Epinephrine is either taken up by sympathetic neurons or rapidly metabolized in the liver and other tissues by both monoamine oxidase (MAO) and catechol-O-methyl-transferase (COMT). The metabolites are readily excreted in the urine.

Norepinephrine (noradrenaline)

Norepinephrine is the primary endogenous post-ganglionic neurotransmitter in the sympathetic nervous system. It stimulates both alpha and beta adrenergic receptors although the alpha stimulation is markedly more pronounced clinically. Intravenously administered norepinephrine will increase intravascular tone from this alpha stimulation and a rise in blood pressure will result. This rise in vascular tone stimulates a vagal reflex which tends to decrease heart rate, this vagal response is usually more profound than the direct beta adrenergic stimulation from norepinephrine. The beta stimulation is, however, significant enough to increase the contractility and as a result, the stroke volume. Additionally, coronary blood flow is higher as a result of the increased systemic blood pressure. The raised stroke volume, in combination with a slower heart rate, often brings about little change in the cardiac output overall. Cardiac output should, however, always be monitored during norepinephrine administration as large increases in blood pressure can result in marked worsening of function in a load sensitive or failing ventricle.

Norepinephrine differs from epinephrine in several important ways. Most notably, there is essentially no beta$_2$ agonist activity, so that at low doses vasodilatation is not seen. The arrhythmogenicity of epinephrine is not a problem with norepinephrine, except potentially with extremely high dose infusions. This is probably also a function of proportionally lesser overall beta receptor stimulation. Similarly to epinephrine in high doses, norepinephrine is a potent vasoconstrictor. It decreases renal blood flow as well as flow to the hepatic, mesenteric, and splanchnic beds. Due to this profound vasoconstrictive property of the drug, it is recommended that norepinephrine be infused only through a central vein, or a large peripheral vein, temporarily, if a central vein is not available. The potential extravasation with peripheral access can result in tissue necrosis and sloughing in the affected area.

Norepinephrine is delivered by infusion. Clinical dosing starts in the low range of $0.5 - 1.0$ μg/min; the infusion rate should then be titrated as needed to maintain the desired blood pressure. The drug is metabolized by the COMT and MAO enzyme systems. It is also taken up by the sympathetic neuron terminals to a significant degree.

Dopamine

Dopamine is an endogenous catecholamine which is a central neurotransmitter and the precursor of norepinephrine and epinephrine. Dopamine is capable of directly stimulating alpha, beta, and dopaminergic receptors and indirectly affecting adrenergic response by inhibiting the reuptake of norepinephrine as well as increasing norepinephrine release (Fig 3-3, page 62). Intravenously administered dopamine cannot cross the blood brain barrier and therefore no CNS effects are seen. At low dosages, dopamine predominantly stimulates dopamine receptors resulting in arterial relaxation in the renal and mesenteric beds. This does bring about increases in the renal blood flow. Although much is quoted concerning the "renal protection" afforded by the administration of low dose dopamine, this has not been well documented. It is known that dopamine has both natriuretic and diuretic properties (Miller, 1984). Therefore, it is often infused in low doses in the setting of renal insufficiency or poor urine output to facilitate clinical management. Dopamine is commonly used in the treatment of cardiac patients receiving other inotropic agents to theoretically offset any renal vasoconstriction caused by the other drugs. This practice remains quite controversial. Low dose administration for primarily dopaminergic receptor stimulation is frequently cited to be 1-5 $\mu g/kg/min$. This is an extremely wide therapeutic range, and it must be emphasized that these values are not well documented in humans. Therefore, each patient must be treated as his or her own control and doses must be carefully and individually titrated for the effect of specific receptor stimulation. At slightly higher dosages than this dopaminergic range, beta adrenergic receptor activity is seen. Dopamine is a positive inotrope in these higher doses both by direct beta stimulation and indirect increases in norepinephrine release. In the higher dosage range tachycardias and arrhythmias can limit therapy and it may be necessary to lower the rates of infusion rate of the drug. At even higher doses alpha receptors are activated and vasoconstriction is clinically apparent.

Dopamine is metabolized rapidly in the liver and other organs by COMT and MAO enzymes. It has a short half life and therefore can be easily titrated to a balance of maximal benefit and minimal side effects. In patients receiving dopamine infusions for periods longer than several days, there is interference with the thyroid hormone feedback axis and thyroid stimulating hormone levels are altered.

Synthetic catecholamines

Synthetic catecholamines are chemically related to the endogenous molecules, distinct in structure primarily by a side group, and as a result, stimulate many of the same receptors. They are all positive inotropes but differ in their effects on the vasculature.

Isoproterenol (Isoprenaline)

Isoproterenol is a pure beta adrenergic receptor agonist. It lacks any alpha or dopaminergic effects. It is an inotrope, so by definition it increases myocardial contractility and oxygen consumption. This pure beta stimulation of both beta$_1$ and beta$_2$ receptors, causes direct increases in heart rate. For this reason, isoproterenol is often a first line therapy in the treatment of profound bradycardias, heart block, other conduction abnormalities, and in denervated hearts as in patients post cardiac transplant. Isoproterenol also causes a marked vasodilatation by unopposed $beta_2$ agonists effects and stimulates the secretion of atrial natriuretic peptide (Schiebinger et al, 1987). In fact, systemic hypotension is often the limiting factor for isoproterenol infusion. In addition, the drug can cause significant arrhythmias in the therapeutic dose range. It is for this reason that it is not used in patients presenting with status asthmaticus despite the profound bronchodilation which is seen with its administration. Tachycardia is perhaps more pronounced than with the other drugs previously mentioned due to both the beta stimulation and a reflex response to the vasodilatation.

Dosing of isoproterenol usually starts at 0.5-1.0 $\mu g/$ min and can be titrated up to several $\mu g/min$ to attain the desired effect. As with the endogenous catecholamines, isoproterenol is metabolized almost immediately by the enzyme COMT, primarily by the liver, but in other tissues as well. In contrast to the previously discussed nonsynthetic catecholamines, it is taken up by sympathetic neurons to a much lesser degree.

Dobutamine

Dobutamine is a synthetic molecule which has a long side chain with an additional aromatic group. Its effects are primarily direct stimulation of beta receptors, $beta_1$ to a greater extent than $beta_2$. Dobutamine, unlike dopamine, does not have any dopaminergic or alpha effects (Fig 3-3, page 62). Clinically, it produces an increase in inotropic state and automaticity of the cardiac conduction system. Although dobutamine can prevent norepinephrine reuptake in neurons to a small degree, a significant rise in blood pressure is not generally seen. In fact, vasodilatation can occur. While some patients with cardiogenic shock may improve with this combination of increased inotropy and pressure unloading, many may actually require concurrent administration of a vasoconstrictor to maintain adequate perfusion pressure for the heart and other vital organs. Tachycardia can be seen with dobutamine, but not to the degree seen with isoproterenol. This effect is a dose-related phenomenon. *Some clinicians advocate using small doses of dopamine in combination* with small doses of dobutamine to get maximal increase in inotropy with a balancing of effects on the vasculature and possibly less tachycardia than with higher doses of either agent used alone. This practice may be beneficial in some patients. However, tachycardia can still be the limiting factor in such therapy. In contrast to the endogenous catecholamines, dobutamine is metabolized by glucuronic acid. Similarly to the other agents, it is metabolized rapidly and this primarily occurs in the liver.

Dopexamine

Dopexamine is also a synthetic catecholamine which is used in congestive heart failure patients, rather than in post cardiac surgery patients. The clinical experience with this agent has been primarily in Europe. It reportedly has both $beta_2$ and dopaminergic agonist properties with minimal $beta_1$ and alpha effects. Therefore, it combines the increased inotropy and unloading of dobutamine with the increased renal blood flow seen with dopamine. Unlike the other catecholamines, dopexamine seems to be able to increase heart rate without any increased arrhythmogenicity. Dopexamine may even have some antiarrhythmogenic effect. All of these features make it potentially a superb agent to treat the post bypass myocardial dysfunction. However, further evaluation of this drug is necessary before it is available for widespread clinical use.

Sympathomimetics

Sympathomimetics are drugs which have a different structure than the catecholamines but do have many of the same physiologic effects. Clinically, the most commonly used sympathomimetics are ephedrine, phenylephrine, and methoxamine. These drugs are classified as phenylisopropylamines, a class of agents with varying abilities to activate alpha and beta receptors as well as to stimulate the central nervous system. Ephedrine, however, is the only of theses commonly used drugs with any significant beta receptor agonist properties and, therefore, it is the only one to be included in this discussion of inotropes.

Ephedrine

Ephedrine is an intravenously administered drug derived from a naturally occurring plant chemical. It has become a common treatment for hypotension in the perioperative period in non cardiac patients. Ephedrine has direct and indirect effects. It stimulates both $beta_1$ and $beta_2$ receptors and the release of norepinephrine at neuronal synapses. Therefore, it dually activates beta receptors increasing contractility, heart rate, and as a result, cardiac output. It also, via the release of norepinephrine and subsequent alpha receptor activity, raises blood pressure. Ephedrine is usually dosed in 5-10 mg intravenous, intermittent boluses. Unlike the previously mentioned agents it is not usually given as a continuous infusion. The physiologic effects of bolus doses last approximately ten minutes. Due to this bolus administration it is more difficult to titrate to effect on a minute to minute basis. As a result, ephedrine is not a commonly used agent in the perioperative cardiac surgical patient population. It is more frequently used in healthy perioperativepatients with a transient need for support. Ephedrine is minimally metabolized by MAO enzymes and is excreted almost unchanged. As with any of the previously mentioned inotropes, it does increase the myocardial consumption of oxygen and can thereby precipitate ischemia in patients who are at risk.

Phosphodiesterase inhibitors

This is a class of drugs which are inotropes through a distinct mechanism from that of the drugs previously discussed (Fig 1-5, page 8). Phosphodiesterases are intracellular enzymes which inactivate cyclic AMP. Therefore, inhibitors of this process prolong the existence and effect of each cyclic AMP molecule. Endogenous catecholamines stimulate beta adrenergic receptors and this receptor activation in turn stimulates the formation of cyclic AMP. Phosphodiesterase inhibitors administered to patients with even normal baseline levels of catecholamines will result in increased levels of inotropy. These drugs have a synergistic effect on the myocardium when delivered in conjunction with exogenous catecholamines. Although these agents have a profound positive inotropic effect, the chronotropic effect is mild in comparison to that of direct increased beta stimulation. In the failing heart, phosphodiesterase inhibitors offer an additional benefit in that they also cause marked systemic vasodilatation. The combination of an increase in contractility and "unloading" of the myocardium have caused this class of drugs to be referred to as inodilators. This can be of profound benefit in a failing heart but also has the theoretical potential for precipitating ischemia in the presence of significant coronary artery disease. The combination of increased myocardial consumption and decreased perfusion pressure can result in an imbalance of oxygen supply and demand. Patients who are at risk of this are difficult to predict, however, because the "unloading" can also decrease the myocardial oxygen requirements by allowing the ventricles to empty to smaller volumes and decreased wall tensions. These drugs are often extremely beneficial but should be used with appropriate caution in patients with known potential for ischemia.

Amrinone, a bipyridine, is the inodilator most used clinically. As with the other drugs in this class, the increase in inotropy is not affected or diminished by drugs which cause adrenergic blockade or by down regulation of receptors as the site of action is beyond the receptor itself. These drugs selectively inhibit phosphodiesterase enzyme fraction III (Levy et al, 1990). Amrinone administration results in profound vasodilatation by the same mechanism of increased cyclic AMP levels in the vascular smooth muscle (Fig 1-9, page 11). This effect often requires some therapy to maintain an adequate blood pressure. This vasodilatation is almost immediate in onset whereas the increased inotropy takes 10-20 minutes to become clinically apparent. The recommended dosing of amrinone is a bolus loading over 10-15 minutes of 0.75-3.0 mg/kg and then an infusion of 100 μg/min titrated upward to desired effect. The maximum suggested daily dose of amrinone should not exceed 10 mg/kg (Schwinn, 1994). The loading dose provides therapeutic concentrations for roughly 60 minutes. Therefore, an infusion is necessary to maintain effect beyond this time period. Amrinone has a longer duration of action than most of the traditional inotropes; the duration of effect depends on dose but varies from 30 minutes to 2 hours.

Amrinone is a relatively safe drug in the perioperative surgical patient population. However, chronic administration shows no long-term beneficial effect and will increase the mortality risk. Also, as with any other positive inotrope, there will be a reduction in efficacy over time. Amrinone can result in several side effects most notably thrombocytopenia in approximately 3% of patients. This is due to a decreased platelet survival time and not a bone marrow or immunological effect of the drug. Other possible effects include fever, hepatic dysfunction, GI upset, and myalgias in non anesthetized patients. Amrinone is contraindicated in patients with an allergy to sulfonamides.

Combination therapy with amrinone and a catecholamine infusion, has become common practice in perioperative cardiac surgery patients. This approach is an attempt to maximize inotropy while minimizing side effects such as tachycardia, ventricular irritability, and vasodilatation. Overall, this group of agents provides an important therapeutic option with a unique mechanism of action for the cardiac anesthesiologist managing cardiac dysfunction.

Milrinone is a derivative of amrinone, therefore also a bipyridine, and is approximately twenty times as potent. The drug has the same inodilator properties as amrinone. However, many clinicians claim that there is significantly less hypotension seen with milrinone administration. The side effects, specifically thrombocytopenia and fever, have only rarely been described with this phosphodiesterase inhibitor. The recommended loading bolus dose is 50 μg/kg over approximately 10 minutes. The infusion rate should be titrated to hemodynamic response, and the suggested range is 0.3-0.75 μg/kg/min. Dosing needs to be adjusted in patients with severe renal impairment as the half-life of milrinone is significantly increased in such patients. In patients with normal renal function the half-life of milrinone is reportedly of the order of 150 minutes.

Milrinone can be prescribed in an oral form although this is not useful in the perioperative period. Long-term treatment has been studied in outpatients with end-stage heart failure. These studies have shown an increase in cardiovascular morbidity and mortality similar to that of chronic administration of other inotropes.

Calcium chloride

Exogenously administered calcium can be useful in improving the contractile state of the myocardium. The use of calcium chloride is quite controversial, however, both because of the transient nature of its effects and the possible problems associated with its use. Increased availability of calcium ions does result in increased excitation-contraction and quickly increases the inotropic state of the myocardium. To this end, calcium is commonly reached for by the cardiac anesthesiologist immediately after cardiopulmonary bypass if there is evidence of myocardial failure or vasodilatation. Often, it is administered as a transient therapy until a longer acting inotropic agent can be delivered or the cardiac function improves over time. It will raise the blood pressure by two mechanisms. It is both an inotrope and a vasoconstrictor. The benefit of this short-lived support must be balanced with the risk of calcium overload, i.e. increases in calcium concentration in the myocardial cells which are likely to occur in ischemic or post-ischemic injury. A rise in calcium ion levels in ischemic cells results in exacerbation of cell injury and increased risk of cell death. It is for this reason that calcium chloride has fallen out of favor in cardiopulmonary resuscitation algorithms. Additionally, calcium has been shown to attenuate the response to epinephrine in both animals and humans recovering from bypass surgery (Zaluga et al, 1988; Zaluga et al, 1990).

Calcium chloride is usually administered in 100 mg increments or 1.36 mmoles of calcium. Several hundred milligrams are often given as a bolus dose. Calcium is also available as calcium gluconate. However, calcium chloride results in higher levels of ionized calcium. Calcium chloride must be given through a central venous access as it may cause sclerosis and can result in marked vascular smooth muscle contraction.

VASODILATORS

Although vasodilators do not increase the inotropic state of the myocardium they facilitate ejection by decreasing the afterload of the heart. In post cardiopulmonary bypass patients vasodilators are often useful in improving myocardial performance especially in those patients who are also relatively vasoconstricted. Vasodilating agents relax arterial smooth muscle and often have a similar effect on the venous system. Careful titration of these agents is necessary as excessive vasodilation can lead to decreased myocardial perfusion and venodilation which can effectively decrease venous return and as a result, stroke volume (Fig 10-3, page 291).

Sodium nitroprusside

Although sodium nitroprusside has been one of the most commonly used vasodilators in the perioperative period, the exact mechanism of action has only recently been explained. Sodium nitroprusside, a nitrate, acts by penetrating the endothelium to form nitric oxide (Fig 6-1, page 142). This, in turn, results in the production of cyclic guanine monophosphate from guanine triphosphate. Cyclic GMP is the intracellular second messenger which activates calcium binding proteins. Intracellular calcium concentration declines and, as a result, vascular smooth muscle relaxes. The effect is almost immediate, the vasodilation occurs within seconds of the drug being administered. Similarly, the dilation disappears almost immediately when the infusion is discontinued. Dosages must be titrated to the effect or the blood pressure desired. Typically, it is given as an infusion, starting in a range of 1-40 µg/min and titrated upward to several hundred µg/min. At low doses, sodium nitroprusside predominantly dilates systemic arteries and arterioles. Its effect is a function of the underlying vascular tone; it is a more potent dilator in vascular beds which are vasoconstricted. As the dose is increased, sodium nitroprusside becomes a venodilator as well.

As a result of this vasodilator activity, the desired effect, a fall in blood pressure will occur. This, in turn, can cause a reflex tachycardia which should be anticipated. Additionally, if venodilation occurs, preload will fall and cardiac output will be reduced. This can often be prevented with concurrent fluid administration. Sodium nitroprusside, by "unloading" the heart, as well as potentially decreasing preload, allows for decreased ventricular wall tension and chamber size. These effects result in decreased myocardial oxygen consumption. However, sodium nitroprusside may potentially result in the "coronary steal phenomenon", as it is also a coronary vasodilator. In patients with steal prone anatomy (Buffington et al, 1988), coronary arteries with stenotic lesions will not dilate, unlike normal vessels. This may increase blood flow to normal, dilated coronaries and reduce flow to areas at risk for ischemia. Therefore, this drug should be used cautiously in patients with significant coronary disease prior to revascularization.

There are several other potential issues of concern with sodium nitroprusside administration. The dilation of vessels also occurs within the lungs. This can cause hypoxia by blunting normal hypoxic vasoconstriction. This effect resolves with cessation of the infusion. Another possible risk of nitroprusside infusion is *cyanide toxicity* which can be life threatening. Cyanide build-up can occur in the setting of rapid or prolonged administration or in the case of impaired liver function. The ferrous ion in nitroprusside reacts rapidly with sulfhydryl-containing compounds in red blood cells to form cyanide (Michenfelder, 1977). The liver then transforms cyanide to thiocyanate which is excreted by the kidneys. If this conversion does not occur, cyanide levels will rise. Cyanide prevents oxygen delivery to the tissues by blocking the final steps of the electron transport chain. This hypoxia results in cell death, tissue injury, and if severe, death of the patient. Therefore, anytime nitroprusside is administered over a period of time, cyanide toxicity must be considered a possible complication. Often the first or only clinical sign of toxicity is a metabolic acidosis. If high cyanide levels are suspected, the infusion must be stopped and a cyanide antidote should be considered. Either thiosulfate (150 mg/kg) or sodium nitrate (5 mg/kg) can be given over 15-30 minutes (Vesey, 1985). The latter compound converts hemoglobin to methemoglobin which then becomes cyanmethemoglobin. This prevents cyanide from blocking oxygen delivery to the tissues. However, unlike hemoglobin, cyanmethemoglobin cannot carry oxygen. Methylene blue (1 mg/kg) can be given, if necessary, to convert cyanmethemoglobin back to hemoglobin, shifting the oxyhemoglobin dissociation curve back to the right and allowing for improved oxygen delivery.

Although the above mentioned issues with nitroprusside are real, it is actually an extremely safe drug to administer, especially in the perioperative period when used in the recommended clinical dosages. It is, in fact, an ideal agent when vasodilation is needed rapidly or transiently.

Hydralazine

Hydralazine is an arterial smooth muscle vasodilator which acts by inhibiting calcium transport. The resulting reduction in blood pressure is usually accompanied by a reflex tachycardia unless a rate slowing agent is concurrently administered. Hydralazine can be administered intravenously in a 2.5-10 mg bolus or orally in a 25-50 mg dose. Unlike nitroprusside, it has little or no effect on venous capacitance even at higher doses. The onset of action occurs within 15 minutes. The vasodilation persists for several hours. These features make hydralazine a useful drug in the postoperative period but it is not a valuable agent for the treatment of intraoperative hypertension. In a small number of patients receiving this drug in large doses or over periods of weeks to months, a lupus like syndrome can be seen. The symptoms disappear within months of discontinuing the drug.

Alpha adrenergic blockers

These drugs vasodilate by blocking the baseline tonic alpha adrenergic stimulation. Post synaptic alpha$_1$ and alpha$_2$ receptors, when activated, cause constriction of vascular smooth muscle. Although there are many alpha adrenergic receptor antagonists known to control blood pressure, very few agents are available for intravenous use in the perioperative patient population. Phentolamine is a pure alpha antagonist which can be given in the intravenous form and has been used in cardiac surgery patients in the past. It does cause arterial as well as venodilation and this, in turn, can bring about increases in heart rate and variable effects on stroke volume and cardiac output. Effects on stroke volume depend on the balance between decreasing afterload and decreasing preload which tend to have opposite effects. In cardiac surgery, phentolamine is used less often than sodium nitroprusside as it is easier to titrate to the desired effect. Phentolamine is currently routinely used in pediatric bypass cases and occasionally in adult cases in the priming solution to treat hypertension and improve flows during the cardiopulmonary bypass itself.

Alpha blockers have been used post cardiopulmonary bypass most commonly in combination therapy with beta blockers to prevent the reflex tachycardia of the alpha blocker. Labetalol, a combination agent is made up of a selective, competitive alpha antagonist and a relatively non selective beta antagonist. The ratio of clinical alpha to beta blockade has been reported as approximately 1:3 to 1:7, depending on oral or intravenous routes of administration.

Nitric oxide

Inhaled nitric oxide, while currently not readily available to the clinical cardiac anesthesiologist, is a relatively new vasodilating agent which may become more widely accepted. Nitric oxide, or endothelium relaxing factor, has recently been shown to be an important second messenger in the relaxation of vascular smooth muscle. Nitric oxide binds to guanylyl cyclase which, in turn, increases cyclic GMP. GMP signals the smooth muscle relaxation (Fig 6-1). In the inhaled form, only the pulmonary vascular beds dilate. The systemic circulation is virtually unaffected due to rapid inactivation. For this reason, NO may prove to be an ideal agent for patients with severe pulmonary hypertension or those who have sustained a right ventricular insult. More extensive work needs to be done to clearly define the role of nitric oxide in the management of perioperative hemodynamics of cardiac surgical patients.

Prostaglandins

PGE_1 is an additional vasodilator which is often used for its effect on the pulmonary vascular when other therapies prove unsuccessful. Similar to the beta adrenergic agents, PGE_1 stimulates adenylyl cyclase in pulmonary and systemic vascular smooth muscle to produce vasodilation. PGE_1 has been used with success for the treatment of acute right ventricular failure due to elevated pulmonary filling pressures. The profound vasodilation achieved with prostaglandin therapy often requires support of the systemic circulation; right atrial PGE_1 administration with concurrent left atrial vasoconstrictor infusion has been well described in the cardiac anesthesia literature. PGE_1 is almost completely metabolized by a single pass through the lungs so at low doses, 0.5-1.0 $\mu g/min$, hypotension may be avoided.

Prostaglandins are beneficial in other ways during cardiopulmonary bypass. Specifically, PGE_1 inhibits white blood cell and platelet aggregation and activation in the lungs. As a result less free radicals and thromboxane are released. This stabilization of platelets seems to reduce postoperative bleeding as well.

VENODILATORS

Although many of the arterial vasodilators also have venodilating properties, a specific venodilator is extremely useful in the management of the patient with cardiac disease. The venodilator most often used in clinical cardiac anesthesia is nitroglycerin. Nitroglycerin is useful in volume overload patients by causing acute drop in preload, allowing ventricular filling pressures to fall. This decreases wall tension and therefore, myocardial oxygen consumption.

Nitroglycerin

Nitroglycerin's mechanism of action is similar to sodium nitroprusside in that it acts on the endothelium and forms nitric oxide which then relaxes vascular smooth muscle. At low doses it dilates only veins. At higher doses it does have some systemic vasodilatory effects. Nitroglycerin acts on venous capacitance vessels as well as epicardial coronary arteries and coronary collaterals. The drug also has the ability to prevent or relax coronary vasospasm. Even in vessels diseased with atherosclerotic plaques, nitroglycerin can cause dilation of the remaining intact wall and allow for greater blood flow through these vessels. Overall, nitroglycerin is extremely useful as it decreases ventricular preload and when titrated appropriately allows for maintained coronary perfusion pressure and dilated coronary arteries and collaterals. The improved balance of oxygen supply and demand make this agent invaluable in the management of patients with coronary disease in the perioperative period.

Nitroglycerin dosing can start as low as 15 μg/min and titrated up to the desired effect, as high as 1000 μg/min in extreme cases. Most of the common side effects of therapy such as headaches and dizziness are not relevant to the cardiac anesthesiologist caring for the patient during surgery. Therapy can result in a precipitous drop in venous return and thereby decrease cardiac output. Therefore, nitroglycerin may need to be administered with intravenous fluids and careful attention to blood pressure. Cardiac anesthesiologists should also be aware that nitroglycerin has been associated with a dose-related increased bleeding perhaps as a result of increased venous blood capacitance (Lichtenthal et al, 1985) or a platelet effect of the increased nitric oxide levels. Patients in which post surgical bleeding is an issue should perhaps not be placed on high doses of nitroglycerin.

Metabolism of this drug takes place in the liver. The half-life is of the order of several minutes. Nitroglycerin and reduced glutathione react to form the nitrate ions which, in turn, oxidizes iron from the ferrous to the ferric state creating methemoglogin (Curry, 1991). Methemoglobin, as discussed with sodium nitroprusside, interferes with oxygen delivery to the tissues. This rarely becomes a significant issue except with high doses of nitroglycerin are administered over many hours to days.

VASOCONSTRICTORS

Vasoconstrictors include any drug which raises blood pressure by increasing tone in arteries and arterioles. Catecholamines, sympathomimetics and calcium chloride, all of which have vasoconstricting as well as other properties, have been discussed previously. Therefore, only pure vasoconstrictors will be described here. This is a very useful class of drugs. However, it must be emphasized that not all cases of hypotension should be treated with vasoconstrictors, especially when fluid resuscitation or inotropic agents are indicated (Fig 11-5, page 333).

Phenylephrine

Phenylephrine is a directly acting vasoconstrictor which as almost a pure alpha adrenergic stimulating agent in clinical concentrations. It does cause some beta stimulation at extremely high concentrations. Its chemical structure is the same as epinephrine without the hydroxyl group on the benzene ring. This small difference, however, results in markedly distinct receptor binding activity. Phenylephrine causes vasoconstriction in most vascular beds, coronary perfusion pressure is actually raised by the systemic increases in tone. Of all of the cardiac vessels, only the large epicardial arteries have a significant quantity of alpha receptors.

Despite this, there is a theoretical possibility of constricting distal coronaries, potentially precipitating ischemia since there are few alpha receptors in distal coronaries. However, ischemia is extremely unlikely to occur in the setting of total increased blood flow and when normal distal vessels are more likely to constrict than diseased vessels (Feigl, 1987).

Phenylephrine can be given as an intravenous bolus in 10-100 μg doses or as an infusion titrated to effect. It is recommended not to exceed doses of 100 μg/kg/min and, of course the clinical scenario must be continually reassessed to evaluate the need for fluids or other agents. Its effect is apparent within seconds and lasts 10-20 minutes. Phenylephrine is metabolized by the enzyme COMT and, therefore can be used safely on patients receiving MAO inhibitor therapy.

SUMMARY

1. *Bypass surgery* challenges the cardiac anesthesiologist to have a comprehensive knowledge base of the available pharmacologic agents.

2. *Effective therapy*, however, requires an understanding of acute and chronic cardiac pathophysiology, the benefits and potential side effects of each medication, and, most importantly, a rational sense of when such intervention is indicated.

3. *A cardiac anesthesiologist* who can master these clinical skills can truly make a great contribution to the medical management of these critically ill patients.

REFERENCES

Bolli R, Zhu WX, Myers ML et al. Beta adrenergic stimulation reverses post-ischemic myocardial dysfunction without producing subsequent functional deterioration. *Am J Cardiol* 1985; 56: 964-968.

Braunwald E, Kloner RA. The stunned myocardium: Prolonged postischemic ventricular dysfunction. *Circulation* 1982; 66: 1146-1149.

Buffington C, Davis K, Gillispie S and Pettinger M. The prevalence of steal-prone coronary anatomy in patients with coronary artery disease: an analysis of the coronary artery surgery study registry. *Anesthesiology* 1988; 69: 721-727.

Curry SC and Arnold-Capell P. Nitroprusside, nitroglycerin, and angiotensin-converting enzyme inhibitors. *Crit Care Clin* 1991; 7: 555-581.

DiNardo JA, Bert A, Schwartz MJ et al. Effects of vasoactive drugs of flows through left internal mammary artery and saphenous vein grafts in man. *J Thorac Cardiovasc Surg* 1991; 102: 730-735.

Ellis SG, Wynn J, Braunwald E et al. Response of reperfusion-salvaged, stunned myocardium to inotropic stimulation. *Am Heart J* 1984; 107: 13-19.

Feigl EO. The paradox of adrenergic coronary vasoconstriction. *Circulation* 1987; 76: 737-745.

Goenen M, Jacquemart JL, Galvez S, et al. Perioperative left ventricular dysfunction and operative risks in coronary bypass surgery. *Chest* 1987; 92: 804-806.

Hoffman BB and Lefkowitz RJ. Catecholamines, sympathomimetic drugs, and adrenergic receptor antagonists. In: Goodman and Gilman's *The Phamacological Basis of Therapeutics*, 9th Edition. McGaw-Hill, New York, 1996 pp 199-248.

Kloner RA and Przyklenk K, Patel B. Altered myocardial states. The stunned and hibernating myocardium. *Am J Med* 1989; 86 (supp 1A): 14-22.

Lederman SN, Wenger TL, Harrell FE et al. Effects of different paced heart rates on canine coronary occlusion and reperfusion arrhythmias. *Am Heart J* 1987; 113: 1365-1369.

Levy JH, Ramsay J, Bailey JM: Pharmacokinetics and pharmacodynamics of phosphodiesterase-III inhibitors. *J Cardiothorac Vasc Anesth* 1990: 6 (suppl 5): 7-11.

Levy JH, Salmenpera MT, Bailey JM, Ramsay J. Postoperative circulatory control, in Kaplan JA (ed): *Cardiac Anesthesia*, ed. 3, Philadelphia, Saunders, 1993, pp 1168-1693.

Lichtenthal PR, Rossi EC, Louis G et al. Dose-related prolongation of the bleeding time by intravenous nitroglycerin. *Anesth Analg* 1985; 64: 30-33.

Michenfelder JD. Cyanide release from sodium nitroprusside in the dog. *Anesthesiology* 1977; 46: 196-202.

Miller, ED. Renal effects of dopamine. *Anesthesiology* 1984; 61: 487-488.

Przyklenk K and Kloner RA. "Reperfusion injury" by oxygen-derived free radicals? *Circ Res* 1989; 64: 86-96.

Royster RL, Butterworth JF IV, Prough DS, et al. Preoperative and intraoperative predictors of inotropic support and long-term outcome in patients having coronary artery bypass grafting. *Anesth Analg* 1991; 72: 729-736.

Royster RL. Myocardial dysfunction following cardiopulmonary bypass: Recovery patterns, predictors of inotropic need, theoretical concepts of inotropic administration. *J Cardiothorac Vasc Anesth* 1993; 7 (suppl 2): 19-23.

Schiebinger, RJ, Baker MZ and Linden J. The effect of adrenergic and muscarinic choliergic agonists on atrial natriuretic peptide secretion by isolated rat atria: a potential role of the autonomic nervous system in modulating atrial natriuretic peptide secretion. *J Clin Invest* 1987; 80: 1687-1691.

Schwinn, DA. Cardiac Pharmacology. In: *Cardiac Anesthesia: Principles and Clinical Practice*, Eds: F Estafanous, P Barash and JB Reves; Lippincott Co., Philadelphia, 1994; pp 21-60.

Swanson DK, Myerowitz PD. Effect of reperfusion temperature and pressure on the functional and metabolic recovery of preserved hearts. *J Thorac Cardiovasc Surg* 1983; 86: 242-251.

Vatner SF, Baig H: Importance of heart rate in determining the effects of sympathomimetic amines on regional myocardial function and blood flow in conscious dogs with acute myocardial ischemia. *Circ Res* 1979; 45: 793-803.

Vesey CJ, Krapez JR, Variey JG, Cole PV. The antidotal action of thiosulfate following acute nitroprusside infusion in dogs. *Anesthesiology* 1985; 62: 415-421.

Zaluga GP, Strickland RA, Butterworth JF et al. Calcium attenuates epinephrine's beta adrenergic effects in postoperative heart surgery patients. *Circulation* 1990; 81: 196-200.

Zaluga GP, Willey S, Malcolm D et al. Hypercalcemia attenuates blood pressure response to epinephrine. *J Pharmacol Exp Ther* 1988; 247: 949-952.

T = table

A